Going for Gaps in Glaucoma

Going for Gaps in Glaucoma

Editors

Miriam Kolko
Barbara Cvenkel

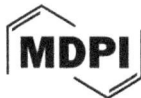

Basel • Beijing • Wuhan • Barcelona • Belgrade • Novi Sad • Cluj • Manchester

Editors
Miriam Kolko
University of Copenhagen
Copenhagen
Denmark

Barbara Cvenkel
University Medical Centre Ljubljana
Ljubljana
Slovenia

Editorial Office
MDPI
St. Alban-Anlage 66
4052 Basel, Switzerland

This is a reprint of articles from the Special Issue published online in the open access journal *Journal of Clinical Medicine* (ISSN 2077-0383) (available at: https://www.mdpi.com/journal/jcm/special_issues/glaucoma_treatment_and_management).

For citation purposes, cite each article independently as indicated on the article page online and as indicated below:

Lastname, A.A.; Lastname, B.B. Article Title. *Journal Name* **Year**, *Volume Number*, Page Range.

ISBN 978-3-0365-9488-0 (Hbk)
ISBN 978-3-0365-9489-7 (PDF)
doi.org/10.3390/books978-3-0365-9489-7

© 2023 by the authors. Articles in this book are Open Access and distributed under the Creative Commons Attribution (CC BY) license. The book as a whole is distributed by MDPI under the terms and conditions of the Creative Commons Attribution-NonCommercial-NoDerivs (CC BY-NC-ND) license.

Contents

Barbara Cvenkel and Miriam Kolko
Going for Gaps in Glaucoma
Reprinted from: *J. Clin. Med.* **2023**, *12*, 5494, doi:10.3390/jcm12175494 1

Fabian Müller, Khaldoon O. Al-Nosairy, Francie H. Kramer, Christian Meltendorf, Nidele Djouoma, Hagen Thieme, et al.
Rapid Campimetry—A Novel Screening Method for Glaucoma Diagnosis
Reprinted from: *J. Clin. Med.* **2022**, *11*, 2156, doi:10.3390/jcm11082156 5

Sze H. Wong and James C. Tsai
Telehealth and Screening Strategies in the Diagnosis and Management of Glaucoma
Reprinted from: *J. Clin. Med.* **2021**, *10*, 3452, doi:10.3390/jcm10163452 19

Anne-Sophie Simons, Julie Vercauteren, João Barbosa-Breda and Ingeborg Stalmans
Shared Care and Virtual Clinics for Glaucoma in a Hospital Setting
Reprinted from: *J. Clin. Med.* **2021**, *10*, 4785, doi:10.3390/jcm10204785 39

Louis Arnould, Alassane Seydou, Christine Binquet, Pierre-Henry Gabrielle, Chloé Chamard, Lionel Bretillon, et al.
Macular Pigment and Open-Angle Glaucoma in the Elderly: The Montrachet Population-Based Study
Reprinted from: *J. Clin. Med.* **2022**, *11*, 1830, doi:10.3390/jcm11071830 63

Adela Magdalena Ciobanu, Vlad Dionisie, Cristina Neagu, Otilia Maria Bolog, Sorin Riga and Ovidiu Popa-Velea
Psychopharmacological Treatment, Intraocular Pressure and the Risk of Glaucoma: A Review of Literature
Reprinted from: *J. Clin. Med.* **2021**, *10*, 2947, doi:10.3390/jcm10132947 75

Barbara Cvenkel and Miriam Kolko
Devices and Treatments to Address Low Adherence in Glaucoma Patients: A Narrative Review
Reprinted from: *J. Clin. Med.* **2023**, *12*, 151, doi:10.3390/jcm12010151 93

Josefine C. Freiberg, Anne Hedengran, Steffen Heegaard, Goran Petrovski, Jette Jacobsen, Barbara Cvenkel and Miriam Kolko
An Evaluation of the Physicochemical Properties of Preservative-Free 0.005% (w/v) Latanoprost Ophthalmic Solutions, and the Impact on In Vitro Human Conjunctival Goblet Cell Survival
Reprinted from: *J. Clin. Med.* **2022**, *11*, 3137, doi:10.3390/jcm11113137 113

Tomaž Gračner
Impact of Short-Term Topical Steroid Therapy on Selective Laser Trabeculoplasty Efficacy
Reprinted from: *J. Clin. Med.* **2021**, *10*, 4249, doi:10.3390/jcm10184249 125

Yu Mizuno, Kazuyuki Hirooka and Yoshiaki Kiuchi
Influence of Overhanging Bleb on Corneal Higher-Order Aberrations after Trabeculectomy
Reprinted from: *J. Clin. Med.* **2022**, *11*, 177, doi:10.3390/jcm11010177 135

Tim J. Enz, James R. Tribble and Pete A. Williams
Comparison of Glaucoma-Relevant Transcriptomic Datasets Identifies Novel Drug Targets for Retinal Ganglion Cell Neuroprotection
Reprinted from: *J. Clin. Med.* **2021**, *10*, 3938, doi:10.3390/jcm10173938 145

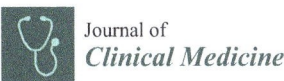

Editorial

Going for Gaps in Glaucoma

Barbara Cvenkel [1,2] and Miriam Kolko [3,4,*]

1. Department of Ophthalmology, University Medical Centre Ljubljana, 1000 Ljubljana, Slovenia; barbara.cvenkel@gmail.com
2. Faculty of Medicine, University of Ljubljana, 1000 Ljubljana, Slovenia
3. Department of Drug Design and Pharmacology, University of Copenhagen, 2100 Copenhagen, Denmark
4. Department of Ophthalmology, Copenhagen University Hospital, Rigshospitalet, 2600 Glostrup, Denmark
* Correspondence: miriamk@sund.ku.dk

Citation: Cvenkel, B.; Kolko, M. Going for Gaps in Glaucoma. *J. Clin. Med.* 2023, 12, 5494. https://doi.org/10.3390/jcm12175494

Received: 18 August 2023
Accepted: 22 August 2023
Published: 24 August 2023

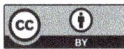

Copyright: © 2023 by the authors. Licensee MDPI, Basel, Switzerland. This article is an open access article distributed under the terms and conditions of the Creative Commons Attribution (CC BY) license (https://creativecommons.org/licenses/by/4.0/).

Glaucoma is the second leading cause of blindness in people over 50 years of age worldwide, and with the ageing population, this number will continue to rise, resulting in a reduced quality of life for these people and an increased social and economic burden on society [1,2]. Since visual impairment due to glaucoma is preventable, timely detection and treatment is critical. This Special Issue of the *Journal of Clinical Medicine* (JCM) contains 10 articles, of which 6 are research articles and 4 are review articles, addressing issues of diagnosis, treatment and new perspectives in the field of glaucoma.

In a paper on rapid campimetry, a novel screening method for glaucoma diagnosis, it was shown to be comparable and even better than 10-2 standard automated perimetry in detecting central macular scotomas [3]. It uses a bright, fast-moving target on a high-contrast background that is perceived as interrupted in the scotoma area. From a distance of 40 cm, the diameter of the moving target depends on the distance to the fixation point and increases with increasing distance from the fixation point. The method is promising for glaucoma screening in the future. It is fast and can be used on a commercially available computer connected to the internet.

Telehealth, i.e., the provision of health care to patients remotely using voice and image communication via a computer or smartphone, was widely used during the coronavirus pandemic. To ensure adequate care for the growing population of glaucoma patients, telehealth and new devices that enable the detection and monitoring of glaucoma will become increasingly important in the future. This review provides an overview of available devices for intraocular pressure measurement, perimetry and fundus photography in a home setting, as well as implemented telehealth programmes for glaucoma screening, monitoring and assessment of glaucoma severity for treatment planning [4]. Ophthalmologists can review results remotely and stratify patients, particularly those with mild to moderate glaucoma and suspected glaucoma, while those with uncontrolled or severe glaucoma should receive an in-person visit. The telehealth approach is cost-effective and particularly beneficial for patients with limited access to healthcare, i.e., in rural areas.

Many eye departments in hospitals are struggling with capacity problems because the increase in newly diagnosed cases is not matched by a proportional increase in the number of ophthalmologists. This inevitably leads to limited access for new patients and an increase in the time between follow-up appointments, leading to the risk that the progression of glaucoma is not detected in time. One solution for the existing number of ophthalmologists is to increase efficiency by offering alternative methods for a safe glaucoma care setting. Simons and colleagues have investigated two alternative schemes for glaucoma care within a hospital, namely shared care and virtual clinics [5]. Both shared care and virtual clinics were found to be safe, cost-effective and acceptable for the care of stable glaucoma patients at low risk of vision loss [5]. The most common non-medical staff involved were optometrists. Patients appreciated the shorter waiting times and did not feel disadvantaged by not seeing a doctor. These two alternative approaches are promising and allow ophthalmologists to assess high-risk patients more quickly without increasing the time intervals for other low-risk glaucoma patients.

Macular pigment plays an important role in visual function and protects the retina from oxidative damage. Macular pigment and glaucoma may be linked through microvascular and oxidative stress processes, both of which have been implicated in the pathogenesis of glaucoma. The Montrachet population-based study, which included participants aged 75 years and older, compared macular pigment optical density and its distribution between eyes with primary open-angle glaucoma and control eyes without optic neuropathy [6]. The macular pigment optical density was determined via the two-wave autofluorescence method using the Heidelberg Retina Angiograph (HRA; Heidelberg Engineering, Heidelberg, Germany) and the macular pigment spatial distribution was generated from the HRA graphs using modified software. Of the 601 eyes, 48 eyes had primary open-angle glaucoma. There were no differences in the macular pigment optical density and its spatial distribution between eyes with primary open-angle and control eyes.

In recent years, the availability and use of psychopharmacological treatments have increased. Ciobanu and co-workers summarise the current knowledge on the risk of psychotropic drug-induced increases in intraocular pressure [7]. Clinicians should be aware of the possibility of psychotropic drug-induced glaucoma and monitor at-risk patients closely, especially if treatment includes tricyclic antidepressants, benzodiazepines and topiramate.

Adherence to IOP-lowering treatment is critical in chronic diseases such as glaucoma, and poor adherence has been associated with faster disease progression [8]. A review paper discusses several strategies to improve adherence, many of which are still in clinical trials [9]. These strategies aim to reduce or avoid the need for eye drops and their side effects. Monitoring devices and smart drug delivery systems, sustained drug delivery systems, lasers, and minimally invasive glaucoma procedures with and without a device in combination with cataract surgery are used for this purpose.

Using an in vitro model, Freiberg and co-workers showed that preservative-free latanoprost ophthalmic solutions differed significantly in their physicochemical properties, including pH, osmolality and surface tension [10]. However, this had no effect on goblet cell viability or mucin release. Future clinical studies are needed to evaluate the long-term efficacy and safety of preservative-free eye drops with different physicochemical properties.

Selective laser trabeculoplasty (SLT) is an established method for lowering intraocular pressure as a first-line treatment or as an adjunct treatment. Treatment with topical steroids or non-steroidal anti-inflammatory drops after SLT is controversial. A retrospective review compared the reduction in intraocular pressure between patients who received topical steroid eye drops for a short time after SLT and those who did not [11]. The success rate was similar in both groups, showing that short-term topical steroid therapy does not affect the efficacy of SLT in patients with primary open-angle glaucoma.

Trabeculectomy has been the reference standard for glaucoma filtration surgery for more than half a century. Antimetabolites used to prevent scarring can cause diffuse filtering blebs that can be uncomfortable, especially if they are high and overhanging. Mizuno and co-workers investigated the effects of overhanging blebs on corneal high-order aberrations using a wavefront analyser [12]. Overhanging blebs after trabeculectomy with a fornix-based conjunctival flap using mitomycin C resulted in an increase in high-order corneal aberrations. The proportion of cornea covered by the bleb correlated positively with the duration of the post-trabeculectomy period and with most of the high-order corneal aberrations causing visual disturbances in the late post-trabeculectomy period.

Lowering intraocular pressure remains the only clinically available treatment, and despite controlled IOP, a proportion of patients progress to blindness. Therefore, efficient neuroprotective therapies would be of great value. The mechanisms underlying retinal ganglion cell degeneration have been studied in several animal models, which, though showing different mechanisms of neuronal damage, may share some common degenerative mechanisms and genetic pathways related to ganglion cell death. Enz and co-workers used three publicly available RNA-sequencing datasets of animal models of glaucoma and screened the shared differentially expressed genes between the three glaucoma models against the Comparative Toxicogenomics Database to identify novel therapeutics [13]. Using a retinal explant model of retinal ganglion cell degeneration, the authors tested a number of these compounds to assess the therapeutic/neuroprotective effects of these drugs. This seems to be a promising approach since, with the increasing use of -omics technologies, there is a wealth of open data in the field of glaucoma that can be explored.

In summary, this Special Issue provides an overview of new treatment strategies and future goals in the management of glaucoma. It also contains new findings that may provide a starting point for new research in this important field.

Author Contributions: Conceptualization, B.C. and M.K.; methodology, B.C. and M.K.; data acquisition, B.C. and M.K.; writing—original draft preparation, B.C. and M.K.; writing—review and editing, B.C. and M.K.; project administration, B.C. and M.K. All authors have read and agreed to the published version of the manuscript.

Conflicts of Interest: B.C. is a consultant and speaker for Thea and Santen. M.K. is a consultant and speaker for Abbvie, Santen and Thea. M.K. receives research support from Thea.

References

1. Blindness, G.B.D.; Vision Impairment, C.; Vision Loss Expert Group of the Global Burden of Disease Study. Causes of blindness and vision impairment in 2020 and trends over 30 years, and prevalence of avoidable blindness in relation to VISION 2020: The Right to Sight: An analysis for the Global Burden of Disease Study. *Lancet Glob. Health* **2021**, *9*, e144–e160. [CrossRef]
2. Traverso, C.E.; Walt, J.G.; Kelly, S.P.; Hommer, A.H.; Bron, A.M.; Denis, P.; Nordmann, J.P.; Renard, J.P.; Bayer, A.; Grehn, F.; et al. Direct costs of glaucoma and severity of the disease: A multinational long term study of resource utilisation in Europe. *Br. J. Ophthalmol.* **2005**, *89*, 1245–1249. [CrossRef] [PubMed]
3. Muller, F.; Al-Nosairy, K.O.; Kramer, F.H.; Meltendorf, C.; Djouoma, N.; Thieme, H.; Hoffmann, M.B.; Hoffmann, F. Rapid Campimetry-A Novel Screening Method for Glaucoma Diagnosis. *J. Clin. Med.* **2022**, *11*, 2156. [CrossRef] [PubMed]
4. Wong, S.H.; Tsai, J.C. Telehealth and Screening Strategies in the Diagnosis and Management of Glaucoma. *J. Clin. Med.* **2021**, *10*, 3452. [CrossRef]
5. Simons, A.S.; Vercauteren, J.; Barbosa-Breda, J.; Stalmans, I. Shared Care and Virtual Clinics for Glaucoma in a Hospital Setting. *J. Clin. Med.* **2021**, *10*, 4785. [CrossRef] [PubMed]
6. Arnould, L.; Seydou, A.; Binquet, C.; Gabrielle, P.H.; Chamard, C.; Bretillon, L.; Bron, A.M.; Acar, N.; Creuzot-Garcher, C. Macular Pigment and Open-Angle Glaucoma in the Elderly: The Montrachet Population-Based Study. *J. Clin. Med.* **2022**, *11*, 1830. [CrossRef]
7. Ciobanu, A.M.; Dionisie, V.; Neagu, C.; Bolog, O.M.; Riga, S.; Popa-Velea, O. Psychopharmacological Treatment, Intraocular Pressure and the Risk of Glaucoma: A Review of Literature. *J. Clin. Med.* **2021**, *10*, 2947. [CrossRef]
8. Newman-Casey, P.A.; Niziol, L.M.; Gillespie, B.W.; Janz, N.K.; Lichter, P.R.; Musch, D.C. The Association between Medication Adherence and Visual Field Progression in the Collaborative Initial Glaucoma Treatment Study. *Ophthalmology* **2020**, *127*, 477–483. [CrossRef] [PubMed]
9. Cvenkel, B.; Kolko, M. Devices and Treatments to Address Low Adherence in Glaucoma Patients: A Narrative Review. *J. Clin. Med.* **2022**, *12*, 151. [CrossRef] [PubMed]
10. Freiberg, J.C.; Hedengran, A.; Heegaard, S.; Petrovski, G.; Jacobsen, J.; Cvenkel, B.; Kolko, M. An Evaluation of the Physicochemical Properties of Preservative-Free 0.005% (w/v) Latanoprost Ophthalmic Solutions, and the Impact on In Vitro Human Conjunctival Goblet Cell Survival. *J. Clin. Med.* **2022**, *11*, 3137. [CrossRef] [PubMed]
11. Gracner, T. Impact of Short-Term Topical Steroid Therapy on Selective Laser Trabeculoplasty Efficacy. *J. Clin. Med.* **2021**, *10*, 4249. [CrossRef] [PubMed]
12. Mizuno, Y.; Hirooka, K.; Kiuchi, Y. Influence of Overhanging Bleb on Corneal Higher-Order Aberrations after Trabeculectomy. *J. Clin. Med.* **2021**, *11*, 177. [CrossRef] [PubMed]
13. Enz, T.J.; Tribble, J.R.; Williams, P.A. Comparison of Glaucoma-Relevant Transcriptomic Datasets Identifies Novel Drug Targets for Retinal Ganglion Cell Neuroprotection. *J. Clin. Med.* **2021**, *10*, 3938. [CrossRef]

Disclaimer/Publisher's Note: The statements, opinions and data contained in all publications are solely those of the individual author(s) and contributor(s) and not of MDPI and/or the editor(s). MDPI and/or the editor(s) disclaim responsibility for any injury to people or property resulting from any ideas, methods, instructions or products referred to in the content.

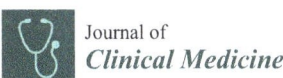

Article

Rapid Campimetry—A Novel Screening Method for Glaucoma Diagnosis

Fabian Müller [1], Khaldoon O. Al-Nosairy [2], Francie H. Kramer [2], Christian Meltendorf [3], Nidele Djouoma [2], Hagen Thieme [2], Michael B. Hoffmann [2,4,*] and Friedrich Hoffmann [5]

1 H & M Medical Solutions GmbH, 14195 Berlin, Germany
2 Ophthalmology Department, Faculty of Medicine, Otto-von-Guericke University, 39120 Magdeburg, Germany
3 Department of Optometry, Berlin University of Applied Sciences and Technology, 10785 Berlin, Germany
4 Center for Behavioral Brain Sciences, 39118 Magdeburg, Germany
5 Ophthalmology Department, Charité—Universitätsmedizin Berlin, 12203 Berlin, Germany
* Correspondence: michael.hoffmann@med.ovgu.de

Abstract: One of the most important functions of the retina—the enabling of perception of fast movements—is largely suppressed in standard automated perimetry (SAP) and kinetic perimetry (Goldmann) due to slow motion and low contrast between test points and environment. Rapid campimetry integrates fast motion (=10°/4.7 s at 40 cm patient–monitor distance) and high contrast into the visual field (VF) examination in order to facilitate the detection of absolute scotomas. A bright test point moves on a dark background through the central 10° VF. Depending on the distance to the fixation point, the test point automatically changes diameter ($\approx 0.16°$ to $\approx 0.39°$). This method was compared to SAP (10-2 program) for six subjects with glaucoma. Rapid campimetry proved to be comparable and possibly better than 10-2 SAP in identifying macular arcuate scotomas. In four subjects, rapid campimetry detected a narrow arcuate absolute scotoma corresponding to the nerve fiber course, which was not identified as such with SAP. Rapid campimetry promises a fast screening method for the detection of absolute scotomas in the central 10° visual field, with a potential for cloud technologies and telemedical applications. Our proof-of-concept study motivates systematic testing of this novel method in a larger cohort.

Keywords: automated static perimetry; rapid campimetry; glaucoma; arcuate scotoma; visual field defect; telemedicine

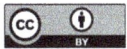

1. Introduction

Peter Piot, Belgian virologist, director of the London School of Hygiene and Tropical Medicine, and COVID-19 advisor to the EU Commission, himself became seriously ill with COVID-19 in mid-March 2020. Since then, the scientific expert on viral diseases has called himself an expert by experience, indicating his new perspectives on viral diseases. New perspectives often enable new insights and promote possible solutions. One of us (F.H.), an ophthalmologist, has recently been diagnosed with normal tension glaucoma, and here, too, the new perspective of an experienced expert could support the development of a new examination method.

Glaucoma is one of the most common causes of irreversible blindness worldwide [1]. It is characterized by progressive optic neuropathy and loss of retinal ganglion cells (RGC) and is associated with visual field (VF) defects. Several approaches are available that allow for reproducible assessment of functional vision loss [2]. Among these, standard automated perimetry (SAP) is a common standard subjective visual field test, but it has limitations, such as response variability [3]. In fact, there have been many recent developments in the field of VF testing in glaucoma and its utility in clinical practice, such as "portable brain-computer interface" [4] or "fundus-tracked perimetry" [5]. Recent evidence from functional and structural testing [6,7] indicates that the macula is affected at early stages of glaucoma. This suggests the importance of central visual field testing, e.g., the 10-2 SAP testing algorithm, for the earlier detection of central VF damage besides its pivotal association with quality of life in affected individuals [8–10]. This motivates further studies to provide better evidence-based guidelines for testing the central 10–20° of the visual field.

Conventional perimetry employed in testing VF limits the detectability of early VF defects in glaucoma and might not be optimal to aid in the salvaging of retinal ganglion cells (RGCs) from permanent damage. Early histological studies revealed that 20–40% of RGCs are lost prior to any detectable VF defects on conventional perimetry [11]. Several psychophysical techniques have been adopted, aiming to spot glaucoma damage at its earliest stages, including tests employing motion perception. Although not widely adopted, several studies have indicated abnormal motion perimetry in glaucoma [12,13], even at early stages, i.e., ocular hypertension [14,15].

In the present work, the perspective of an experienced expert (F.H.) served to explore a novel examination method for better understanding and earlier detection of VF defects based on the following case observation: In March 2017, F.H. observed a visual field defect on his right eye while rubbing the left eye. At the desk, a scotoma was identified as lying within the central 10° of the VF and was established as an arcuate scotoma in the superior temporal visual field, in analogy to locating the blind spot with a moving coin while fixating at a central point (Figure 1a). In June 2019, a second arcuate scotoma became apparent in the same eye (Figure 1a), it was unnoticed by Octopus 301 SAP (30°, Figure 1b) and was confirmed by Humphrey Field Analyzer (HFA3) 10-2 testing, applying 68 test points in the central 10° visual field (Figure 1c). Attempts to make the perceived visual field loss subjectively more salient utilized the observation that a small light, travelling rapidly through the visual field defect, was perceived as interrupted in the area of the scotoma. This insight was translated into the VF-testing method, i.e., rapid campimetry, which is described in the present paper. As proof-of-concept, it was applied in an additional five subjects with advanced glaucoma-related visual field defects.

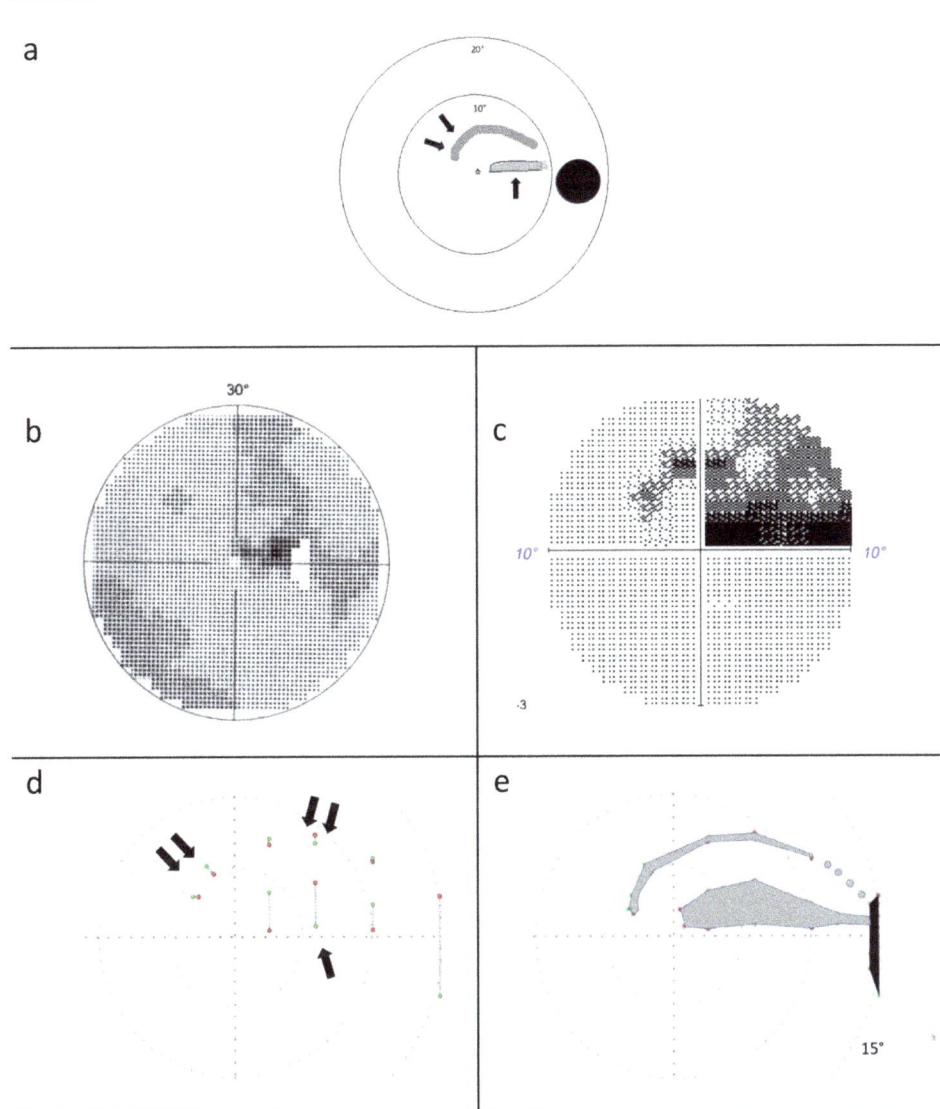

Figure 1. F.H. Visual field findings. (**a**) Sketch of the grey, drawn scotoma in the visual field of the right eye subjectively perceived by F.H. (first scotoma—one arrow, second scotoma—two arrows). (**b**) 30° field of view examined with Octopus 301. The scotoma is dark grey in the temporal upper field of view, the blind spot is shown in white. (**c**) 10° central visual field examined with the Humphrey Field Analyzer (HFA3). The absolute scotoma is black in the temporal superior visual field, and the relative scotoma is dark grey in the temporal and nasal superior visual fields. (**d**) Red and green dots, connected by a grey line, represent the beginning and end of the scotoma in the paramacular visual field after the screening procedure. One arrow marks the first scotoma, two arrows marks the second. (**e**) The 15° central visual field findings of scotoma delineation campimetry. After finding the two scotomas in the screening procedure, the exact scotoma borders were determined. The four grey spots

between the arcuate scotoma and blind spot (black) represent the presumed scotoma course. In this area, the test point is thicker than the narrow scotoma and therefore does not become invisible. When the test dot moves quickly, a brightness difference is perceived here, indicating the defect.

2. Materials and Methods

2.1. Subjects

Five glaucoma patients (see Table 1 for demographic data), besides F.H., with central visual field defects were enrolled in this proof-of-concept study, which followed the tenets of the Helsinki Declaration and was approved by the local university hospital, after giving written informed consent. All subjects already had established glaucoma and met the inclusion criteria for open-angle glaucoma (n = 6, age 50 years or older) with an open anterior chamber and typical glaucomatous optic disc damage defined by a vertical cup ratio ≥ 0.7, retinal nerve fibre layer defect or localized rim depression, and glaucomatous visual field defects [16].

Table 1. Demographic data of the subjects.

	Gender	Age [Years]	BCVA [logMAR] OD	BCVA [logMAR] OS	MD 10-2 OD [dB]	MD 10-2 OS [dB]
S1	m	81	0.0	0.2	0.29	−15.48
S2	f	80	0.80	0.4	−14.52 *	−1.73 *
S3	m	55	−0.1	−0.1	1.20	−3.64
S4	m	70	0.0	0.1	−10.77	−1.03
S5	f	62	0.0	0.0	−0.40	−13.30

S: Subject; m: male; f: female; BCVA: Best corrected visual acuity; OD: right eye; OS: left eye; logMAR: logarithm of minimal angle of resolution; MD: mean visual field deviation of 10-2 SITA standard VF; dB: Decibels; * 10-2 SITA fast protocol.

2.2. Standard Automated Perimetry Check (SAP)

Visual field defects were assessed using the 10-2 standard algorithm (subjects 1, 3, 4, 5 and F.H.) or 10-2 SITA Fast (subject 2) of the Humphrey Field Analyzer 3 (Carl Zeiss Meditec AG, Jena, Germany). The test stimulus was 4 mm² in size (equivalent to a size III Goldmann stimulus, i.e., 0.43°) and presented for 0.2 s.

2.3. Rapid Campimetry

Following the observation that a small light passed rapidly through the visual field defect is perceived as interrupted in the area of the defect, the central 10° visual field is tested in rapid campimetry with a bright test dot (140 cd/m²) on a dark screen (0.8 cd/m²) at a viewing distance of 40 cm (Figure 2). The visual field of the campimetry is extended temporally to 15° adjacent to the area of the blind spot to ensure that the patient understands the principle of the test by signalling the disappearance of the dot in the area of the blind spot. In the centre of the screen, there is a clearly visible cross as a fixation target (1.39° diameter) with lower brightness than the test marker.

The size of the test point was chosen to be as small as possible, such that it would not overlap the scotoma, while having good visibility at the same time. Because of the decreasing resolution from the centre to the periphery, the size of the test point increased with increasing distance from the fixation target. The optimal test point size was determined subjectively in pilot experiments (Table 2) and was 1.05 mm (0.16°) near the fixation point at a distance of 40 cm between the subject and the screen, and increased by 0.11 mm per degree, such that it had a size of 2.72 mm (0.39°) in the blind spot region. As the test point moves vertically, diagonally, and horizontally through the visual field, the size of the test spot changes automatically depending on the distance from the fixation point.

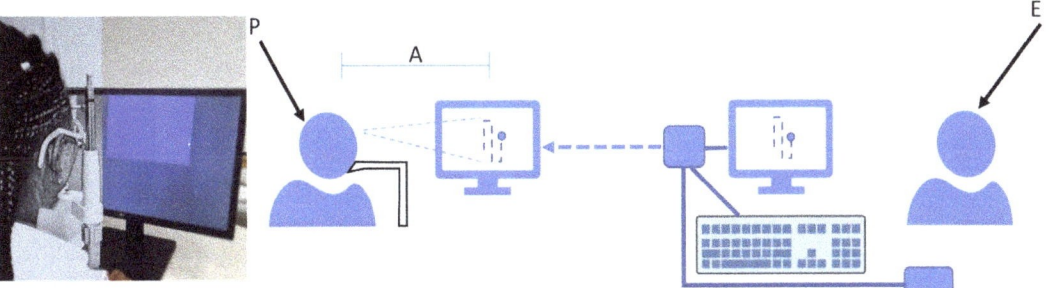

Figure 2. Rapid campimetry testing environment. Left Panel: Snapshot of the actual campimetry setting (with increased room lighting for better visualisation) with a volunteer fixating the centre of the testing area; left part of the image is masked to disable identification. Right panel: a sketch showing a person (P) looking at the monitor with a 40 cm distance (A) while an examiner (E) controls and runs the test on a different monitor.

Table 2. Various test point sizes in relation to position.

Distance [°] From Fixation Point	Diameter [mm] of the Test Point	Angle Diameter [°] of the Test Point
0.0°	1.05	0.16°
1.0°	1.16	0.17°
2.5°	1.33	0.19°
5.0°	1.61	0.23°
7.5°	1.88	0.27°
10.0°	2.17	0.31°
12.5°	2.45	0.35°
15.0°	2.72	0.39°

The most important difference in rapid campimetry in comparison to other visual-field testing methods is the running speed of the test point. The optimal running speed was determined subjectively on a narrow scotoma at a point approximately 8° from the fixation point, marked by a black ring (Figure 3). Different running speeds ranging from 0.18 cm/s to 24 cm/s were subjectively tested and the optimal speed was selected with which the scotoma was most reliably identified.

Using a too fast, 24 cm/s, or too slow, 0.18 cm/s, speed to run the test point disables the detection of the scotoma. Subjectively judged, the optimal speed of the test point seems to be ≈3 cm/s at 40 cm viewing distance from the screen. Here, it can be overlooked that the flat examination surface of the monitor results in an outward slowing of the velocity, since this variance at 10° results in about a 4% difference in velocity between the flat and curved surfaces. If the test point travels through the field of view at this speed along the seven vertical, diagonal, and horizontal paths mentioned in Figure 3, for a total length of ≈70 cm, then the test run passes through >1000 pixels ("test points"), depending on the resolution of the monitor (dpi). The specific screen area tested in rapid campimetry was 21.4 cm (442 pixels horizontally) by 14.1 cm (295 pixels vertically) and thus, for the test point progression of rapid campimetry (see below), ≈1400 test points. Due to the very fast update of the test point on the monitor (60 Hz), a subject perceives an uninterrupted line of light, that is, a point moving on the examination field of the monitor without interruption. The examination is completed within less than 30 s and the presence of absolute scotomas in the central 10° visual field can be largely excluded, if subjects see the test point uninterruptedly during the examination run.

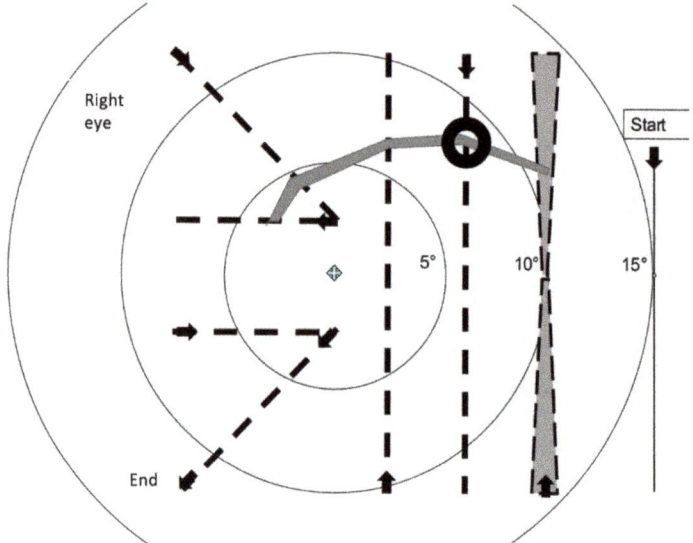

Figure 3. The path tested in the screening procedure of rapid campimetry is shown in dashed lines. In the arc scotoma marked by a black ring, 8° from the fixation point, the optimum test point speed was determined. The test point changes its diameter with the distance from the fixation point; the greater the distance, the greater its diameter. In the outer of the three vertical test lines, the used size change is overdrawn. If one wants to determine the examined area in this area, then the area is calculated as the sum of two identical trapezoids.

The test point trajectory is, in principle, arbitrary. However, for better comparability of the results for "rapid campimetry", a certain pattern is specified for the test point course. Within less than a minute, the test point first runs at 15° through the blind spot, then on three vertical, two diagonal and two horizontal lines through the central 10° visual field (Figure 3). The pattern of this test point course was chosen to follow the nerve fibre course traversing arcuate scotomas as perpendicularly as possible. As Aulhorn wrote, this is the best way to accurately determine glaucomatous scotoma boundaries [17].

The testing screen is coupled with an observation screen to enable monitoring of the test point by the examiner during examination. If the subject signals the disappearance or reappearance of the test point, these points of the scotoma rim are marked and the coordinates of these points are stored. In the examination result, the two points (scotoma start and end) are connected by a grey line symbolizing the scotoma, as shown in Figure 1d.

At the end of the test session, the examiner recognizes the suspected scotoma at the marked points at which the test point became invisible (off points) or visible again (on points). The scotoma can subsequently be delineated as in ordinary kinetic perimetry ("scotoma delineation campimetry"; duration approximately 1–10 min for one eye depending on the size of the VF defects) by moving the test point vertically, as, for example, shown in Figure 1e. Identifying the scotoma boundary accurately is facilitated by reducing the running speed of the test point, e.g., by a factor of 4 or 8.

If the examined area of each test point run is to be determined and set in relation to the square visual field with the horizontal and vertical diameter of the 10° area, and if the edge length of this square is 14.1 cm, then the total area to be examined is 198.81 cm^2. The path tested in the screening procedure is shown in dashed lines in Figure 3. The test point changes its diameter with distance from the fixation point; the greater the distance from the fixation point, the greater its diameter. In the outer of the three vertical test lines, the size change used is exaggerated for clarity. The examined area is calculated approximately as the sum of two identical trapezoids, which are shifted vertically. Minimal deviations result from the fact that the test point change is linear only for lines running directly from the fixed point. The two trapezoids therefore have very slightly curved lines in the direction of travel. If they are placed next to each other, they approximately form a rectangle with half the running distance of the test point and the sum of the largest diameter of the test point at the top and the smallest diameter in the middle of the path. The area tested in rapid campimetry then adds up to a total of 13.41 cm^2 of the total 198.81 cm^2 from the three vertical, two identical diagonal, and two identical horizontal paths of the test point, and thus 6.75% of the paracentral visual field to be examined (Table 3).

Table 3. Area calculation of the tested visual field fractions during the test run.

	Greatest Test Point Thickness [cm]	Smallest Test Point Thickness [cm]	Sum of Both Test Point Thicknesses [cm]	Half the Running Distance of the Test Point [cm]	Area [cm^2]
Vertical 1	0.26	0.22	0.48	7	3.35
Vertical 2	0.24	0.18	0.42	7	2.93
Vertical 3	0.22	0.13	0.35	7	2.47
Diagonal 1 + 2	0.24	0.14	0.38	7.44	2.81
Horizontal 1 + 2	0.19	0.14	0.33	5.6	1.85
Total					13.41

3. Results

The case observation of F.H.'s scotomas is shown in Figure 1. The novel method of rapid campimetry verified the two subjectively observed scotomas. Figure 1d shows the result at the end of the test run of the rapid campimetry, and Figure 1e shows the result of the scotoma delineation campimetry. The red and green dots connected with a grey dotted line represent the scotoma's start and end.

Five additional subjects (detailed in Methods) with a glaucomatous VF defect were included in this study to compare VF defects between SAP and rapid campimetry. Unintentionally, all five subjects had no SAP evidence of a VF defect in the fellow eye, which thus served as reference.

In general, there was an excellent agreement between rapid campimetry and SAP. All eyes without VF defects presented without abnormalities in either test (Figure 4). Similarly, the area and extent of the grey/black shaded regions of the VF defects in SAP corresponded to the scotoma line delineated by the rapid campimetry (Figure 5).

In combination with scotoma delineation campimetry, the following results are obtained for each subject compared to SAP: In subject 1, HFA detected scotomas in the upper visual field and normal sensitive retina between these scotomas. Scotoma delineation campimetry found instead a continuous arcuate scotoma in the same location. In subject 2, both HFA and campimetry demonstrated comparable findings showing an upper quadrant scotoma (Figure 5). In the lower visual hemifield of the left eye of subject 3, there was a relative scotoma in the centre of the arcuate scotoma, which scotoma delineation campimetry identified as an absolute scotoma. In subject 4, both campimetry and SAP depicted a similar arcuate scotoma in the superior VF of the right eye. Finally, subject 5 has an upper arcuate scotoma at a site of relative scotoma that rapid campimetry classified as an absolute scotoma.

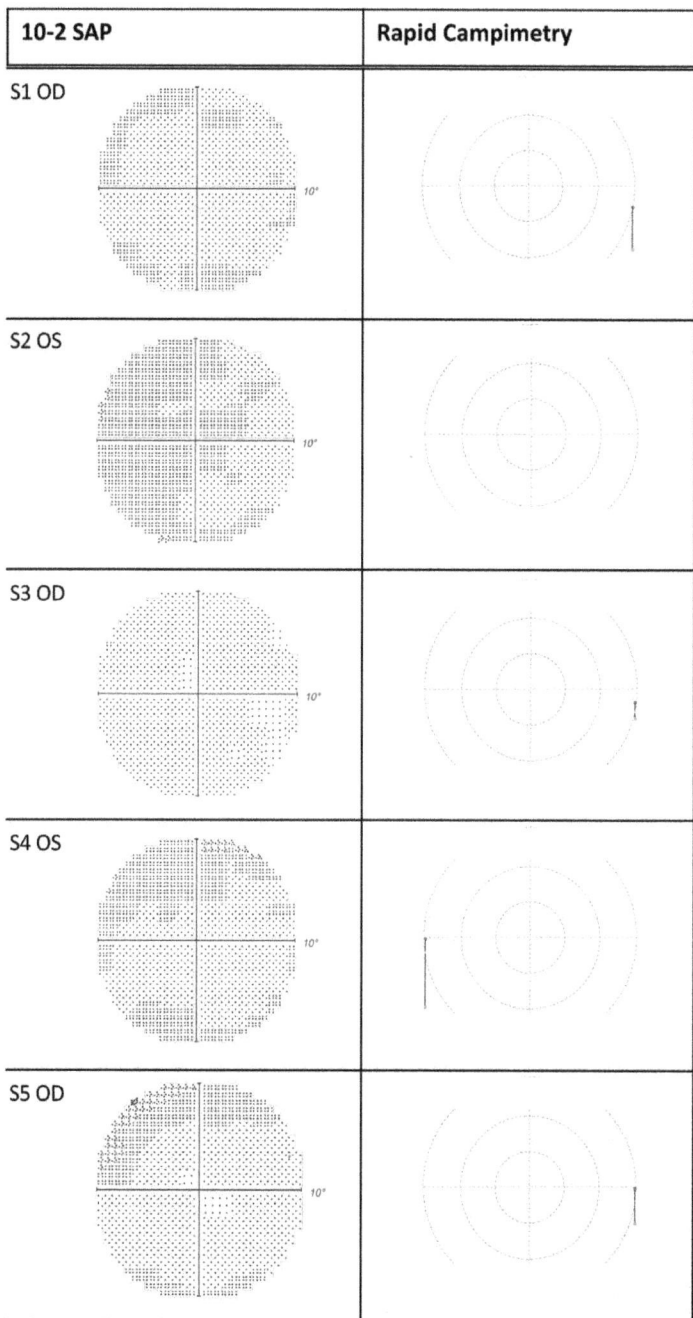

Figure 4. Eyes with normal visual field of subjects 1–5. The blind spot was detectable at 15° for all subjects except subject 2 (S2) with rapid campimetry. SAP = standard automated perimetry. OD = right eye; OS = left eye; S: subject; SAP: standard automated perimetry.

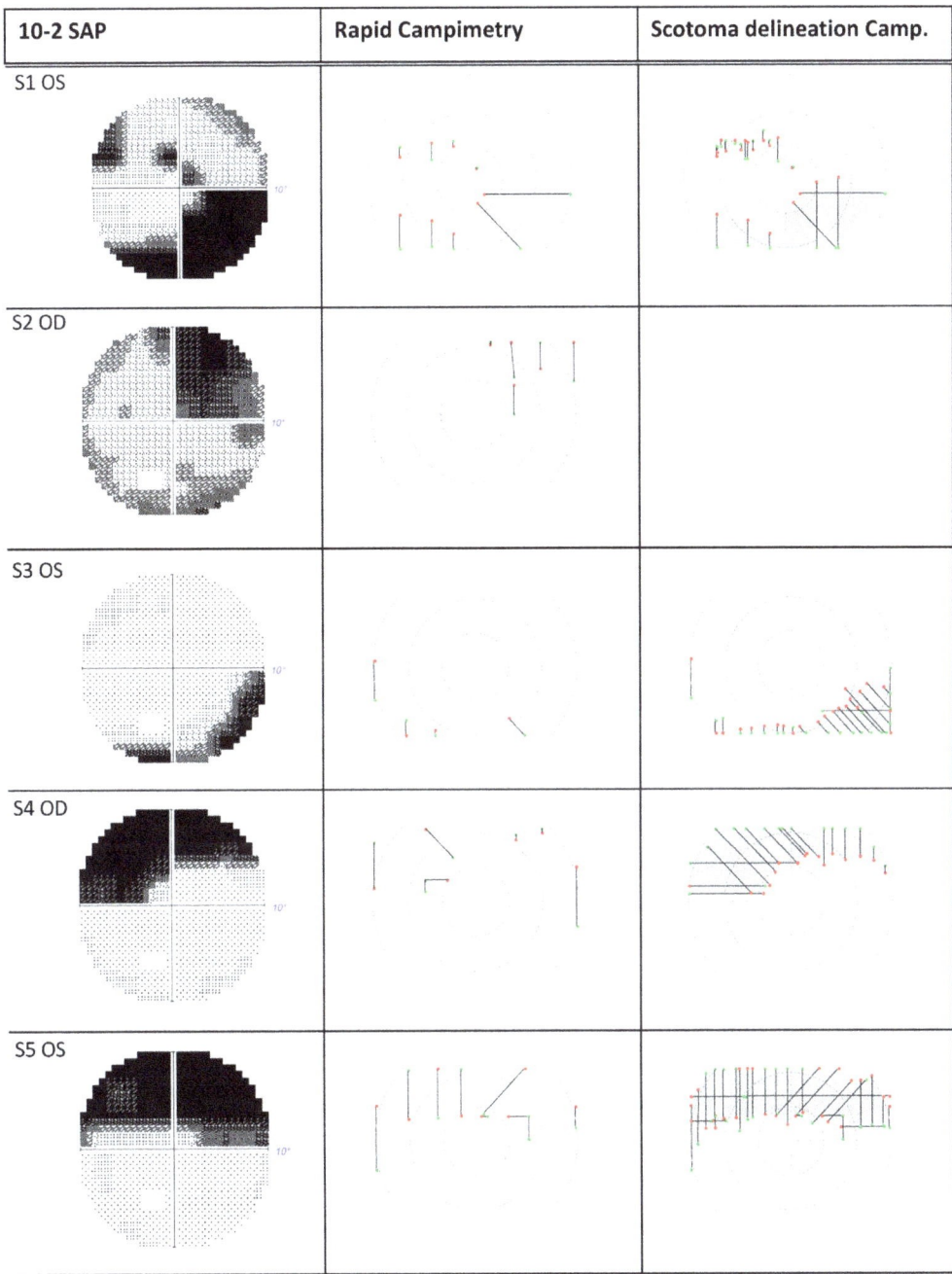

Figure 5. Eyes with visual field defects of subjects 1–5 compared between 10-2 SAP vs. rapid campimetry and scotoma delineation campimetry. SAP = standard automated perimetry. OD = right eye; OS = left eye; S: subject.

4. Discussion

The aim of this proof-of-concept study was to compare the novel visual field examination technique, rapid campimetry, with the established standard automated perimetry (SAP) in a case series regarding the detection of glaucomatous defects. In this six-subject sample, we found strong agreement between SAP and rapid campimetry in identifying VF defects in all eyes.

4.1. Increasing Attention via Fast Stimulus Movement

In the established SAP, the response behavior of the examinees is strongly dependent on their attention, since they are supposed to judge the appearance of a test point just at the threshold of perception and in weak contrast with the surroundings. The image change occurs so weakly or slowly that it is easily overlooked, but it is necessary in this form to define the threshold of perception [18]. One of the most important functions of the retina, namely, enabling the perception of rapid movement, was important in evolution because detection of the movement of a prey animal or enemy provided a survival advantage [19]. The perception of fast motion, however, is not tested in threshold perimetry. Notably, in order to identify retinal areas without light perception, i.e., whether there are absolute scotomas, fast motion can be used in combination with high contrast, with several key advantages, such as hardly strained participant attention.

4.2. Proportion of the Examined Visual Field Area in the Paracentral Visual Field

Another important difference between the different VF testing methods is the portion of the visual field actually examined. Testing the central VF using either Octopus, G1 program (17 points), or HFA3, 10-2 program (68 points) and employing Goldmann point size III, i.e., 4 mm^2 [4], the area examined only covers 3.1% and <1.0% of the central visual field, respectively. Here, at the examination distance of 30 cm, the 10° area of the central visual field is 87.58 cm^2 with a radius of 5.28 cm with minimal error variability due to the spherical surface deviation. These values explain why the arcuate scotoma was not found in F.H. with the Octopus perimeter. More accurate results can be expected with rapid campimetry where 6.75% of the paracentral visual field is tested.

4.3. Accuracy of Rapid Campimetry

To further test the accuracy of rapid campimetry vs. other standard perimetry, i.e., HFA3, we assessed whether glaucomatous VF defects were comparable in both techniques. Here, the examination of glaucomatous VF defects of five participants demonstrated agreement in the findings. In addition, rapid campimetry appeared to detect scotomata areas that were missed in the standard HFA3 test. The findings of subjects 1, 3, and 5, as well as F.H. suggest a superiority of the rapid campimetry vs. HFA3: For example, for F.H., the HFA found a relative scotoma in the upper visual field, whereas the campimetry instead found an absolute narrow arcuate scotoma at the same location (Figure 1e). As shown in Table 2, the angular diameter of the test point at the edge of the central 10° field of view is 0.31° compared to the conventional perimeter test mark III with a diameter of 0.43° at any point in the VF [18]. This latter large test mark cannot totally disappear in the narrow, approximately 0.35°-wide scotoma of Figure 1e, and cannot be perceived as an absolute scotoma, but only as a relative one. Finding these narrow scotomas appears to be facilitated by rapid campimetry's technique of a continuous vertical light line of ≈1400 closely spaced test points that overlap during motion and intersect all nerve fibres running to the blind spot.

4.4. Detection of Arc Scotomas

The method of rapid campimetry is similar to the campimetry described by Rönne and developed by his teacher Bjerrum, where a 1 cm-sized test point with angular diameter of 0.29° moves slowly on a black rod at 4 m^2 square black wall at 1–2 m distance [20]. In rapid campimetry, the dimensions are reduced and tailored to today's technology, as well as having the crucial feature of rapid movement. According to Rönne, the first early defects in glaucoma usually present in the Bjerrum area as small paramacular scotomas, which may be arcuately connected to the blind spot [20]. An explanation for arcuate scotomas is easily given by comparing the nerve fibre course in the retina with the shape and location of the arcuate scotomas where glaucoma damages individual optic nerve bundles and leads to interruption of the input from the corresponding retinal sites, leaving other bundles intact [21]. With today's standard examination methods, arcuate scotomas are hardly detected as such early stages, although their presence is theoretically probable [21].

Recently, finer patterns than the standard 24-2 VF tests, e.g., a $6 \times 6°$ grid, have been applied, and studies have confirmed that multiple macular VF defects can occur in glaucoma, of which arcuate scotoma is the most common [22,23]. These VF defects could also correspond to structural damage [24]. More recently, a new testing paradigm, the 24-2C, has been developed, in which 10 asymmetrically distributed test points from the 10-2 grid are integrated into the 24-2 grid so that both the central and peripheral visual fields can be tested. Nevertheless, testing the central 10 degrees supports higher resolution in terms of a detailed description of VF defects and better structure–function agreement [25].

4.5. Automation of Test Point Movement in the Paramacular Visual Field

Glaucoma is a group of progressive optic neuropathies characterized by degeneration of retinal ganglion cells [26]. The probable consequence of such ganglion cell degeneration is absolute rather than relative scotoma. Aulhorn, in reviewing 961 visual fields of glaucoma subjects, found that very early scotomas, despite their small extent, are usually absolute and very rarely relative [17]. In principle, the shape of a scotoma can be described well with kinetic perimetry, but small paramacular scotomas can be easily missed [17]. The requirement for slow test point movement can be met by the instrument only if large movement distances on the examiner's side correspond to a small visual angle on the subject's side. This is only possible, however, if very large-area examination screens are used for direct test point guidance, as for example with the Bjerrum wall, or if a translation mechanism is used for indirect test point movement [17].

The combination of the two demands may seem absurd, to increase the running speed of the test point for a safer scotoma detection on the one hand, and to move the test point as slowly as possible for an accurate definition of the scotoma margins on the other hand. However, both demands belong together, and only together do they fulfill their task perfectly. With the automatic test point movement, which can be slowed down by a factor of 4 or 8, the rapid campimetry meets Aulhorn's demand of translation mechanics in the paramacular range. In this way, it is possible to translate the advantages of Bjerrum's and Rönne's campimetry [20] into a novel technique and to combine it with the attentional enhancement of the fast movement.

4.6. Limitations of the Study

Our case-series study has a number of limitations which need to be addressed in a follow-up study on a larger participant cohort. The study was designed to provide proof-of-concept of rapid campimetry and was not designed to assess the sensitivity and specificity of the approach. For the latter purpose, a systematic investigation with a greater sample size is essential, including patients with different disease states and healthy controls. Further, potentially confounding effects of visual pathologies, e.g., optic media opacities, deserve attention in future studies. Finally, the quality of the fixation and its relation to the campimetry outcome has not been addressed in the present study, where patients were instructed to fixate the central target during testing and repeatedly reminded of the importance of central fixation. Online tracking of eye movements and fixation monitoring would help to assess whether maintaining central fixation is an issue during rapid campimetry testing.

4.7. Outlook

In addition to glaucoma screening, there are a number of fields where rapid campimetry might be of value. One potential application of the new examination method leads back to the beginning of the text—the COVID-19 pandemic, which has alerted us to the importance of telemedicine. Rapid campimetry is enabled via the internet and leverages the potential of cloud technologies, as a commercially available computer connected to the internet enables rapid campimetry virtually anywhere in the world with very low barriers to entry compared to current investigative methods. Possibly, this novel method could also help correlate morphologic differences of certain scotomas with their cause through more accurate scotoma description: Lachenmayr, for example, points out that in addition to mechanical nerve fibre damage due to intraocular pressure, there is vascular damage with typically classic nerve fibre bundle defects that manifests as arcuate scotoma [18]. Furthermore, migraine is considered a risk factor for glaucoma [27], which raises the question of whether visual field defects associated with migraine aura can be morphologically distinguished from typical glaucoma-related scotomas.

4.8. Conclusions

Our present proof-of-concept study suggests that rapid campimetry has advantages in glaucoma-screening compared to SAP. However, follow-up assessments are needed that investigate greater sample sizes of patients and healthy controls to assess the value of rapid campimetry as a screening and diagnostic tool for VF defect detection in glaucoma. In short, this method appears to be comparable to standard perimetry in the detection of central VF defects in glaucoma, and holds promise of applicability in ophthalmology as a screening and telemedicine tool.

5. Patents

European patent pending: Nr. EP21151704.0, EP21176171.3, EP21196409.3—PCT/EP2022/050765 "Verfahren und Einrichtung zum Messen des Gesichtsfeldes einer Person".

Author Contributions: Conceptualization, F.H. and F.M.; methodology, F.H. and F.M.; investigation, F.H., F.M., K.O.A.-N. and C.M.; software, F.M.; writing—original draft preparation, F.H. and F.M.; writing—review and editing, F.M., K.O.A.-N., F.H.K., C.M., N.D., H.T., M.B.H. and F.H. All authors have read and agreed to the published version of the manuscript.

Funding: This work was supported by funding of the German research foundation (DFG, HO2002/20-1) to MBH.

Institutional Review Board Statement: The study was conducted according to the guidelines of the Declaration of Helsinki, and approved by Ethics Committee of Faculty of medicine, Otto-von-Guericke University, Magdeburg (No: 151/16).

Informed Consent Statement: Informed consent was obtained from all subjects involved in the study.

Data Availability Statement: Upon request.

Acknowledgments: Dedication: to Elfriede Aulhorn (†), my (F.H.) mentor.

Conflicts of Interest: Fabian Müller received no support for the present manuscript but he had funding for the patenting with H & M Medical Solutions GmbH. Other authors had none. The authors declare no conflict of interest.

References

1. Tham, Y.-C.; Li, X.; Wong, T.Y.; Quigley, H.A.; Aung, T.; Cheng, C.-Y. Global Prevalence of Glaucoma and Projections of Glaucoma Burden through 2040: A Systematic Review and Meta-Analysis. *Ophthalmology* **2014**, *121*, 2081–2090. [CrossRef] [PubMed]
2. Al-Nosairy, K.O.; Hoffmann, M.B.; Bach, M. Non-invasive Electrophysiology in Glaucoma, Structure and Function—A Review. *Eye* **2021**, *35*, 2374–2385. [CrossRef] [PubMed]
3. Chauhan, B.C.; Garway-Heath, D.F.; Goñi, F.J.; Rossetti, L.; Bengtsson, B.; Viswanathan, A.C.; Heijl, A. Practical Recommendations for Measuring Rates of Visual Field Change in Glaucoma. *Br. J. Ophthalmol.* **2008**, *92*, 569–573. [CrossRef] [PubMed]

4. Nakanishi, M.; Wang, Y.-T.; Jung, T.-P.; Zao, J.K.; Chien, Y.-Y.; Diniz-Filho, A.; Daga, F.B.; Lin, Y.-P.; Wang, Y.; Medeiros, F.A. Detecting Glaucoma with a Portable Brain-Computer Interface for Objective Assessment of Visual Function Loss. *JAMA Ophthalmol.* **2017**, *135*, 550–557. [CrossRef]
5. Wu, Z.; Medeiros, F.A. Recent Developments in Visual Field Testing for Glaucoma. *Curr. Opin. Ophthalmol.* **2018**, *29*, 141–146. [CrossRef]
6. Hood, D.C.; Raza, A.S.; de Moraes, C.G.V.; Liebmann, J.M.; Ritch, R. Glaucomatous Damage of the Macula. *Prog. Retin Eye Res.* **2013**, *32*, 1–21. [CrossRef]
7. Bach, M.; Sulimma, F.; Gerling, J. Little Correlation of the Pattern Electroretinogram (PERG) and Visual Field Measures in Early Glaucoma. *Doc. Ophthalmol.* **1997**, *94*, 253–263. [CrossRef]
8. Blumberg, D.M.; De Moraes, C.G.; Prager, A.J.; Yu, Q.; Al-Aswad, L.; Cioffi, G.A.; Liebmann, J.M.; Hood, D.C. Association between Undetected 10-2 Visual Field Damage and Vision-Related Quality of Life in Patients with Glaucoma. *JAMA Ophthalmol.* **2017**, *135*, 742–747. [CrossRef]
9. De Moraes, C.G.; Hood, D.C.; Thenappan, A.; Girkin, C.A.; Medeiros, F.A.; Weinreb, R.N.; Zangwill, L.M.; Liebmann, J.M. 24-2 Visual Fields Miss Central Defects Shown on 10-2 Tests in Glaucoma Suspects, Ocular Hypertensives, and Early Glaucoma. *Ophthalmology* **2017**, *124*, 1449–1456. [CrossRef]
10. Park, H.-Y.L.; Hwang, B.-E.; Shin, H.-Y.; Park, C.K. Clinical Clues to Predict the Presence of Parafoveal Scotoma on Humphrey 10-2 Visual Field Using a Humphrey 24-2 Visual Field. *Am. J. Ophthalmol.* **2016**, *161*, 150–159. [CrossRef]
11. Quigley, H.A.; Dunkelberger, G.R.; Green, W.R. Retinal Ganglion Cell Atrophy Correlated with Automated Perimetry in Human Eyes with Glaucoma. *Am. J. Ophthalmol.* **1989**, *107*, 453–464. [CrossRef]
12. Bullimore, M.A.; Wood, J.M.; Swenson, K. Motion Perception in Glaucoma. *Investig. Ophthalmol. Vis. Sci.* **1993**, *34*, 3526–3533.
13. Wall, M.; Ketoff, K.M. Random Dot Motion Perimetry in Patients with Glaucoma and in Normal Subjects. *Am. J. Ophthalmol.* **1995**, *120*, 587–596. [CrossRef]
14. Silverman, S.E.; Trick, G.L.; Hart, W.M., Jr. Motion Perception Is Abnormal in Primary Open-Angle Glaucoma and Ocular Hypertension. *Investig. Ophthalmol. Vis. Sci.* **1990**, *31*, 722–729.
15. Wall, M.; Jennisch, C.S.; Munden, P.M. Motion Perimetry Identifies Nerve Fiber Bundlelike Defects in Ocular Hypertension. *Arch. Ophthalmol.* **1997**, *115*, 26–33. [CrossRef]
16. European Glaucoma Society Terminology and Guidelines for Glaucoma, 5th Edition. *Br. J. Ophthalmol.* **2021**, *105*, 1–169. [CrossRef]
17. Aulhorn, E. Subjective Examination Methods in Glaucoma Diagnosis. *Buch Augenarzt* **1976**, *69*, 128–139.
18. Lachenmayr, B.; Vivell, P.M.O. *Perimetrie*; Thieme: Stuttgart, Germany, 1992.
19. Pembury Smith, M.Q.R.; Ruxton, G.D. Camouflage in Predators. *Biol. Rev. Camb. Philos. Soc.* **2020**, *95*, 1325–1340. [CrossRef]
20. Rönne, H. Über das Gesichtsfeld beim Glaukom. *Klin Mbl Augenheilkunde* **1909**, *47*, 12–33.
21. Goldmann, H. Demonstration unseres neuen Projektionskugelperimeters samt theoretischen und klinischen Bemerkungen über Perimetrie. *OPH* **1946**, *111*, 187–192. [CrossRef]
22. Schiefer, U.; Papageorgiou, E.; Sample, P.A.; Pascual, J.P.; Selig, B.; Krapp, E.; Paetzold, J. Spatial Pattern of Glaucomatous Visual Field Loss Obtained with Regionally Condensed Stimulus Arrangements. *Invest. Ophthalmol. Vis. Sci.* **2010**, *51*, 5685–5689. [CrossRef]
23. Traynis, I.; De Moraes, C.G.; Raza, A.S.; Liebmann, J.M.; Ritch, R.; Hood, D.C. Prevalence and Nature of Early Glaucomatous Defects in the Central 10° of the Visual Field. *JAMA Ophthalmol.* **2014**, *132*, 291–297. [CrossRef] [PubMed]
24. Hood, D.C.; Raza, A.S.; de Moraes, C.G.V.; Odel, J.G.; Greenstein, V.C.; Liebmann, J.M.; Ritch, R. Initial Arcuate Defects within the Central 10 Degrees in Glaucoma. *Invest. Ophthalmol. Vis. Sci.* **2011**, *52*, 940–946. [CrossRef]
25. Phu, J.; Kalloniatis, M. Comparison of 10-2 and 24-2C Test Grids for Identifying Central Visual Field Defects in Glaucoma and Suspect Patients. *Ophthalmology* **2021**, *128*, 1405–1416. [CrossRef]
26. Weinreb, R.N.; Aung, T.; Medeiros, F.A. The Pathophysiology and Treatment of Glaucoma. *JAMA* **2014**, *311*, 1901–1911. [CrossRef] [PubMed]
27. Cursiefen, C.; Wisse, M.; Cursiefen, S.; Jünemann, A.; Martus, P.; Korth, M. Migraine and Tension Headache in High-Pressure and Normal-Pressure Glaucoma. *Am. J. Ophthalmol.* **2000**, *129*, 102–104. [CrossRef]

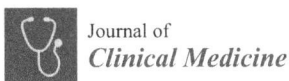

Review

Telehealth and Screening Strategies in the Diagnosis and Management of Glaucoma

Sze H. Wong * and James C. Tsai

Department of Ophthalmology, Icahn School of Medicine at Mount Sinai, New York Eye and Ear Infirmary of Mount Sinai, New York, NY 10003, USA; jtsai@nyee.edu
* Correspondence: swong@nyee.edu

Abstract: Telehealth has become a viable option for glaucoma screening and glaucoma monitoring due to advances in technology. The ability to measure intraocular pressure without an anesthetic and to take optic nerve photographs without pharmacologic pupillary dilation using portable equipment have allowed glaucoma screening programs to generate enough data for assessment. At home, patients can perform visual acuity testing, web-based visual field testing, rebound tonometry, and video visits with the physician to monitor for glaucomatous progression. Artificial intelligence will enhance the accuracy of data interpretation and inspire confidence in popularizing telehealth for glaucoma.

Keywords: telehealth; glaucoma; screening; monitoring

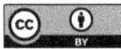

1. Introduction

Glaucoma is a progressive disease of the optic nerve and a leading cause of irreversible vision loss. Globally, in 2013, the prevalence of glaucoma was 3.54% among people aged 40–80, affecting 64.3 million [1]. It was estimated that by 2040, this number will increase to 111.8 million [1]. The demand for ophthalmologists to take care of glaucoma patients is expected to exceed the supply. In 2018, the Association of American Medical Colleges (AAMC) forecasted that there will be worsening shortages of physicians in the United States, with an estimated shortfall of 33,800 to 72,700 specialists by 2030 [2]. The report did not state what the estimated shortfall of ophthalmologists will be per se, but the trend is expected to be similar. The reasons for this shortfall include the stagnant number of ophthalmology residency and glaucoma fellowship positions, the increasing number of retiring ophthalmologists, and the aging population. In order to ensure adequate care for the increasing population of glaucoma patients, each ophthalmologist will have to accommodate a greater number of patients, eventually leading to overbooked clinic schedules, long wait times for patients, and crowded waiting rooms. The increasingly long wait times for the next available appointment can be detrimental to patient care. New strategies, such as the use of telehealth, will be increasingly important to limit clinic visits to patients who absolutely need to be seen, without compromising the care of patients with a stable disease.

Telehealth, as defined by Merriam-Webster, is health care provided remotely to a patient in a separate location using a two-way voice and visual communication. A computer or smartphone is needed to establish this communication. Because of the coronavirus disease 2019 (COVID-19) pandemic, the use of telehealth has accelerated due to patients' fear of contracting COVID-19 and the reduced number of in-person appointments given. Telehealth has also provided a convenient way for people living in rural regions to access their doctors.

There are three main purposes of telehealth in the field of glaucoma. One, is to screen for patients who have glaucoma, or are glaucoma suspects (i.e., those who have optic nerve appearances suspicious but not definitive for glaucoma). Two, for those newly diagnosed with glaucoma, to determine the severity of the disease and treatment plan. Three, for those diagnosed in the past, to monitor for disease progression and change management as needed. Each purpose requires a different set of equipment, as discussed below.

2. Equipment

2.1. Visual Acuity Test

Visual acuity is checked conventionally with a Snellen chart of letters placed 20 feet or 6 m away. If the patient has a refractive error, one should wear glasses corrected for distance. For each eye, the visual acuity of the smallest line the patient can read (at least half the letters correctly) is recorded. For the patient to perform this at home, one can either purchase a Snellen chart and hang it 20 feet away, print out a Snellen chart online and follow its instructions, or use a smartphone app. Of note, small Snellen charts, such as those on the smartphone, are referenced at reading distance, and would require presbyopic patients (typically those age 40 or above) to wear their reading glasses. A literature review [3] of mobile vision acuity applications revealed that the Peek Acuity application (Peek Vision Ltd., Berkhamsted, England) performed best, with a test–retest variability of ±0.029 Logarithm of the Minimum Angle of Resolution (LogMAR) for 95% confidence interval limits and a mean difference of 0.055 LogMAR when compared with visual acuity measured in clinic.

2.2. Intraocular Pressure Measurement

Knowing the intraocular pressure (IOP) is crucial for the diagnosis and management of glaucoma. The Early Manifest Glaucoma Trial (EMGT) demonstrated that reducing the IOP by 25% lowered the risk of glaucoma progression by 50% over 6 years [4]. Measuring IOP via telehealth is a challenge because measurement requires the instillation of an anesthetic eye drop with fluorescein and the use of a Goldmann applanator attached to a slit lamp, which is equipment that can only be used in the clinic by a skilled technician or physician. Portable IOP measuring devices with reasonable accuracy are available for use. In the setting of a glaucoma screening outside of clinic, the Tono-Pen®, the Pulsair Air Puff tonometer, the iCare rebound tonometer, the Ocular Response Analyzer, and the Diaton transpalpebral tonometer are suitable devices that technicians can use. At home, patients can rely on the iCare HOME. Intraocular sensors such as the Eyemate® and Injectsense can provide IOP data throughout the day as well. If no equipment is available, the IOP range can be estimated by palpation.

2.2.1. Tono-Pen® (Reichert; Depew, New York, NY, USA)

This is a hand-held electronic device that measures the force needed to applanate the cornea via a plunger. Prior to measurement, a topical anesthetic is applied to the eye, and a sanitized disposable cover is placed over the device tip. The operator then lightly taps the central cornea with the device tip multiple times until 10 measurements are recorded. The average IOP of the 10 measurements, along with a statistical confidence indicator, are displayed. The Tono-Pen® is easy to use and has reasonable accuracy when compared with Goldmann applanation, the gold standard for IOP measurement. A masked, randomized study on 270 eyes showed that Tono-Pen® measurements were 1.7 mm Hg higher than Goldmann applanation for IOPs from 6 to 24 mm Hg [5]. Another study looked at 197 eyes with glaucoma or ocular hypertension and found that Tono-Pen® measurements had a high correlation ($r \geq 0.86$) with Goldmann applanation. However, at high IOPs ($\geq$30 mm Hg), Tono-Pen® tended to underestimate Goldmann; and at low IOPs ($\leq$9 mm Hg), Tono-Pen® tended to overestimate [6]. Another study [7] of 142 eyes reported a correlation of coefficient of 0.84 between Tono-Pen® and Goldmann measurements. This study likewise subdivided the eyes into IOP ranges. For eyes with low IOPs (4–10 mm Hg), the Tono-Pen® measured an average 1.78 mm Hg higher than Goldmann applanation. For eyes with IOP in the normal range (11–20 mm Hg), the Tono-Pen® measured an average 0.07 mm Hg lower than Goldmann applanation. For eyes with elevated IOPs (21–30 mm

Hg), the Tono-Pen® measured an average 1.27 mm Hg lower than Goldman applanation. Additionally, for eyes with very elevated IOPs (31–45 mm Hg), the Tono-Pen® measured an average 4.15 mm Hg lower than Goldmann applanation. The higher the IOP, the more the Tono-Pen® underestimates. Tono-Pen IOP measurements have also been shown to be increased by a greater central corneal thickness (CCT) and a greater corneal resistance factor (CRF) [8–13]. However, for most eyes, the Tono-Pen® has reasonable accuracy. The Tono-Pen® is particularly useful for patients with a corneal edema or scar, as Goldmann applanation can underestimate the IOP in the presence of a spongy, edematous cornea and overestimate the IOP in the presence of a calcified scar; the Tono-Pen® is less affected by corneal edema and the device tip can be easily directed away from the scar when measuring. Another distinct of advantage of the Tono-Pen® is that the patient does not need to be upright. If the patient can only remain supine due to a medical condition or cannot position one's head vertically due to neck or spinal disease, the Tono-Pen® can still be used, as long as the operator ensures that the device tip taps the cornea perpendicularly. Other devices require the head to be upright for accurate measurement.

2.2.2. Air Puff Non-Contact Tonometer

This is a non-contact way to measure IOP. An electric device delivers a puff of air, and the force required to applanate the cornea is recorded. Multiple measurements are taken and the average IOP measured is calculated. Because there is no physical contact to the eye, a topical anesthetic is not required and there is no risk of corneal abrasion or infection from the equipment. The device is automated and easy to use. The noncontact tonometers available on the market include the Pulsair Desktop Tonometer (Keeler; Malvern, PA, USA), the CT-80 (Topcon; Tokyo, Japan), the NT-530/510 (NIDEK; Gamagori, Japan), and the TX-20 (Canon; Tokyo, Japan). Many studies found that noncontact tonometer IOP measurements are in moderate agreement with that of Goldmann applanation; as a result, the authors concluded that air puff tonometers can serve as good screening tools but are not accurate enough to substitute for Goldmann applanation [14–18]. Of note, there is an air puff tonometer that is compact and weighs approximately 2.5 kg called the Pulsair IntelliPuff (Keeler; Malvern, PA, USA). It is portable and can be easily brought to a glaucoma screening venue. Hubanova et al. [19] compared IOP measurements between the IntelliPuff tonometer and Goldmann applanation on 137 eyes and found that there was good agreement with an intraclass correlation coefficient of 0.86. The IntelliPuff tonometer overestimated the IOP by 1.5 ± 1.8 mm Hg in normotensive eyes and 2.3 ± 4.8 mm Hg in hypertensive eyes. Air puff is particularly useful in young children who do not tolerate eye drops well or are particularly anxious, as anesthetic eye drops are not required and there is no tip or probe that contacts the eye. However, some patients do not find the air puffs comfortable and would prefer other methods of measurement.

2.2.3. iCare (iCare Finland Oy; Helsinki, Finland)

This is a hand-held device that bounces a light-weight probe off the cornea. The contact is gentle enough that no topical anesthetic is needed. The IOP displayed is a function of the probe's deceleration at contact and the contact time, as measured by an induction-based coil system. The first generation TA01i model and the second generation ic100 model require the patient to be upright for measurement. Nakakura et al. [20] compared measurements of the iCare TA01i, iCare ic100, and Goldmann applanation on 106 eyes, and found that both iCare models measured significantly lower IOPs than Goldmann applanation (12.2 ± 2.9, 11.7 ± 3.0, and 16.9 ± 3.2 mm Hg, respectively). Furthermore, both iCare models' IOP measurements were correlated with central corneal thickness ($r = 0.50$). In contrast, Gao et al. [21] compared TA01i iCare measurements to that of Goldmann applanation on 672 eyes and found no significant differences between the two (18.30 ± 5.10 and 18.52 ± 4.46 mm Hg, respectively; $p = 0.19$), with a correlation coefficient $r = 0.806$. However, for eyes with IOP ≥ 23 mm Hg by Goldmann applanation, the iCare measurements were significantly lower (1.66 mm Hg, $p = 0.007$) than that of Goldmann applanation. Central corneal thickness had a stronger correlation with iCare measurements ($r = 0.39$) than with Goldmann applanation ($r = 0.19$). Subramaniam et al. [22] compared IOP measurements of iCare ic100 with Goldmann applanation in 1000 eyes and reported an intraclass correlation coefficient of 0.73. The ic100 measurements were significantly lower than Goldmann applanation measurements (12.1 vs. 16.2 mm Hg), even when the data were subdivided into different ranges of IOP. In January 2020, the iCare ic200 model was granted marketing authorization in the United States; it allows for IOP measurement even when the patient is reclined or supine. Badakere et al. [23] compared the ic200 with Goldmann applanation in 156 eyes and found that the ic200 readings were on average 1.27 mm Hg higher, but with no statistically significant difference.

A unique benefit of a portable tonometer that does not require a topical anesthetic is that home measurements can be performed. The iCare HOME is a device that allows for easy self-measurement. After loading a single-use probe, the device is placed in front of the eye at an appropriate distance (adjustable with the device's forehead and cheek supports). A hold of a button allows for six consecutive measurements, and the average measurement, along with the time of measurement, are saved in the device. When the patient returns the device to the clinic, these measurement data can be extracted and a diurnal IOP graph can be generated. Being able to take multiple measurements throughout the day at home is particularly useful in glaucoma patients with disease progression than normal IOPs measured in clinic. In this scenario, glaucoma specialists must determine whether the disease progression is a result of the "normal IOP" measured in clinic being above the target IOP to halt progression, or whether there are IOP elevations not detected because they occurred outside of clinic hours. The iCare HOME is a useful device that can answer this question. A comparison [24] of the iCare HOME measurement by the patient versus Goldmann applanation reported a high correlation ($r = 0.846$); the iCare HOME on average measured 0.70 mm Hg greater than Goldmann applanation ($p < 0.001$), and this difference increased by 1.2% for every 10% increase in central corneal thickness. Importantly, 98% of the 128 participants were able to use the iCare HOME.

2.2.4. Ocular Response Analyzer (Reichert; Depew, NY, USA)

This is a desktop device that uses a stream of air to applanate the cornea. No topical anesthetic is needed. Infrared light is emitted onto the cornea, and an infrared light detector measures a peak in light intensity when the cornea is flat. At this state, the inward applanation pressure is measured. The force of air then increases so that the cornea becomes concave, and then decreases until the cornea is flat again. At this state, the outward applanation pressure is measured. The entire measurement process takes about 20 milliseconds. The inward applanation pressure is greater than the outward applanation pressure, and this difference is the biomechanical property of the cornea termed corneal hysteresis. The device displays the inward intraocular pressure measurement (which should be identical to Goldmann tonometry) and the intraocular pressure measurement corrected by corneal hysteresis. Ehrlich et al. [25] and Ogbuehi et al. [26] compared ocular response analyzer (ORA) IOP measurements with those of Goldmann tonometry and found no statistically significant difference between them. However, a number of studies [27–31] found that the ORA significantly overestimated IOP when compared with Goldmann applanation. The importance of the ORA lies in its ability to measure corneal hysteresis, which is a known risk factor for glaucoma progression [32]. Eyes with a corneal hysteresis < 10 are 2.9 times more likely to have moderate to severe glaucoma than eyes with a corneal hysteresis ≥ 10; thus, corneal hysteresis can serve as a screening tool for glaucoma [33].

2.2.5. Sensimed Triggerfish® Contact Lens (Sensimed; Lausanne, Switzerland)

This soft contact lens, approved by the United States Food and Drug Administration (FDA), has a sensor that takes automated recordings for 24 h of the corneoscleral junction's dimensional changes, which are thought to correlate with changes in IOP. The lens is composed of silicone and has a high oxygen transmissibility to prevent hypoxia of the cornea. The sensor transmits data wirelessly to a circular antenna taped to the periorbital region. The antenna then sends the data via a cable to a recorder that the user wears hanging from the neck. The contact lens has been shown to be safe and well-tolerated, with a fair amount of reproducibility in diurnal IOP patterns [34]. A clinical trial [35] of 33 patients compared the slope of IOP increase from wake to sleep position measured by the contact lens sensor in one eye versus that of which was measured by the pneumatonometer in the contralateral eye; there was a high correlation coefficient of 0.914, suggesting that the contact lens sensor is accurate in detecting IOP changes.

A unique advantage of using a contact lens is it allows for the generation of a diurnal curve, even when the user is sleeping. This device can detect IOP elevations outside of clinic hours that may provide clues as to why a patient's glaucoma is progressing despite normal IOPs measured in clinic. In fact, a multicenter study that included 445 patients showed that certain variables measured by the contact lens, such as the night bursts ocular pulse frequency standard deviation and night bursts ocular pulse amplitude standard deviation correlated with prior rates of visual field progression [36].

2.2.6. Other Contact Lenses in Development

Researchers in South Korea developed a soft contact lens that measures IOP using a strain sensor [37]. The contact lens was tested on rabbit and human eyes, and it demonstrated reliable and accurate IOP measurements. Different from Triggerfish®, this contact lens sends data wirelessly to a smartphone; thus, allowing for the real-time monitoring of IOP and eliminating the need to carry a bulky recording device.

2.2.7. Eyemate® (Implandata Ophthalmic Products GmbH; Hannover, Germany)

This is a CE-certified IOP sensor placed into the ciliary sulcus during cataract surgery or Boston keratoprosthesis Type 1 (BI-KPro) implantation. Similarly to an intraocular lens, the sensor is foldable and can be injected into the eye through a corneal incision. This 11.2 mm wide silicone implant consists of eight pressure-sensitive capacitors in a single application-specific integrated circuit and a microcoil antenna arranged circumferentially. In order to obtain IOP measurements, a handheld reader device is placed at a short distance in front of the eye. The device emits a high frequency field that powers the sensor, and <2 s is needed for the sensor to measure the IOP and send the data to the reader device. A clinical trial demonstrated the successful implantation of Eyemate® in six patients; pupillary distortion and pigment dispersion were observed and some IOP measurements were significantly different from that of Goldmann applanation [38]. Another clinical trial involved 12 patients who underwent BI-KPro surgery and Eyemate® implantation; IOP measurements were found to correlate with surgical manometry ($r = 0.87$) with a mean difference of 3.9 ± 8.6 mm Hg [39]. The Eyemate® intraocular sensor is the first of its kind and can potentially revolutionize IOP monitoring for post cataract surgery or post BI-KPro surgery patients.

2.2.8. Injectsense (Injectsense, Inc.; Emeryville, CA, USA)

This is an IOP sensor, smaller than a grain of rice, that can be implanted transsclerally via an injection. Similarly to an intravitreal injection, implantation of the sensor can be performed in clinic using an injector that pierces the sclera and pars plana. The device self-anchors in the sclera and acts as a plug to prevent the egress of vitreous humor. The sensor measures the IOP at preset time intervals and stores the data. The patient is instructed to wear a pair of smart glasses once a week in order to recharge the sensor and download the stored IOP data, which are then automatically uploaded to a physician-accessible cloud database. This device is limited to investigational use at this time.

2.2.9. Diaton Transpalpebral Tonometer (DevelopAll Inc.; New York, NY, USA)

This is a digital device that measures IOP through the upper eyelid without contact with the cornea. The patient lies in a recumbent position looking up at a 45-degree angle.

A measurer pulls up the upper eyelid so that the lid margin is at the corneal limbus. The tonometer tip is placed perpendicular to the eyelid and parallel to the lid margin. A measurement is conducted when the tonometer tip touches the eyelid. The advantages of this device are measurements that can be performed by anyone after a brief training session, a topical anesthetic is not needed and it causes minimal patient discomfort. When compared with Goldmann applanation, Diaton demonstrated a moderate correlation acceptable for glaucoma screening but not as a substitute for Goldmann applanation in the management of glaucoma patients [40–43].

2.2.10. Finger Palpation

A crude method for the patient to estimate IOP is via finger palpation on the eye through the upper eyelid and describe whether the eye feels such as a tomato (low IOP), grape (normal IOP), or apple (high IOP). This is especially useful for patients who had recent glaucoma surgery and may experience extremes in IOP. An abnormally soft or firm eye would usually require a visit to the clinic soon.

2.3. Anterior Segment Photography

Although photography does not offer as much clarity as an in-person examination on the slit lamp, it can provide important information relevant to the diagnosis of the type of glaucoma and to monitor for postoperative complications. For example, the camera may capture the presence of white material along with pupillary margin, indicative of pseudoexfoliation, or an opacity within the pupil, indicative of a dense cataract.

In the setting of a screening program where a slit lamp is not available, a digital single-lens reflex camera (DSLR) with maximum zoom can be used to capture images. For those who had glaucoma surgery, of which the surgical site is in the superior or inferior conjunctiva, the technician would need to shift the eyelid away and have the patient look at the opposite direction to capture images of these areas. The advantages of the DSLR camera include its high resolution, wide range of magnification, and the ability to adjust the flash intensity. Tweaking the settings allow for high quality images of the anterior segment. It has even been demonstrated that when a DSLR camera's infrared-blocking filter is replaced with a piece of glass, iris transillumination defects of the iris can be photographed clearly [44].

At home, a cell phone camera can be used to capture a gross image of the eye, but the resolution and magnification are not high enough to visualize the anterior chamber. A smartphone adapter attached over the camera is needed for adequate magnification and near focusing in order to obtain clinically useful images. One such adapter is the Paxos Scope (DigiSight Technologies; San Francisco, CA, USA) which was found to be easy to use and was able to image a variety of anterior segment pathologies [45].

2.4. Iridocorneal Angle Imaging

To identify whether a patient is at risk for angle closure glaucoma, the ophthalmologist performs an examination technique called gonioscopy, in which a lens with side mirrors is placed on the cornea. The mirrors allow for the visualization of the anterior chamber angle, which contains the trabecular meshwork, the start of the aqueous humor's drainage pathway. When a large part of the trabecular meshwork is not visible due to the steepening of the iris, the patient is considered high risk for angle closure, and peripheral laser iridotomy is recommended.

In a setting where an ophthalmologist is not present to perform the gonioscopy, an anterior segment optical coherence tomography (ASOCT) can be used to measure the iridocorneal angle. Optical coherence tomography (OCT) uses near-infrared light to capture a high-resolution cross-sectional image of biologic tissue by the principal of interferometry. ASOCT parameters associated with angle closure include smaller anterior chamber dimensions (width, area, and volume) [46,47], a greater iris thickness and area [48], and a larger lens vault [49,50]. A regression model consisting of these parameters can diagnose angle closure with an area under the receiver operating characteristic curve (AUC) > 0.95 [51]. A validated scoring system can be incorporated into the ASOCT image analysis software to identify eyes with angle closure [52]. If a suspiciously narrow iridocorneal angle is seen in a screening program, pharmacologic pupillary dilation should be deferred (as dilation can induce acute angle closure glaucoma) and the patient should be sent to an ophthalmologist for a gonioscopy to verify the diagnosis. Of note, ASOCT is a desktop device that is not portable and is only available in the clinic setting.

Ultrasound biomicroscopy (UBM) uses a high frequency transducer (35–100 MHz) to obtain high resolution images of the anterior segment and measurements of the anterior chamber depth, angle, and the lens vault. Compared with the ASOCT, UBM has a greater penetration range, allowing for the visualization of the ciliary body. This increased range is particularly useful to visualize the plateau iris, cyclodialysis cleft, anterior choroidal effusions, or any masses beneath the iris. The disadvantage of the UBM is a transmission medium, such as a bag of fluid or gel, between the ultrasound probe and the eye is needed. In order to obtain clinically useful images, the technician needs to be well-trained.

A direct visualization of the iridocorneal angle can be performed using a gonioscopy camera. The Gonioscope GS-1 (NIDEK; Gamagori, Japan) is a desktop device that acquires 360-degree color photographs of the angle. The patient's eye is anesthetized and coated with gel, and the device's attached 16-mirror gonioprism contacts the cornea. The system then automatically captures images at different focus points from each gonioprism mirror; it takes approximately 1.5 min to photograph both eyes. Images in focus are then selected and a 360-degree fused panoramic image of the angle can be generated. A more portable gonioscope is the EyeCam (Clarity Medical Systems; Pleasanton, CA, USA), which consists of a handheld camera that can be used to visualize the angle when the probe is held against the eye coated with a coupling gel [53]. The Nanyang Technological University and Singapore Eye Research Institute similarly developed the GonioPEN, a smaller pen-like probe that can obtain images of the angle [54].

2.5. Fundus Photography

When evaluating a patient for glaucoma, being able to visualize the optic nerve head is key. Traditionally, photographs of the optic nerve head can only be taken with a desktop camera after the pupil is pharmacologically dilated. In recent years, handheld cameras have been developed that can take fundus photographs, even without dilation. In addition to glaucomatous nerve damage, these cameras allow for the diagnosis of macular pathology and other retinal diseases as well. The portable fundus cameras on the market include the Pictor Prestige (Volk; Mentor, OH, USA), VISUSCOUT® 100 (Zeiss; Oberkochen, Germany), SIGNAL (Topcon; Tokyo, Japan), and VERSACAM™ α (NIDEK; Tokyo, Japan). They are generally gun-shaped with a base charger, weighs approximately 1 pound, has a 40 to 50-degree fundus angle of view (with a pupil at least 3 mm in diameter), has autofocus or manual focus modes, has a touchscreen that displays the photograph taken, and has Wi-Fi connectivity to send images online.

An alternative to using the fundus camera is to rely on a smartphone camera attachment. The D-Eye Retinal Camera (D-EYE Srl, Padova, Italy) is an attachment that can obtain images of the optic nerve, even without pupillary dilation. The camera attachment requires the smartphone to be as close to the eye as possible, and the smartphone's video mode is turned on so that the split-second frame of which the optic nerve is centered within the field of view and is in focus is captured. This method of obtaining optic nerve photographs requires practice and an adequately large undilated pupil. The image resolution is limited by the smartphone camera. A prospective study demonstrated that vertical cup/disc ratios graded from D-Eye smartphone ophthalmoscopy agreed with those from slit lamp examination in 72.4% of primary open angle glaucoma patients and 66.7% of ocular hypertension patients [55]. Another study revealed that pharmacologic pupillary dilation improved D-Eye's vertical cup/disc ratio measurement significantly [56].

2.6. Optical Coherence Tomography of the Retinal Nerve Fiber Layer

In the past, serial optic nerve head photography was the only way to document structural changes indicative of glaucoma. In recent years, however, optical coherence tomography (OCT) has taken over as a more precise and objective tool in the diagnosis and monitoring of glaucoma. OCT relies on near-infrared light to obtain a cross-sectional image of the retina and optic nerve head. Different layers of the retina can be isolated in the scan, as there is an increased reflectivity in the nerve fiber layer and the plexiform layers and decreased reflectivity in the cell and nuclear layers. OCT performs a retinal nerve fiber layer (RNFL) analysis by measuring the RNFL thickness at a circle, 3.4–3.5 mm in diameter, centered around the optic nerve head. In the presence of a glaucoma, areas of RNFL loss are seen, typically in the superotemporal and inferotemporal regions of the circle. The OCT compares the RNFL thickness pattern with that of a normative database of the same age group and flags any areas below the reference range with a color-coded scheme. The OCT is a powerful tool in the early detection of glaucoma, as RNFL thinning can be seen, even before peripheral visual field loss occurs. Furthermore, when serial OCT scans are taken, the RNFL thickness of each region can be plotted on a trend line to assess for disease progression over time.

OCT is a desktop device only available in clinic. Companies are working to develop a portable version, but the closest to that at this time is the Envisu C2300 (Leica; Wetzlar, Germany), which consists of a handheld OCT scanhead attached to a cart of equipment. The Envisu C2300 is particularly useful for patients who cannot sit up to reach a desktop device. In the future, a portable home OCT machine for glaucoma patients may be available, given that Notal Vision (Manassas, VA, USA) has developed one for the detection of neovascular age-related macular degeneration (AMD) progression at home.

2.7. Visual Field

Glaucoma is known as the "sneak thief of sight" because of its tendency to affect the peripheral visual field first. As a result, many patients do not realize that they have glaucoma until the visual field loss encroaches centrally. In clinic, standard automated perimetry (SAP) is performed to detect visual field loss. The patient places his/her head on a chinrest in front of a white bowl. While fixating on a target, he/she is instructed to push a button whenever a spot of light is seen. The machine will display light stimuli at various locations and intensities. In the end, the machine will map out spots that the patient did significantly worse relative to his/her age group.

Because SAP is a large device only available in clinic, it cannot be used in a screening program outside or at home. Alternatives of SAP include online perimetry performed on a computer, tablet, or with virtual reality glasses.

2.7.1. Peristat Online Perimetry

This is a visual field test accessed at keepyoursight.org and is performed on a computer with a 17-inch or larger monitor. In the beginning, the patient is asked to adjust his/her distance from the monitor until a flashing light temporal to the fixation point disappears (i.e., enters the blind spot). The patient is then asked to fixate at a central point. Stimuli are presented at various locations across a 24-degree horizontal by 20-degree vertical field with various intensities, and the patient is asked to push the spacebar whenever one is seen. The test takes less than 5 min per eye. Similarly to SAP, the Peristat test generates a report with reliability indices and a grayscale visual field image; the results are emailed to the doctor who ordered the test.

A prospective study [57] comparing Peristat Online Perimetry with Humphrey Visual Field 24-2 test reported Spearman rank correlations ranging from 0.55 to 0.77 for abnormal points in both tests. Peristat Online Perimetry demonstrated a high diagnostic ability, with the AUC ranging from 0.77 to 0.81 for mild glaucoma and 0.85 to 0.87 for moderate to severe glaucoma.

2.7.2. Melbourne Rapid Fields (MRF)

This is a web-based program that relies on a touchscreen tablet. Voice prompts of multiple languages are available. The subject is asked to sit 33 cm away from the screen and fixate at a crosshair target. There is a square area that the subject is supposed to tap whenever a stimulus is seen. The stimuli are presented as dots of various intensities in different locations, similar to SAP. When using a small tablet, the fixation target may shift to a corner of the screen to widen the visual field area tested (to up to 30 degrees from fixation). The MRF test takes approximately 3–4 min per eye, which is significantly shorter than the Humphrey Visual Field 24-2 SITA-standard program (average 6–7 min per eye) [58,59]. After completion of the MRF test, a report is generated, showing the reliability indices, the sensitivity value of each spot, the total deviation map, the pattern deviation map, and the visual field gray scale. Multiple studies have shown that MRF has a low retest variability and high correlation with the Humphrey Field Analyzer [58–61].

2.7.3. Virtual Reality Headsets

In recent years, virtual reality (VR) systems have become available to the public for entertainment, especially video gaming. VR headsets have gyroscopes that detect head movement and gaze trackers, allowing the user to immerse into a 3D virtual environment that shifts according to his/her head and eye movements. This technology is particularly useful in visual field testing because it eliminates the problem of fixation loss. The accuracy of a conventional visual field test relies on the subject to fixate at the target for the duration of the test. This is no longer necessary with a VR system, because the stimulus position can be adjusted based on the change in fixation. Tsapakis et al. [62] had 20 patients use virtual reality glasses hooked up to a computer. They ran a software that used a fast-threshold 3-decibel step staircase algorithm to test 52 points scattered across 24 degrees of visual field from fixation. The patients were asked to click the mouse whenever a stimulus was seen. This VR visual field test had a high correlation coefficient of 0.808 when compared with the Humphrey Visual Field. VR visual field systems that are commercially available include the Advanced Vision Analyzer (Elisar; New City, NY, USA), the C3 Field Analyzer (Remidio; Glen Allen, VA, USA), the PalmScan VF2000 Visual Field Analyzer (Micro Medical Devices; Calabasas, CA, USA), Virtual Field (Virtual Field; New York, NY, USA), VirtualEye Perimeter (BioFormatix; San Diego, CA, USA), VisuALL (OllEyes Inc, Summit, NJ, USA), and Vivid Vision Perimetry (Vivid Vision, San Francisco, CA, USA).

In addition to fixation loss, current visual field tests rely on patients to minimize the false-positive rate (meaning hitting the clicker when there is no stimulus presented) and the false-negative rate (meaning not hitting the clicker when the stimulus should be seen, based on previous responses). To eliminate the "human factor" of visual field testing, a VR headset called NGoggle was developed to detect multifocal steady-state visual-evoked potentials when a stimulus is presented. The headset consists of a wireless electroencephalogram, an electrooculogram, and a head-mounted display. In a study where glaucoma was diagnosed based on stereo photographs of the optic discs, Nakanishi et al. [63] found that the NGoggle had a higher AUC (0.92) than SAP mean deviation (0.81), SAP mean sensitivity (0.80), and SAP mean pattern standard deviation (0.77), suggesting that NGoggle may be better at detecting glaucoma than SAP. A VR headset that can detect visual-evoked potentials may prove to be more accurate and efficient than the current gold standard of SAP, setting a paradigm shift in visual field testing.

2.8. Artificial Intelligence

In ophthalmology, deep learning in artificial intelligence (AI) has become a hot topic as it demonstrated remarkable accuracy in the detection of disease. Deep learning is a machine learning technique that uses multiple layers of an artificial neural network to extract high-level features from raw data and generate an output. This design is inspired by how neurons connect with each other in the human brain. In order for the machine to generate a highly accurate neural network, it needs to be fed a massive set of data that encompass all variations. To make the diagnosis of glaucoma and recommend the appropriate management plan via telehealth, the ophthalmologist takes into account the IOP, visual field test report, fundus photography, OCT, and other available test results. Having a specialist review the data may not be necessary in the future, as artificial intelligence technology becomes more powerful with the ability to self-learn such as a human.

A number of deep learning AI systems have been developed to diagnose glaucoma based on optic disc photographs. The European Optic Disc Assessment Study [64] compared the performance of the Pegasus v1.0 (Visulytix Ltd., London, UK) AI software with that of ophthalmologists and optometrists in diagnosing glaucoma from stereoscopic optic disc photographs. Pegasus was able to diagnose with an accuracy of 83.4%, which was statistically similar to the accuracies of ophthalmologists (80.5%) and optometrists (80%). Eyes that truly had glaucoma were identified by glaucoma specialists who saw reproducible visual field scotomas that matched the appearance of the optic discs. Several other studies demonstrated that certain deep learning parameters can achieve high accuracy with AUC > 0.9 and sensitivity and specificity levels > 90%; false-positive and false-negative results were commonly due to pathologic myopia [65–70]. Even with the use of different fundus cameras, deep learning artificial intelligence was able to achieve an AUC > 0.9, provided that image augmentation was performed [71]. Al-Aswad et al. [72] used data from the Singapore Malay Eye Study to determine how the Pegasus deep learning system performed compared with ophthalmologists in diagnosing glaucoma solely based on fundus photographs. They found that Pegasus outperformed five out of six ophthalmologists and took only 10% of the time the ophthalmologists did in diagnosing glaucoma. Remarkably, Medeiros et al. [73] showed that by training a deep learning algorithm to match disc photographs with OCT RNFL scans, the machine was able to predict the average RNFL thickness based on the fundus photograph with a high Pearson correlation coefficient of 0.832 and a mean difference of 7.39 microns. In fact, when deep learning artificial intelligence was used on fundus disc photographs taken over time, it was able to identify eyes with worsening glaucoma based on a decreasing predicted RNFL thickness [74,75].

In addition to the analysis of fundus photographs, deep learning artificial intelligence can be trained to diagnose glaucoma based on OCT RNFL and the ganglion cell-inner plexiform layer (GCIPL) scans with high accuracy (AUC > 0.9) [76–81]. In fact, one study showed that a deep learning model trained with OCT images outperformed SAP and mean circumpapillary RNFL thickness in detecting glaucoma [76]. If the deep learning algorithms are exposed to OCT nerve images paired with visual field data, the machine is able to predict visual field parameters accurately [82,83].

Deep learning can also play a role in diagnosing angle closure based on OCT anterior segment images. Fu et al. [84] developed a deep learning system to detect angle closure and tested it on 8270 OCT anterior segment images (of which 895 had angle closure as classified by clinicians). The system achieved an AUC of 0.96 with a sensitivity of 0.90 and specificity of 0.92. Xu et al. [85] applied deep learning methods on 4036 OCT anterior segment images (of which 2093 had closed angles) in the Chinese–American Eye Study and found that the ResNet-18 classifier achieved an AUC of 0.952.

Machine learning of visual field data may have utility in diagnosing pre-perimetric glaucoma. Asaoka et al. [86] reported that a deep feed-forward neural network classifier had an AUC of 92.6% in diagnosing pre-perimetric glaucoma based on Humphrey Visual Field 30-2 data. In addition to diagnosis, deep learning has been shown to predict future visual field progression. Wen et al. [87] used various deep learning algorithms on more than 30,000 Humphrey Visual Field 24-2 reports and found that the Cascade-Net5 performed the best in forecasting visual fields up to 5 years later, with a pointwise mean absolute error (2.47 dB), significantly less than that of the rate of progression linear models (3.77–3.96 dB) and the pointwise regressed linear model (3.29 dB). Yousefi et al. [88] reported that machine learning analysis detected visual field progression earlier (at 3.5 years) than global (at 5.2 years), region-wise (at 4.5 years), and point-wise (at 3.9 years) linear regression analyses.

3. Setups for Telehealth Programs

As discussed previously, telehealth can serve three purposes: (1) screen for glaucoma, (2) evaluate the severity of glaucoma to determine the treatment plan, and (3) to monitor disease progression. How each of these purposes can be achieved should depend on the equipment/facilities available, the patient population (the prevalence of certain types of glaucoma can vary), and the socioeconomic and/or geographic barriers to face-to-face ophthalmologic care.

A number of telehealth screening programs have been implemented and can serve as templates tailored to the needs of the community. For example, the Philadelphia Telemedicine Glaucoma Detection and Follow-up Study [89] executed a program of which people at risk for glaucoma could be screened at a primary care practice or a Federally Qualified Health Center. At the first visit, the participant's medical and family history were recorded. An ophthalmic technician used a nonmydriatic, portable fundus camera to take two fundus photographs (macula and optic nerve) and one anterior segment photograph per eye. The technician measured IOP using the iCare tonometer. If the IOP was ≥30 mm Hg, the participant was referred to an ophthalmologist immediately. All information obtained was sent to glaucoma and retina specialists for reading. If a participant had an IOP of 22–29 mm Hg, an abnormal finding (such as a suspicious optic nerve appearance), or an unreadable image, he/she were contacted to schedule an eye examination at the same primary care practice or health center within 6 months. At visit two, the subjects underwent a slit lamp examination by a glaucoma specialist, along with SAP. The equipment was brought in by a community outreach van. Based on the assessment at this visit, follow-up testing, appointment, or treatment was recommended. This screening program was conducted over 5 years. Of the 902 people screened, 37% had an abnormal image, 17.2% had an unreadable image, and 6.9% had ocular hypertension; therefore, 59.4% were asked to attend visit 2. Of the people asked to attend visit 2, 64.7% showed up. Of those who showed up, 10.9% had glaucoma, 7.2% had ocular hypertension, and 45.8% were glaucoma suspects. Taken together, 24.6% of the original 902 people screened had glaucoma, ocular hypertension, or were glaucoma suspects in this urban, multiethnic population.

Similar to the Philadelphia screening program, the Manhattan Vision Screening and Follow-up Study in Vulnerable Populations (NYC-SIGHT) [90] is a community-based screening program to be conducted for 5 years, specifically for residents in New York City Housing Authority developments. Because of the COVID-19 pandemic, participants will have medical history obtained and a visual function questionnaire asked over the phone and will be screened for COVID-19 symptoms before being allowed at the community screening site. At the screening, visual acuity check, IOP measurement, and nonmydriatic fundus photography are performed. Participants who fail the vision screening will be scheduled to see an optometrist on-site for a refraction and a nondilated eye examination by a portable slit lamp and a direct ophthalmoscope. Participants with a high IOP, an abnormal fundus image, or a concerning examination finding will be referred to an ophthalmologist in the clinic.

The Michigan Screening and Intervention for Glaucoma and Eye Health Through Telemedicine (MI-SIGHT) [91] and the Alabama Screening and Intervention for Glaucoma and Eye Health Through Telemedicine (AL-SIGHT) [92] programs are designed to be more comprehensive at the first visit. Similarly to the Philadelphia program, federally qualified health centers are used, and people with specific risk factors for glaucoma are eligible. In the Alabama program, an ophthalmic technician checks the visual acuity, performs auto-refraction, measures IOP with iCare rebound tonometer, and takes images using a combined OCT and fundus camera machine (Maestro2, Topcon Medical Systems, Oakland, NJ, USA) and a smartphone with an adapter (D-Eye retinal camera), and performs visual field testing using the Humphrey Visual Field Analyzer and Melbourne Rapid Fields application on a tablet. In the Michigan program, an ophthalmic technician checks the visual acuity and performs refraction, assesses the iridocorneal angle with penlight, assess ocular motility, measures IOP with iCare tonometer, and dilates the participant if

IOP < 30 mm Hg and/or angles are not narrow. Fundus photographs and OCT RNFL images are obtained when the pupils are dilated. In both programs, the data are sent to an ophthalmologist for review in order to determine the appropriate follow-up.

Rather than screening the community for glaucoma, a telemedicine program [93] in Northern Alberta served as a glaucoma consult service. Patients seen by an optometrist, ophthalmologist, or family physician were referred to the program if they had risk factors for glaucoma or suspicious-looking optic discs or visual field test. At each office, a tonometer, corneal pachymeter, visual field machine, and a retinal camera were available for use by technicians. A glaucoma specialist at the University of Alberta then reviewed the data remotely and gave recommendations for management and follow-up.

In addition to screening for glaucoma, telemedicine can be used to monitor for the development of glaucoma. The Kaiser Permanente Eye Monitoring Center conducted a 2-year telemedicine program [94] to monitor low-risk glaucoma suspects. Each year, a technician checked the visual acuity, measured the IOP using a handheld applanation tonometer, and took OCT RNFL images at a local ophthalmology clinic. Different from other telemedicine programs, the data were sent to a trained technician first, rather than a glaucoma specialist. If there was a decline in visual acuity of at least two lines, an IOP elevation $\geq$ 5 mm Hg, or a significant change in the RNFL thickness in the superotemporal or inferotemporal region (defined as $\geq$10-micron reduction or transition into the abnormal red range), the technician would send the patient data to a glaucoma specialist for review remotely. Of the 225 glaucoma suspects enrolled in the program, five were referred for examination by an ophthalmologist due to concern for progression on OCT. Of those five patients, two were started on glaucoma medications. This program demonstrated that telemedicine is a viable option for monitoring glaucoma suspects and can capture the small number of patients who develop glaucoma and need treatment.

Telehealth programs can be used to monitor patients with an established diagnosis of glaucoma as well. Rutgers New Jersey Medical School conducted a program [95] on patients who had glaucoma or were glaucoma suspects. The patients went through the tele-glaucoma setup in the following order: (1) medical history intake; (2) IOP measurement with puff tonometer; (3) auto-refraction; (4) OCT imaging of the iridocorneal angle (and central corneal thickness measurement), cup/disc ratio, RNFL, and ganglion cell complex; (5) nonmydriatic color photography of the anterior segment and fundus, as well as auto-fluorescence imaging of the fundus. A glaucoma specialist then reviewed the data remotely and gave recommendations on management and follow-up. To compare the accuracy of the data and assess the program with a clinical examination, the subjects underwent a comprehensive eye examination on the same day by an ophthalmologist. IOP was measured by Goldmann applanation and the slit lamp was used to examine the anterior segment and fundus. OCT and visual field testing were performed under the discretion of the ophthalmologist. When comparing the tele-glaucoma program with the clinical examination, there were strong correlations in IOP measurements and cup/disc ratios. The recommended follow-up time was shorter for the tele-glaucoma program (2.7 months vs. 3.9 months). The clinical examination was better at identifying exotropia, iridotomy, iris neovascularization, and trabeculectomy. The tele-glaucoma program was better at identifying narrow angles, age-related macular degeneration, macular edema, diabetic retinopathy, retinal vein occlusion, choroidal nevus, and splinter hemorrhages.

A similar study [96] in London compared a "virtual clinic" staffed by an ophthalmic nurse versus an examination by an ophthalmologist for patients with open angle glaucoma. In the nurse clinic, a technician checked visual acuity, conducted SAP, took fundus photos, and performed scanning laser ophthalmoscopy with Heidelberg Retina Tomography. The nurse performed Goldmann applanation tonometry and a slit lamp examination of the anterior segment. The patient then was examined by an ophthalmologist and the assessment was recorded. One year later, the same ophthalmologists who took part in the study were asked to review the data from the nurse "virtual clinic" a year ago and classify whether the patient was stable or unstable based on just these data. The study found that 3.4%

of patients were misclassified as "stable" by review of the "virtual clinic" data when in fact they were "unstable" according to the in-person assessment by the ophthalmologist. The authors concluded that 3.4% was an acceptably low misclassification rate and that a "virtual clinic" run by ophthalmic nurses can be a viable option for managing relatively stable glaucoma patients.

A review of these glaucoma telehealth programs shows that a variety of setups can be used to screen for glaucoma and monitor for disease progression. At the bare minimum, a technician should record the patient's medical history, visual acuity, IOP, and take a fundus photograph. Technological advances have allowed IOP measurements without the use of topical anesthetic and fundus imaging without pharmacologic pupillary dilation. SAP to detect visual field scotomas and OCT to detect structural nerve fiber layer loss can provide additional valuable data, but these bulky machines are unlikely available outside of the ophthalmology clinic setting. As deep learning artificial intelligence technology matures, fundus imaging may be all that is needed to accurately predict RNFL thickness and visual field loss. Artificial intelligence will play a significant role in reducing the amount of equipment required for glaucoma screening and monitoring through telehealth. A summary of the components of a glaucoma telehealth examination is listed in Table 1. Even at its current state, without reliance on artificial intelligence, telehealth has shown to be cost-effective. An analysis of remote glaucoma screening in rural Alberta, Canada revealed that teleglaucoma costs an average of CAD 867 per patient, which was dramatically less than the average CAD 4420 per patient for in-person screening [97]. In order to control healthcare costs while providing access to care, especially in rural regions, telehealth will become an important tool in the screening and monitoring of chronic diseases such as glaucoma.

Table 1. Components of a glaucoma telehealth examination.

	Utility	Disadvantages
Visual Acuity	Changes can be due to a new central scotoma, refractive error, cataract, and other ocular pathologies.	Glaucoma typically presents with peripheral visual field loss which visual acuity does not assess. Only very advanced glaucoma affects visual acuity.
Intraocular Pressure (IOP)	A very important parameter to assess the efficacy of treatment and a major risk factor for disease progression.	Goldmann applanation, the gold standard for measuring IOP, is only performed in clinic. Portable tonometers can significantly differ from Goldmann measurements for IOPs outside the normal range.
Anterior Segment Photography	In lieu of the slit lamp examination, the camera can capture abnormalities of the external and anterior parts of the eye.	The camera may miss subtle pathologies such as a pigment deposition on the corneal endothelium or iris neovascularization. In addition, it cannot capture the anterior chamber cell and flare.
Iridocorneal Angle Imaging	Identifies eyes with anatomic narrow angles at risk for acute angle closure glaucoma.	Angle camera devices and UBM require instillation of topical anesthetic.
Fundus Photography	Captures images of the optic nerve head and macula. Progressive cupping of the optic nerve is a sign of uncontrolled glaucoma.	Although many cameras do not require pharmacologic dilation, the brightness and resolution of the images may be affected by pupil size.
Ocular Coherence Tomography (OCT)	Measures retinal nerve fiber layer thickness using near-infrared light. A reference database is available for comparison. An abnormally thin nerve fiber layer or progressive thinning is a sign of uncontrolled glaucoma.	The device is not portable and is only available in clinic.

Table 1. *Cont.*

	Utility	Disadvantages
Visual Field	Testing is important to detect early peripheral visual field loss and to monitor for expansion of the scotoma. The amount of visual field loss determines the severity of disease and plays a role in setting the target IOP.	Traditional standard automated perimetry is not portable and is only available in clinic. Visual field monitoring at home can only be performed using a web-based program on a computer, a tablet, or with virtual reality glasses.
Artificial Intelligence (Deep Learning)	By self-learning via an artificial neural network, the technology has demonstrated remarkable accuracy in diagnosing glaucoma and monitoring for disease progression using fundus images, OCT, and visual field.	It is still under development and not available to the public yet.

4. How the Coronavirus Pandemic Shaped Telehealth

In December 2019, a novel respiratory illness COVID-19 emerged in Wuhan, China. Because of the disease's highly contagious nature, it quickly spread globally, and a pandemic was declared by the World Health Organization on 11 March 2020. Governments worldwide imposed lockdowns to stop the spread of disease, as COVID-19 overwhelmed hospital systems with vast numbers of people requiring ventilators. In the United States, state governments issued stay-at-home orders and social distancing guidelines. People were asked to work from home and to avoid venturing outside except for essential activities. On 18 March 2020, the American Academy of Ophthalmology (AAO) recommended the cessation of elective surgery and routine clinic visits to protect patients from catching COVID-19 and to conserve personal protective equipment (PPE).

Because many ophthalmology practices closed their offices, telehealth through video visits became a necessary way for patients to see their doctors. In the United States, the Centers for Medicare and Medicaid Services (CMS) relaxed the requirements to bill for telehealth visits; thus, allowing practices to be reimbursed for remote patient care. Many practices implemented a telemedicine program for the first time and had to develop protocols to address patient needs virtually. Saleem et al. [98] depicted a workflow diagram as a reference to implement an ophthalmology telemedicine program. Essentially, the front desk staff reaches out to patients who had their appointments canceled and offers them a telephone or video visit for non-urgent problems. If the patient describes an issue that appears to be an emergency, the physician is contacted to determine whether the problem can be addressed remotely or the patient must be examined in person.

A major hurdle in managing glaucoma patients through video visits is that glaucoma, for the most part, is an asymptomatic disease, unless there is a substantial increase in IOP causing eye pain or rapid visual field loss causing noticeable constriction in vision. A video visit does not allow for IOP measurement, visual field testing, or the visualization of the optic nerve. A crude method for the patient to estimate IOP is via finger palpation on the eye through the eyelid. A more accurate way than digital palpation is for the patient to use the iCare HOME rebound tonometer on him/herself. The tonometer is easy to use, comfortable, and requires no topical anesthetic. Because the device is expensive, companies such as MyEYES (myeyes.net) and Enlivened (enlivened.com) offer rentals for a fee. Patients are taught how to use the device and borrow it for one or more weeks. The downside, however, is that the IOP readings are not displayed; the patient must return the device to the office to extract the IOP diurnal curve. An alternative to using the iCare HOME is to wear the Sensimed Triggerfish® Contact Lens, which makes automated corneoscleral dimensional measurements for 24 h. However, the patient is required to have a circular antenna taped around the eye, wear a recording device hanging from the neck, and return to the office the next day to extract the diurnal curve. A new contact lens being developed in South Korea allows for convenient IOP monitoring using a smartphone.

Implantable devices such as the Eyemate® and Injectsense can provide IOP monitoring as well. If there is concern for visual field progression, the patient can use the computer-based Peristat Online Perimetry, the tablet-based Melbourne Rapid Fields program, or virtual reality perimetry to generate a visual field report and send it to the physician.

As pandemic lockdown restrictions loosened, ophthalmology practices reopened with the implementation of new protocols for the safety of the patients and staff members. Vinod et al. [99] described methods that practices used to enforce social distancing and enhance safety, such as limiting the number of appointments, rearranging chairs in the waiting rooms, asking patients to remain in their cars outside the clinic until they are called, mandating everyone to wear masks, and installing large breath shields on slit lamps. However, some patients are still uncomfortable with in-person examinations and prefer telehealth until the pandemic ends.

5. Conclusions

As demand for glaucoma care increases, there will be a need for telehealth. Just as radiologists review scans remotely, ophthalmologists can review results and risk-stratify patients. A glaucoma suspect can be monitored remotely, provided that one has access to an OCT or visual field machine yearly. A patient with well-controlled mild to moderate glaucoma can also be monitored remotely if one has IOP measurements performed regularly and that an in-person dilated examination is performed annually. A patient with uncontrolled or severe glaucoma should have face-to-face visits, as there is much less room for error and a high likelihood of needing laser or surgical procedures. This algorithm for remote monitoring is illustrated in Figure 1. Essentially, face-to-face examinations can be limited to confirmation of diagnosis, management of patients with uncontrolled or severe glaucoma, and patients with new, concerning ocular symptoms. The telehealth approach is cost-effective and can increase patient satisfaction by decreasing waiting time during visits. Telehealth is particularly beneficial for patients in rural areas who have limited access to care and in the setting of a pandemic, when social distancing is enforced and the number of appointments is severely limited to reduce disease spread. Deep learning artificial intelligence will play an increasing role in the diagnosis and management of glaucoma using data extracted from telehealth.

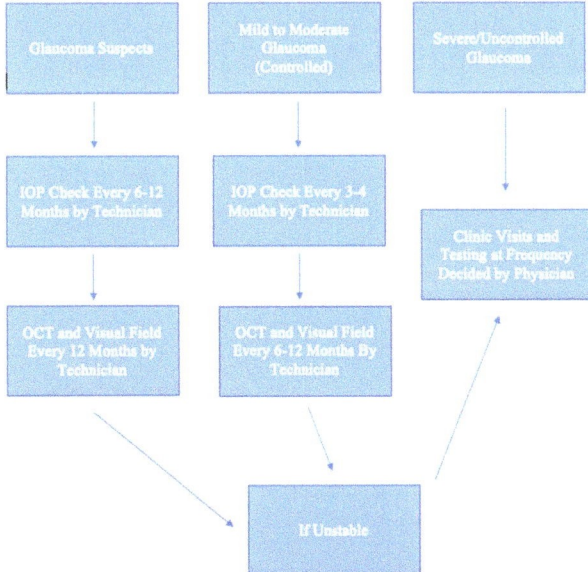

Figure 1. Algorithm for Remote Monitoring. IOP: intraocular pressure. OCT: Optical coherence tomography.

Author Contributions: Conceptualization, S.H.W. and J.C.T.; methodology, S.H.W. and J.C.T.; software, S.H.W.; validation, S.H.W. and J.C.T.; formal analysis, S.H.W.; investigation, S.H.W. and J.C.T.; resources, S.H.W. and J.C.T.; data curation, S.H.W. and J.C.T.; writing—original draft preparation, S.H.W.; writing—review and editing, S.H.W. and J.C.T.; visualization, S.H.W. and J.C.T.; supervision, J.C.T.; project administration, J.C.T.; funding acquisition, J.C.T. All authors have read and agreed to the published version of the manuscript.

Funding: This work was supported in part by a Challenge Grant award from Research to Prevent Blindness, New York.

Institutional Review Board Statement: Not applicable.

Informed Consent Statement: Not applicable.

Data Availability Statement: Not applicable.

Conflicts of Interest: S.H.W. declares no conflict of interest. J.C.T. is a consultant for Eyenovia, ReNetX Bio, and SmartLens and has equity interest in Ocutrx and SmartLens. The funder had no role in the design of the study; in the collection, analyses, or interpretation of data; in the writing of the manuscript, or in the decision to publish the results.

Consultant: Eyenovia: ReNetX Bio, SmartLens. Equity Interest: Ocutrx, SmartLens.

References

1. Tham, Y.-C.; Li, X.; Wong, T.Y.; Quigley, H.A.; Aung, T.; Cheng, C.-Y. Global Prevalence of Glaucoma and Projections of Glaucoma Burden through 2040: A Systematic Review and Meta-Analysis. *Ophthalmology* **2014**, *121*, 2081–2090. [CrossRef] [PubMed]
2. Dall, T.; Reynolds, R.; Chakrabarti, R.; Jones, K.; Iacobucci, W. The Complexities of Physician Supply and Demand: Projections From 2018 to 2033. *Assoc. Am. Med Coll.* **2020**, 1–92.
3. Samanta, A.; Mauntana, S.; Barsi, Z.; Yarlagadda, B.; Nelson, P.C. Is Your Vision Blurry? A Systematic Review of Home-Based Visual Acuity for Telemedicine. *J. Telemed. Telecare* **2020**. [CrossRef] [PubMed]
4. Heijl, A.; Leske, M.C.; Bengtsson, B.; Hyman, L.; Bengtsson, B.; Hussein, M. Early Manifest Glaucoma Trial Group Reduction of Intraocular Pressure and Glaucoma Progression: Results from the Early Manifest Glaucoma Trial. *Arch. Ophthalmol* **2002**, *120*, 1268–1279. [CrossRef]
5. Minckler, D.S.; Baerveldt, G.; Heuer, D.K.; Quillen-Thomas, B.; Walonker, A.F.; Weiner, J. Clinical Evaluation of the Oculab Tono-Pen. *Am. J. Ophthalmol.* **1987**, *104*, 168–173. [CrossRef]
6. Kao, S.F.; Lichter, P.R.; Bergstrom, T.J.; Rowe, S.; Musch, D.C. Clinical Comparison of the Oculab Tono-Pen to the Goldmann Applanation Tonometer. *Ophthalmology* **1987**, *94*, 1541–1544. [CrossRef]
7. Frenkel, R.E.; Hong, Y.J.; Shin, D.H. Comparison of the Tono-Pen to the Goldmann Applanation Tonometer. *Arch. Ophthalmol.* **1988**, *106*, 750–753. [CrossRef] [PubMed]
8. Bao, B.; Diaconita, V.; Schulz, D.C.; Hutnik, C. Tono-Pen versus Goldmann Applanation Tonometry: A Comparison of 898 Eyes. *Ophthalmol. Glaucoma* **2019**, *2*, 435–439. [CrossRef]
9. Bhartiya, S.; Bali, S.J.; Sharma, R.; Chaturvedi, N.; Dada, T. Comparative Evaluation of TonoPen AVIA, Goldmann Applanation Tonometry and Non-Contact Tonometry. *Int. Ophthalmol.* **2011**, *31*, 297–302. [CrossRef]
10. Dohadwala, A.A.; Munger, R.; Damji, K.F. Positive Correlation between Tono-Pen Intraocular Pressure and Central Corneal Thickness. *Ophthalmology* **1998**, *105*, 1849–1854. [CrossRef]
11. Hsu, S.-Y.; Sheu, M.-M.; Hsu, A.-H.; Wu, K.-Y.; Yeh, J.-I.; Tien, J.-N.; Tsai, R.-K. Comparisons of Intraocular Pressure Measurements: Goldmann Applanation Tonometry, Noncontact Tonometry, Tono-Pen Tonometry, and Dynamic Contour Tonometry. *Eye* **2009**, *23*, 1582–1588. [CrossRef] [PubMed]
12. Razeghinejad, M.R.; Salouti, R.; Khalili, M.R. Intraocular Pressure Measurements by Three Different Tonometers in Children with Aphakic Glaucoma and a Thick Cornea. *Iran. J. Med. Sci.* **2014**, *39*, 11–19. [PubMed]
13. Tonnu, P.-A.; Ho, T.; Newson, T.; El Sheikh, A.; Sharma, K.; White, E.; Bunce, C.; Garway-Heath, D. The Influence of Central Corneal Thickness and Age on Intraocular Pressure Measured by Pneumotonometry, Non-Contact Tonometry, the Tono-Pen XL, and Goldmann Applanation Tonometry. *Br. J. Ophthalmol.* **2005**, *89*, 851–854. [CrossRef]
14. Bang, S.P.; Lee, C.E.; Kim, Y.C. Comparison of Intraocular Pressure as Measured by Three Different Non-Contact Tonometers and Goldmann Applanation Tonometer for Non-Glaucomatous Subjects. *BMC Ophthalmol.* **2017**, *17*, 199. [CrossRef] [PubMed]
15. García-Resúa, C.; Giráldez Fernández, M.J.; Yebra-Pimentel, E.; García-Montero, S. Clinical Evaluation of the Canon TX-10 Noncontact Tonometer in Healthy Eyes. *Eur. J. Ophthalmol.* **2010**, *20*, 523–530. [CrossRef]
16. Kutzscher, A.E.; Kumar, R.S.; Ramgopal, B.; Rackenchath, M.V.; Devi, S.; Nagaraj, S.; Moe, C.A.; Fry, D.M.; Stamper, R.L.; Keenan, J.D. Reproducibility of 5 Methods of Ocular Tonometry. *Ophthalmol. Glaucoma* **2019**, *2*, 429–434. [CrossRef] [PubMed]
17. Mansoori, T.; Balakrishna, N. Effect of Central Corneal Thickness on Intraocular Pressure and Comparison of Topcon CT-80 Non-Contact Tonometry with Goldmann Applanation Tonometry. *Clin. Exp. Optom.* **2018**, *101*, 206–212. [CrossRef]

18. Tonnu, P.-A.; Ho, T.; Sharma, K.; White, E.; Bunce, C.; Garway-Heath, D. A Comparison of Four Methods of Tonometry: Method Agreement and Interobserver Variability. *Br. J. Ophthalmol.* **2005**, *89*, 847–850. [CrossRef] [PubMed]
19. Hubanova, R.; Aptel, F.; Zhou, T.; Arnol, N.; Romanet, J.-P.; Chiquet, C. Comparison of Intraocular Pressure Measurements with the Reichert Pt100, the Keeler Pulsair Intellipuff Portable Noncontact Tonometers, and Goldmann Applanation Tonometry. *J. Glaucoma* **2015**, *24*, 356–363. [CrossRef]
20. Nakakura, S.; Mori, E.; Fujio, Y.; Fujisawa, Y.; Matsuya, K.; Kobayashi, Y.; Tabuchi, H.; Asaoka, R.; Kiuchi, Y. Comparison of the Intraocular Pressure Measured Using the New Rebound Tonometer Icare Ic100 and Icare TA01i or Goldmann Applanation Tonometer. *J. Glaucoma* **2019**, *28*, 172–177. [CrossRef]
21. Gao, F.; Liu, X.; Zhao, Q.; Pan, Y. Comparison of the ICare Rebound Tonometer and the Goldmann Applanation Tonometer. *Exp. Ther. Med.* **2017**, *13*, 1912–1916. [CrossRef] [PubMed]
22. Subramaniam, A.G.; Allen, P.; Toh, T. Comparison of the Icare Ic100 Rebound Tonometer and the Goldmann Applanation Tonometer in 1000 Eyes. *Ophthalmic Res.* **2021**, *64*, 321–326. [CrossRef] [PubMed]
23. Badakere, S.V.; Chary, R.; Choudhari, N.S.; Rao, H.L.; Garudadri, C.; Senthil, S. Agreement of Intraocular Pressure Measurement of Icare Ic200 with Goldmann Applanation Tonometer in Adult Eyes with Normal Cornea. *Ophthalmol. Glaucoma* **2021**, *4*, 89–94. [CrossRef]
24. Takagi, D.; Sawada, A.; Yamamoto, T. Evaluation of a New Rebound Self-Tonometer, Icare HOME: Comparison with Goldmann Applanation Tonometer. *J. Glaucoma* **2017**, *26*, 613–618. [CrossRef] [PubMed]
25. Ehrlich, J.R.; Haseltine, S.; Shimmyo, M.; Radcliffe, N.M. Evaluation of Agreement between Intraocular Pressure Measurements Using Goldmann Applanation Tonometry and Goldmann Correlated Intraocular Pressure by Reichert's Ocular Response Analyser. *Eye* **2010**, *24*, 1555–1560. [CrossRef]
26. Ogbuehi, K.C.; Almubrad, T.M. Evaluation of the Intraocular Pressure Measured with the Ocular Response Analyzer. *Curr. Eye Res.* **2010**, *35*, 587–596. [CrossRef]
27. Martinez-de-la-Casa, J.M.; Garcia-Feijoo, J.; Fernandez-Vidal, A.; Mendez-Hernandez, C.; Garcia-Sanchez, J. Ocular Response Analyzer versus Goldmann Applanation Tonometry for Intraocular Pressure Measurements. *Investig. Ophthalmol. Vis. Sci.* **2006**, *47*, 4410–4414. [CrossRef]
28. Renier, C.; Zeyen, T.; Fieuws, S.; Vandenbroeck, S.; Stalmans, I. Comparison of Ocular Response Analyzer, Dynamic Contour Tonometer and Goldmann Applanation Tonometer. *Int. Ophthalmol.* **2010**, *30*, 651–659. [CrossRef]
29. Kotecha, A.; White, E.; Schlottmann, P.G.; Garway-Heath, D.F. Intraocular Pressure Measurement Precision with the Goldmann Applanation, Dynamic Contour, and Ocular Response Analyzer Tonometers. *Ophthalmology* **2010**, *117*, 730–737. [CrossRef]
30. Vandewalle, E.; Vandenbroeck, S.; Stalmans, I.; Zeyen, T. Comparison of ICare, Dynamic Contour Tonometer, and Ocular Response Analyzer with Goldmann Applanation Tonometer in Patients with Glaucoma. *Eur. J. Ophthalmol.* **2009**, *19*, 783–789. [CrossRef]
31. Carbonaro, F.; Andrew, T.; Mackey, D.A.; Spector, T.D.; Hammond, C.J. Comparison of Three Methods of Intraocular Pressure Measurement and Their Relation to Central Corneal Thickness. *Eye* **2010**, *24*, 1165–1170. [CrossRef] [PubMed]
32. Medeiros, F.A.; Meira-Freitas, D.; Lisboa, R.; Kuang, T.-M.; Zangwill, L.M.; Weinreb, R.N. Corneal Hysteresis as a Risk Factor for Glaucoma Progression: A Prospective Longitudinal Study. *Ophthalmology* **2013**, *120*, 1533–1540. [CrossRef] [PubMed]
33. Schweitzer, J.A.; Ervin, M.; Berdahl, J.P. Assessment of Corneal Hysteresis Measured by the Ocular Response Analyzer as a Screening Tool in Patients with Glaucoma. *Clin. Ophthalmol.* **2018**, *12*, 1809–1813. [CrossRef] [PubMed]
34. Mansouri, K.; Medeiros, F.A.; Tafreshi, A.; Weinreb, R.N. Continuous 24-Hour Monitoring of Intraocular Pressure Patterns with a Contact Lens Sensor: Safety, Tolerability, and Reproducibility in Patients with Glaucoma. *Arch. Ophthalmol.* **2012**, *130*, 1534–1539. [CrossRef] [PubMed]
35. Mansouri, K.; Weinreb, R.N.; Liu, J.H.K. Efficacy of a Contact Lens Sensor for Monitoring 24-h Intraocular Pressure Related Patterns. *PLoS ONE* **2015**, *10*, e0125530. [CrossRef]
36. De Moraes, C.G.; Mansouri, K.; Liebmann, J.M.; Ritch, R. Association between 24-hour intraocular pressure monitored with contact lens sensor and visual field progression in older adults with glaucoma. *JAMA Ophthalmol.* **2018**, *136*, 779–785. [CrossRef]
37. Kim, J.; Park, J.; Park, Y.-G.; Cha, E.; Ku, M.; An, H.S.; Lee, K.-P.; Huh, M.-I.; Kim, J.; Kim, T.-S.; et al. A Soft and Transparent Contact Lens for the Wireless Quantitative Monitoring of Intraocular Pressure. *Nat. Biomed. Eng.* **2021**, *5*, 772–782. [CrossRef]
38. Koutsonas, A.; Walter, P.; Roessler, G.; Plange, N. Implantation of a Novel Telemetric Intraocular Pressure Sensor in Patients with Glaucoma (ARGOS Study): 1-Year Results. *Investig. Ophthalmol. Vis. Sci.* **2015**, *56*, 1063–1069. [CrossRef]
39. Enders, P.; Hall, J.; Bornhauser, M.; Mansouri, K.; Altay, L.; Schrader, S.; Dietlein, T.S.; Bachmann, B.O.; Neuhann, T.; Cursiefen, C. Telemetric Intraocular Pressure Monitoring after Boston Keratoprosthesis Surgery Using the Eyemate-IO Sensor: Dynamics in the First Year. *Am. J. Ophthalmol.* **2019**, *206*, 256–263. [CrossRef] [PubMed]
40. Li, Y.; Shi, J.; Duan, X.; Fan, F. Transpalpebral Measurement of Intraocular Pressure Using the Diaton Tonometer versus Standard Goldmann Applanation Tonometry. *Graefes Arch. Clin. Exp. Ophthalmol.* **2010**, *248*, 1765–1770. [CrossRef]
41. Risma, J.M.; Tehrani, S.; Wang, K.; Fingert, J.H.; Alward, W.L.M.; Kwon, Y.H. The Utility of Diaton Tonometer Measurements in Patients with Ocular Hypertension, Glaucoma, and Glaucoma Tube Shunts: A Preliminary Study for Its Potential Use in Keratoprosthesis Patients. *J. Glaucoma* **2016**, *25*, 643–647. [CrossRef]
42. Bali, S.J.; Bhartiya, S.; Sobti, A.; Dada, T.; Panda, A. Comparative Evaluation of Diaton and Goldmann Applanation Tonometers. *Ophthalmologica* **2012**, *228*, 42–46. [CrossRef] [PubMed]

43. Doherty, M.D.; Carrim, Z.I.; O'Neill, D.P. Diaton Tonometry: An Assessment of Validity and Preference against Goldmann Tonometry. *Clin. Exp. Ophthalmol.* **2012**, *40*, e171–e175. [CrossRef]
44. Chan, E.C.; Roberts, D.K.; Loconte, D.D.; Wernick, M.N. Digital Camera System to Perform Infrared Photography of Iris Transillumination. *J. Glaucoma* **2002**, *11*, 426–428. [CrossRef] [PubMed]
45. Ludwig, C.A.; Murthy, S.I.; Pappuru, R.R.; Jais, A.; Myung, D.J.; Chang, R.T. A Novel Smartphone Ophthalmic Imaging Adapter: User Feasibility Studies in Hyderabad, India. *Indian J. Ophthalmol.* **2016**, *64*, 191–200. [CrossRef] [PubMed]
46. Nongpiur, M.E.; Sakata, L.M.; Friedman, D.S.; He, M.; Chan, Y.-H.; Lavanya, R.; Wong, T.Y.; Aung, T. Novel Association of Smaller Anterior Chamber Width with Angle Closure in Singaporeans. *Ophthalmology* **2010**, *117*, 1967–1973. [CrossRef]
47. Wu, R.-Y.; Nongpiur, M.E.; He, M.-G.; Sakata, L.M.; Friedman, D.S.; Chan, Y.-H.; Lavanya, R.; Wong, T.-Y.; Aung, T. Association of Narrow Angles with Anterior Chamber Area and Volume Measured with Anterior-Segment Optical Coherence Tomography. *Arch. Ophthalmol.* **2011**, *129*, 569–574. [CrossRef]
48. Wang, B.; Sakata, L.M.; Friedman, D.S.; Chan, Y.-H.; He, M.; Lavanya, R.; Wong, T.-Y.; Aung, T. Quantitative Iris Parameters and Association with Narrow Angles. *Ophthalmology* **2010**, *117*, 11–17. [CrossRef] [PubMed]
49. Nongpiur, M.E.; He, M.; Amerasinghe, N.; Friedman, D.S.; Tay, W.-T.; Baskaran, M.; Smith, S.D.; Wong, T.Y.; Aung, T. Lens Vault, Thickness, and Position in Chinese Subjects with Angle Closure. *Ophthalmology* **2011**, *118*, 474–479. [CrossRef] [PubMed]
50. Tan, G.S.; He, M.; Zhao, W.; Sakata, L.M.; Li, J.; Nongpiur, M.E.; Lavanya, R.; Friedman, D.S.; Aung, T. Determinants of Lens Vault and Association with Narrow Angles in Patients from Singapore. *Am. J. Ophthalmol.* **2012**, *154*, 39–46. [CrossRef]
51. Foo, L.-L.; Nongpiur, M.E.; Allen, J.C.; Perera, S.A.; Friedman, D.S.; He, M.; Cheng, C.-Y.; Wong, T.Y.; Aung, T. Determinants of Angle Width in Chinese Singaporeans. *Ophthalmology* **2012**, *119*, 278–282. [CrossRef]
52. Nongpiur, M.E.; Haaland, B.A.; Perera, S.A.; Friedman, D.S.; He, M.; Sakata, L.M.; Baskaran, M.; Aung, T. Development of a Score and Probability Estimate for Detecting Angle Closure Based on Anterior Segment Optical Coherence Tomography. *Am. J. Ophthalmol.* **2014**, *157*, 32–38. [CrossRef]
53. Perera, S.A.; Baskaran, M.; Friedman, D.S.; Tun, T.A.; Htoon, H.M.; Kumar, R.S.; Aung, T. Use of EyeCam for Imaging the Anterior Chamber Angle. *Investig. Ophthalmol. Vis. Sci.* **2010**, *51*, 2993–2997. [CrossRef]
54. Shinoj, V.K.; Murukeshan, V.M.; Baskaran, M.; Aung, T. Integrated Flexible Handheld Probe for Imaging and Evaluation of Iridocorneal Angle. *J. Biomed. Opt.* **2015**, *20*, 016014. [CrossRef]
55. Russo, A.; Mapham, W.; Turano, R.; Costagliola, C.; Morescalchi, F.; Scaroni, N.; Semeraro, F. Comparison of Smartphone Ophthalmoscopy with Slit-Lamp Biomicroscopy for Grading Vertical Cup-to-Disc Ratio. *J. Glaucoma* **2016**, *25*, e777–e781. [CrossRef] [PubMed]
56. Wintergerst, M.W.M.; Brinkmann, C.K.; Holz, F.G.; Finger, R.P. Undilated versus Dilated Monoscopic Smartphone-Based Fundus Photography for Optic Nerve Head Evaluation. *Sci. Rep.* **2018**, *8*, 10228. [CrossRef]
57. Lowry, E.A.; Hou, J.; Hennein, L.; Chang, R.T.; Lin, S.; Keenan, J.; Wang, S.K.; Ianchulev, S.; Pasquale, L.R.; Han, Y. Comparison of Peristat Online Perimetry with the Humphrey Perimetry in a Clinic-Based Setting. *Transl. Vis. Sci. Technol.* **2016**, *5*, 4. [CrossRef] [PubMed]
58. Prea, S.M.; Kong, Y.X.G.; Mehta, A.; He, M.; Crowston, J.G.; Gupta, V.; Martin, K.R.; Vingrys, A.J. Six-Month Longitudinal Comparison of a Portable Tablet Perimeter with the Humphrey Field Analyzer. *Am. J. Ophthalmol.* **2018**, *190*, 9–16. [CrossRef] [PubMed]
59. Johnson, C.A.; Thapa, S.; George Kong, Y.X.; Robin, A.L. Performance of an IPad Application to Detect Moderate and Advanced Visual Field Loss in Nepal. *Am. J. Ophthalmol.* **2017**, *182*, 147–154. [CrossRef]
60. Kong, Y.X.G.; He, M.; Crowston, J.G.; Vingrys, A.J. A Comparison of Perimetric Results from a Tablet Perimeter and Humphrey Field Analyzer in Glaucoma Patients. *Transl. Vis. Sci. Technol.* **2016**, *5*, 2. [CrossRef]
61. Schulz, A.M.; Graham, E.C.; You, Y.; Klistorner, A.; Graham, S.L. Performance of IPad-Based Threshold Perimetry in Glaucoma and Controls. *Clin. Exp. Ophthalmol.* **2018**, *46*, 346–355. [CrossRef] [PubMed]
62. Tsapakis, S.; Papaconstantinou, D.; Diagourtas, A.; Droutsas, K.; Andreanos, K.; Moschos, M.M.; Brouzas, D. Visual Field Examination Method Using Virtual Reality Glasses Compared with the Humphrey Perimeter. *Clin. Ophthalmol.* **2017**, *11*, 1431–1443. [CrossRef] [PubMed]
63. Nakanishi, M.; Wang, Y.-T.; Jung, T.-P.; Zao, J.K.; Chien, Y.-Y.; Diniz-Filho, A.; Daga, F.B.; Lin, Y.-P.; Wang, Y.; Medeiros, F.A. Detecting Glaucoma with a Portable Brain-Computer Interface for Objective Assessment of Visual Function Loss. *JAMA Ophthalmol.* **2017**, *135*, 550–557. [CrossRef]
64. Rogers, T.W.; Jaccard, N.; Carbonaro, F.; Lemij, H.G.; Vermeer, K.A.; Reus, N.J.; Trikha, S. Evaluation of an AI System for the Automated Detection of Glaucoma from Stereoscopic Optic Disc Photographs: The European Optic Disc Assessment Study. *Eye* **2019**, *33*, 1791–1797. [CrossRef]
65. Hemelings, R.; Elen, B.; Barbosa-Breda, J.; Lemmens, S.; Meire, M.; Pourjavan, S.; Vandewalle, E.; Van de Veire, S.; Blaschko, M.B.; De Boever, P.; et al. Accurate Prediction of Glaucoma from Colour Fundus Images with a Convolutional Neural Network That Relies on Active and Transfer Learning. *Acta Ophthalmol.* **2020**, *98*, e94–e100. [CrossRef]
66. Lee, J.; Kim, Y.; Kim, J.H.; Park, K.H. Screening Glaucoma with Red-Free Fundus Photography Using Deep Learning Classifier and Polar Transformation. *J. Glaucoma* **2019**, *28*, 258–264. [CrossRef]

67. Li, F.; Yan, L.; Wang, Y.; Shi, J.; Chen, H.; Zhang, X.; Jiang, M.; Wu, Z.; Zhou, K. Deep Learning-Based Automated Detection of Glaucomatous Optic Neuropathy on Color Fundus Photographs. *Graefes Arch. Clin. Exp. Ophthalmol.* **2020**, *258*, 851–867. [CrossRef]
68. Li, Z.; He, Y.; Keel, S.; Meng, W.; Chang, R.T.; He, M. Efficacy of a Deep Learning System for Detecting Glaucomatous Optic Neuropathy Based on Color Fundus Photographs. *Ophthalmology* **2018**, *125*, 1199–1206. [CrossRef]
69. Liu, H.; Li, L.; Wormstone, I.M.; Qiao, C.; Zhang, C.; Liu, P.; Li, S.; Wang, H.; Mou, D.; Pang, R.; et al. Development and Validation of a Deep Learning System to Detect Glaucomatous Optic Neuropathy Using Fundus Photographs. *JAMA Ophthalmol.* **2019**, *137*, 1353–1360. [CrossRef] [PubMed]
70. Li, Z.; Guo, C.; Lin, D.; Nie, D.; Zhu, Y.; Chen, C.; Zhao, L.; Wang, J.; Zhang, X.; Dongye, M.; et al. Deep Learning for Automated Glaucomatous Optic Neuropathy Detection from Ultra-Widefield Fundus Images. *Br. J. Ophthalmol.* **2020**. [CrossRef]
71. Asaoka, R.; Tanito, M.; Shibata, N.; Mitsuhashi, K.; Nakahara, K.; Fujino, Y.; Matsuura, M.; Murata, H.; Tokumo, K.; Kiuchi, Y. Validation of a Deep Learning Model to Screen for Glaucoma Using Images from Different Fundus Cameras and Data Augmentation. *Ophthalmol. Glaucoma* **2019**, *2*, 224–231. [CrossRef] [PubMed]
72. Al-Aswad, L.A.; Kapoor, R.; Chu, C.K.; Walters, S.; Gong, D.; Garg, A.; Gopal, K.; Patel, V.; Sameer, T.; Rogers, T.W.; et al. Evaluation of a Deep Learning System For Identifying Glaucomatous Optic Neuropathy Based on Color Fundus Photographs. *J. Glaucoma* **2019**, *28*, 1029–1034. [CrossRef]
73. Medeiros, F.A.; Jammal, A.A.; Thompson, A.C. From Machine to Machine: An OCT-Trained Deep Learning Algorithm for Objective Quantification of Glaucomatous Damage in Fundus Photographs. *Ophthalmology* **2019**, *126*, 513–521. [CrossRef] [PubMed]
74. Lee, T.; Jammal, A.A.; Mariottoni, E.B.; Medeiros, F.A. Predicting Glaucoma Development with Longitudinal Deep Learning Predictions from Fundus Photographs. *Am. J. Ophthalmol.* **2021**, *225*, 86–94. [CrossRef]
75. Medeiros, F.A.; Jammal, A.A.; Mariottoni, E.B. Detection of Progressive Glaucomatous Optic Nerve Damage on Fundus Photographs with Deep Learning. *Ophthalmology* **2021**, *128*, 383–392. [CrossRef]
76. Christopher, M.; Belghith, A.; Weinreb, R.N.; Bowd, C.; Goldbaum, M.H.; Saunders, L.J.; Medeiros, F.A.; Zangwill, L.M. Retinal Nerve Fiber Layer Features Identified by Unsupervised Machine Learning on Optical Coherence Tomography Scans Predict Glaucoma Progression. *Investig. Ophthalmol. Vis. Sci.* **2018**, *59*, 2748–2756. [CrossRef] [PubMed]
77. Kim, K.E.; Kim, J.M.; Song, J.E.; Kee, C.; Han, J.C.; Hyun, S.H. Development and Validation of a Deep Learning System for Diagnosing Glaucoma Using Optical Coherence Tomography. *J. Clin. Med.* **2020**, *9*, 2167. [CrossRef]
78. Lee, J.; Kim, Y.K.; Park, K.H.; Jeoung, J.W. Diagnosing Glaucoma with Spectral-Domain Optical Coherence Tomography Using Deep Learning Classifier. *J. Glaucoma* **2020**, *29*, 287–294. [CrossRef] [PubMed]
79. Thompson, A.C.; Jammal, A.A.; Berchuck, S.I.; Mariottoni, E.B.; Medeiros, F.A. Assessment of a Segmentation-Free Deep Learning Algorithm for Diagnosing Glaucoma From Optical Coherence Tomography Scans. *JAMA Ophthalmol.* **2020**, *138*, 333–339. [CrossRef]
80. Wang, P.; Shen, J.; Chang, R.; Moloney, M.; Torres, M.; Burkemper, B.; Jiang, X.; Rodger, D.; Varma, R.; Richter, G.M. Machine Learning Models for Diagnosing Glaucoma from Retinal Nerve Fiber Layer Thickness Maps. *Ophthalmol. Glaucoma* **2019**, *2*, 422–428. [CrossRef] [PubMed]
81. Zheng, C.; Xie, X.; Huang, L.; Chen, B.; Yang, J.; Lu, J.; Qiao, T.; Fan, Z.; Zhang, M. Detecting Glaucoma Based on Spectral Domain Optical Coherence Tomography Imaging of Peripapillary Retinal Nerve Fiber Layer: A Comparison Study between Hand-Crafted Features and Deep Learning Model. *Graefes Arch. Clin. Exp. Ophthalmol.* **2020**, *258*, 577–585. [CrossRef]
82. Christopher, M.; Bowd, C.; Belghith, A.; Goldbaum, M.H.; Weinreb, R.N.; Fazio, M.A.; Girkin, C.A.; Liebmann, J.M.; Zangwill, L.M. Deep Learning Approaches Predict Glaucomatous Visual Field Damage from OCT Optic Nerve Head En Face Images and Retinal Nerve Fiber Layer Thickness Maps. *Ophthalmology* **2020**, *127*, 346–356. [CrossRef]
83. Hashimoto, Y.; Asaoka, R.; Kiwaki, T.; Sugiura, H.; Asano, S.; Murata, H.; Fujino, Y.; Matsuura, M.; Miki, A.; Mori, K.; et al. Deep Learning Model to Predict Visual Field in Central 10° from Optical Coherence Tomography Measurement in Glaucoma. *Br. J. Ophthalmol.* **2021**, *105*, 507–513. [CrossRef]
84. Fu, H.; Baskaran, M.; Xu, Y.; Lin, S.; Wong, D.W.K.; Liu, J.; Tun, T.A.; Mahesh, M.; Perera, S.A.; Aung, T. A Deep Learning System for Automated Angle-Closure Detection in Anterior Segment Optical Coherence Tomography Images. *Am. J. Ophthalmol.* **2019**, *203*, 37–45. [CrossRef] [PubMed]
85. Xu, B.Y.; Chiang, M.; Chaudhary, S.; Kulkarni, S.; Pardeshi, A.A.; Varma, R. Deep Learning Classifiers for Automated Detection of Gonioscopic Angle Closure Based on Anterior Segment OCT Images. *Am. J. Ophthalmol.* **2019**, *208*, 273–280. [CrossRef]
86. Asaoka, R.; Murata, H.; Iwase, A.; Araie, M. Detecting Preperimetric Glaucoma with Standard Automated Perimetry Using a Deep Learning Classifier. *Ophthalmology* **2016**, *123*, 1974–1980. [CrossRef] [PubMed]
87. Wen, J.C.; Lee, C.S.; Keane, P.A.; Xiao, S.; Rokem, A.S.; Chen, P.P.; Wu, Y.; Lee, A.Y. Forecasting Future Humphrey Visual Fields Using Deep Learning. *PLoS ONE* **2019**, *14*, e0214875. [CrossRef]
88. Yousefi, S.; Kiwaki, T.; Zheng, Y.; Sugiura, H.; Asaoka, R.; Murata, H.; Lemij, H.; Yamanishi, K. Detection of Longitudinal Visual Field Progression in Glaucoma Using Machine Learning. *Am. J. Ophthalmol.* **2018**, *193*, 71–79. [CrossRef] [PubMed]
89. Hark, L.A.; Myers, J.S.; Pasquale, L.R.; Razeghinejad, M.R.; Maity, A.; Zhan, T.; Hegarty, S.E.; Leiby, B.E.; Waisbourd, M.; Burns, C.; et al. Philadelphia Telemedicine Glaucoma Detection and Follow-up Study: Intraocular Pressure Measurements Found in a Population at High Risk for Glaucoma. *J. Glaucoma* **2019**, *28*, 294–301. [CrossRef] [PubMed]

90. Hark, L.A.; Kresch, Y.S.; De Moraes, C.G.; Horowitz, J.D.; Park, L.; Auran, J.D.; Gorroochurn, P.; Stempel, S.; Maruri, S.C.; Stidham, E.M.; et al. Manhattan Vision Screening and Follow-up Study in Vulnerable Populations (NYC-SIGHT): Design and Methodology. *J. Glaucoma* **2021**, *30*, 388–394. [CrossRef]
91. Newman-Casey, P.A.; Musch, D.C.; Niziol, L.M.; Elam, A.R.; Zhang, J.; Moroi, S.E.; Johnson, L.; Kershaw, M.; Saadine, J.; Winter, S.; et al. Michigan Screening and Intervention for Glaucoma and Eye Health Through Telemedicine (MI-SIGHT): Baseline Methodology for Implementing and Assessing a Community-Based Program. *J. Glaucoma* **2021**, *30*, 380–387. [CrossRef] [PubMed]
92. Rhodes, L.A.; Register, S.; Asif, I.; McGwin, G.; Saaddine, J.; Nghiem, V.T.H.; Owsley, C.; Girkin, C.A. Alabama Screening and Intervention for Glaucoma and Eye Health Through Telemedicine (AL-SIGHT): Study Design and Methodology. *J. Glaucoma* **2021**, *30*, 371–379. [CrossRef]
93. Verma, S.; Arora, S.; Kassam, F.; Edwards, M.C.; Damji, K.F. Northern Alberta Remote Teleglaucoma Program: Clinical Outcomes and Patient Disposition. *Can. J. Ophthalmol.* **2014**, *49*, 135–140. [CrossRef]
94. Modjtahedi, B.S.; Chu, K.; Luong, T.Q.; Hsu, C.; Mattox, C.; Lee, P.P.; Nakla, M.L.; Fong, D.S. Two-Year Outcomes of a Pilot Glaucoma Suspect Telemedicine Monitoring Program. *Clin. Ophthalmol.* **2018**, *12*, 2095–2102. [CrossRef]
95. Chandrasekaran, S.; Kass, W.; Thangamathesvaran, L.; Mendez, N.; Khouri, P.; Szirth, B.C.; Khouri, A.S. Tele-Glaucoma versus Clinical Evaluation: The New Jersey Health Foundation Prospective Clinical Study. *J. Telemed. Telecare* **2020**, *26*, 536–544. [CrossRef] [PubMed]
96. Clarke, J.; Puertas, R.; Kotecha, A.; Foster, P.J.; Barton, K. Virtual Clinics in Glaucoma Care: Face-to-Face versus Remote Decision-Making. *Br. J. Ophthalmol.* **2017**, *101*, 892–895. [CrossRef]
97. Thomas, S.; Hodge, W.; Malvankar-Mehta, M. The Cost-Effectiveness Analysis of Teleglaucoma Screening Device. *PLoS ONE* **2015**, *10*, e0137913. [CrossRef]
98. Saleem, S.M.; Pasquale, L.R.; Sidoti, P.A.; Tsai, J.C. Virtual Ophthalmology: Telemedicine in a COVID-19 Era. *Am. J. Ophthalmol.* **2020**, *216*, 237–242. [CrossRef] [PubMed]
99. Vinod, K.; Sidoti, P.A. Glaucoma Care during the Coronavirus Disease 2019 Pandemic. *Curr. Opin. Ophthalmol.* **2021**, *32*, 75–82. [CrossRef]

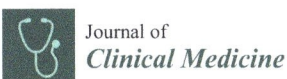

Review

Shared Care and Virtual Clinics for Glaucoma in a Hospital Setting

Anne-Sophie Simons [1,*], Julie Vercauteren [2], João Barbosa-Breda [3,4,5] and Ingeborg Stalmans [1,3]

1. Department of Ophthalmology, University Hospitals Leuven, 3000 Leuven, Belgium; ingeborg.stalmans@uzleuven.be
2. Faculty of Medicine, KU Leuven, 3000 Leuven, Belgium; julie.vercauteren@student.kuleuven.be
3. Research Group Ophthalmology, Department of Neurosciences, KU Leuven, 3000 Leuven, Belgium; joao_breda@hotmail.com
4. Cardiovascular R&D Center, Faculty of Medicine of the University of Porto, 4200-319 Porto, Portugal
5. Department of Ophthalmology, Centro Hospitalar e Universitário São João, 4200-319 Porto, Portugal
* Correspondence: anne-sophie.simons@uzleuven.be; Tel.: +32-(0)-476238306

Abstract: Glaucoma patients require lifelong management, and the prevalence of glaucoma is expected to increase, resulting in capacity problems in many hospital eye departments. New models of care delivery are needed to offer requisite capacity. This review evaluates two alternative schemes for glaucoma care within a hospital, i.e., shared care (SC) and virtual clinics (VCs), whereby non-medical staff are entrusted with more responsibilities, and compares these schemes with the "traditional" ophthalmologist-led outpatient service (standard care). A literature search was conducted in three large bibliographic databases (PubMed, Embase, and Trip), and the abstracts from the prior five annual meetings of the Association for Research in Vision and Ophthalmology were consulted. Twenty-nine were included in the review (14 on SC and 15 on VCs). Patients with low risk of vision loss were considered suitable for these approaches. Among the non-medical staff, optometrists were the most frequently involved. The quality of both schemes was good and improved with the non-medical staff being trained in glaucoma care. No evidence was found on patients feeling disadvantaged by the lack of a doctor visit. Both schemes increased the hospital's efficiency. Both SC and VCs are promising approaches to tackle the upcoming capacity problems of hospital-based glaucoma care.

Keywords: glaucoma; ocular hypertension; outpatient clinic; shared care; allied health personnel; collaborative care; patient care; virtual clinic; virtual system; user computer interface

1. Introduction

Glaucoma is the leading cause for irreversible visual loss worldwide [1]. Periodic assessments are necessary to detect progression at an early stage and to adjust treatment in order to prevent further damage. Once diagnosed with glaucoma, even when asymptomatic, the patient requires lifelong management [2].

The prevalence of glaucoma is expected to increase. The elderly population is growing, and the prevalence of glaucoma increases with age [3]. Advances in diagnostic technologies also allow for earlier detection [4–6]. Furthermore, in the case of the UK, the National Institute for Health and Care Excellence (NICE) released guidance on the diagnosis and management of glaucoma [7], which resulted in an increase in the total number of referrals to hospitals [8,9]. Many hospital eye departments fear capacity problems, since the increase in newly diagnosed cases is not followed by a proportional increase in the number of ophthalmologists [10–12]. Ophthalmologists will be obliged to stretch the time intervals between follow-up (FU) appointments, with the risk of not detecting glaucoma progression early on [13]. Moreover, patients with a known higher risk of blindness will be prioritized, thereby reducing access for new patients [14].

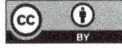

One solution is to increase the number of ophthalmologists, which is not feasible in most cases [15]. Another solution is to increase efficiency; studies have identified both shared care (SC) and virtual clinics (VCs) as alternative methods offering a safe, efficient and accepted framework for glaucoma care [16]. For the care of other chronic diseases, such as asthma [17] or diabetes [18], SC schemes have already been demonstrated to be safe, cost-effective and acceptable. VCs have been demonstrated to be beneficial in the care of suspected melanoma [19] and chronic kidney diseases [20].

The aim of this paper was to review the existing literature concerning SC and VCs running in a hospital-based setting. For each scheme, the implementation was investigated, including the role delegation between the different Health Care Providers (HCPs) and the envisioned type of patients. The quality, the productivity and the acceptance of the care delivered were also examined.

2. Methods

2.1. Study Selection

A literature search was performed using the MEDLINE (PubMed), Embase and Trip databases to identify articles concerning SC and VCs published between January 2000 and July 2021. Relevant abstracts from the annual meeting of the Association for Research in Vision and Ophthalmology (ARVO) of the previous five years were also included.

Two different search queries were made, both using the keywords [glaucoma], [ocular hypertension] and [outpatient clinic]. One search query additionally included the keywords [shared care], [allied health personnel], [collaborative care] and [patient care]. The second search query additionally include the keywords [virtual clinic], [virtual system], and [user computer interface].

Moreover, in order to expand the search, we conducted backward citation tracking, by examining the included article's reference lists.

2.2. Inclusion and Exclusion Criteria

The following inclusion criteria were used: (1) studies evaluating the organization of the glaucoma care pathway; (2) studies evaluating an alternative way of practice, i.e., SC and/or VCs; (3) patients with the diagnosis of glaucoma or suspected glaucoma, or patients at risk of developing glaucoma, e.g., having ocular hypertension (OHT); (4) the staff, working at the clinic, had to be at least one medical Glaucoma Expert (GE) and one non-medical HCP; (5) the clinic operating in a hospital-based setting.

The following exclusion criteria were used: (1) studies evaluating referral patterns from a community-based clinic; (2) studies evaluating case-finding by screening the general population; (3) only optometrists running the clinic; (4) only doctors running the clinic; (5) studies evaluating the care delivered by non-medical HCPs against the care delivered by general ophthalmologists without training or experience in the subspecialty of glaucoma; (6) tele-medicine; (7) virtual reality; (8) the clinic operating in a community-based setting only; (9) the following types of publications (editorials, commentaries, letters); (10) animal studies or in-vitro studies. Only publications in English were considered.

2.3. Terminology

2.3.1. Glaucoma Subtypes

One of the most prevalent subtypes is open-angle glaucoma, where the anterior chamber angle is open and the intra-ocular pressure (IOP) is usually elevated, i.e., above 21 mm Hg [21].

Another subtype is closed-angle glaucoma, where the anterior chamber angle is closed. Despite being less prevalent worldwide, closed-angle glaucoma carries a much higher risk of blindness because narrow/closed angles can lead to very high IOP levels in a short period of time [22].

A glaucoma suspect is characterized by having glaucomatous visual field defects or glaucomatous structural optic nerve defects (and not both) [23]. OHT is a condition of having a documented IOP > 21 mm Hg without evidence of visual or structural glaucomatous damage [24].

2.3.2. HCP Working in the Clinic

In this review, ophthalmologists will be referred to as Glaucoma Experts (GEs). No specific criteria for the training were used, since this certification process has only been established in recent years through the collaboration between the European Board of Ophthalmology (EBO) and the European Glaucoma Society (EGS) [25].

The non-medical staff may consist of ophthalmic nurse practitioners (ONP), orthoptists, optometrists and ophthalmic technicians, with different training and responsibilities [26].

Kappa (κ) values were used to measure the chance-corrected agreement between HCPs on a scale of 0.00 to 1.00, indicating no to perfect agreement, respectively. The nomenclature of Landis and Koch was adopted for denominating different kappa ranges as follows: 0.00–0.20 as "slight", 0.21–0.40 as "fair", 0.41–060 as "moderate", 0.61–0.80 as "substantial" and 0.81–1.00 as "almost perfect" agreement [27].

2.3.3. Organization of the Clinic

In standard care (StC) of glaucoma, patients have their appointment with a GE who makes the diagnosis, sets up a management plan during the initial assessment, and decides on a possible change of the management plan during follow-up.

In SC, the non-medical staff assesses patients during most appointments alone. At regular intervals, or earlier if the patient meets the referral criteria, an appointment is planned with the GE, who will examine the patient face-to-face, as is the case in the StC.

In a VC, both HCPs assess the patient at each appointment, with the non-medical staff assessing the patient in a face-to-face consultation and the GE examining the patient remotely, by virtually reviewing the data collected by the non-medical staff.

3. Results of Shared Care Studies

3.1. Study Selection

From the 400 articles identified, 13 were selected, complemented with one additional article obtained from the reference lists. The processes of identification, screening, duplicates removal and full-text assessment are shown in Figure 1.

3.2. Description of the Included Articles

Illustration of the baseline characteristics of the selected articles, including study design, year, location, hospital, SC clinic and population (Table 1).

3.2.1. Recommendations for Shared Glaucoma Care

Two articles provided a model of reference and recommendations on how glaucoma care could benefit from involving the non-medical staff [28,29]. The recommendations of the Australian and New Zealand Glaucoma Interest Group and the Royal Australian and New Zealand College of Ophthalmologists (ANGIG&RANZCO) [28] followed the National Health and Medical Research Council (NHMRC) guidelines [30], and the recommendations from the Canadian Glaucoma Society Committee (CGSC) [29] followed the Canadian Ophthalmology glaucoma clinical practice guidelines (COSgcpg) [31]. For their risk assessment, however, they used the same guidelines [32]. They did not examine the performance of the non-medical staff nor the performance of a SC scheme in general.

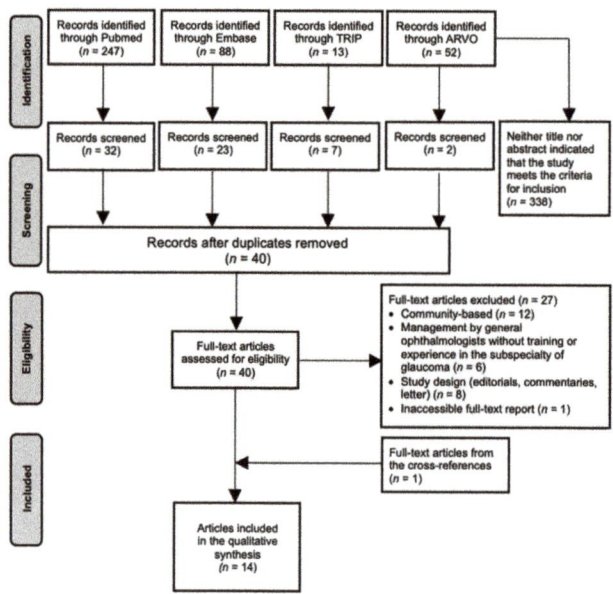

Figure 1. Study selection PRISMA flow chart on Shared Care. Abbreviations: ARVO = Annual Meeting of the Association for Research in Vision and Ophthalmology; n = amount.

3.2.2. Implementation and Performance of SC Clinics

These articles compared the performance of the non-medical staff with that of the GE, or compared SC in general with StC [33–44]. All articles concentrated on an actual clinic performing SC, including the glaucoma follow-up unit in the Rotterdam Eye Hospital (SC-GFU) [36–38], the Mayo clinic (SC-MC) [33–35], the Moorfield Eye Hospital (SC-MEH) [40,42], the Queen's medical centre (SC-QMC) [39], the Stable Glaucoma Clinic in New Zealand (SC-SGC) [43], the Glaucoma Management Clinic in Australia (SC-GMC) [44] and one established between the Royal Victorian Eye & Ear Hospital and the Australian College of Optometry (SC-RVAC) [41]. The corresponding StC clinic in each hospital is referred as "StC—(name of the corresponding clinic/hospital)".

3.3. The Organization: Implementing SC for Glaucoma

3.3.1. The Role of the GE

As a common rule, new patients had to be assessed by a GE, who decided on their diagnosis, set the target intra-ocular pressure (tIOP) and implemented a management plan. The recommendations of both the ANGIG&RANZCO [28] and the CGSC [29] formed an exception as they considered the GE's initial assessment unnecessary when a new patient was initially assessed by the non-medical staff and judged to be of low-to-moderate risk [29], without significant ocular risk factors [28]. After the initial assessment, the GE still examined the patient, however less frequently than in StC.

3.3.2. The Role of the Non-Medical Staff

The prerequisite skills of the non-medical staff working in the corresponding SC scheme are listed in Table 2.

Table 1. Baseline Characteristics "Shared Care".

First Author, Year	Country	Hospital	SC/Recommendation	Study Sample	NG/OSR vs. FU-Patients
White et al., 2014	Australia and New Zealand	/	ANGIG& RANZCO	/	FU-patients
Bentley et al., 2019	Australia	RVEEH	SC-RVAC	1024 patients	FU-patients
Canadian Glaucoma Society Committee, 2011	Canada	/	CGSC	/	FU-patients
Holtzer-Goor et al., 2010	The Netherlands	REH	CS-GFU	815 patients (2100 visits) SC-GFU: 405 (1181 visits) StC-GFU: 410 (919 visits)	FU-patients
Holtzer-Goor et al., 2016	The Netherlands	REH	CS-GFU	815 patients (2100 visits) SC-GFU: 405 (1181 visits) StC-GFU: 410 (919 visits)	FU-patients
Lemij et al., 2010	The Netherlands	REH	CS-GFU	815 patients (2100 visits) SC-GFU: 405 (1181 visits) StC-GFU: 410 (919 visits)	FU-patients
Damento et al., 2018	USA	MC	SC-MC	358 patients	FU-patients
Winkler et al., 2017	USA	MC	SC-MC	591 patients	FU-patients
Shah et al., 2018	USA	MC	SC-MC	200 patients (299 eyes)	FU-patients
Banes et al., 2000	UK	MEH	SC-MEH	54 patients (102 eyes)	FU-patients
Banes et al., 2006	UK	MEH	SC-MEH	349 patients	FU-patients
Ho et al., 2011	UK	QMC	SC-QMC	140 patients	FU-patients
Bhota et al., 2019	New Zealand	SGC	SC-SGC	509 patients (760 visits)	FU-patients
Phu et al., 2019	Australia	GMC	SC-GMC	101 patients	FU-patients

Abbreviations: SC = shared care clinic; StC = standard care clinic; FU = follow-up; NG/OSR = new glaucoma/ocular hypertension suspect referrals; ANGIG&RANZCO = recommendations of the Australian and New Zealand Glaucoma Interest Group and the Royal Australian and New Zealand College of Ophthalmologists; SC-RVAC = shared care clinic, established between the Royal Victorian Eye & Ear Hospital and the Australian College of Optometry; CGSC = recommendations from the Canadian Glaucoma Society Committee; RVEEH = Royal Victorian Eye & Ear Hospital; GFU = Glaucoma Follow-up Unit; MC = Mayo Clinic's campus in Rochester; MEH = Moorfield Eye Hospital; QMC = Queen's medical center; REH = Rotterdam Eye Hospital; USA = United States of America; UK = United Kingdom, SGC = Stable Glaucoma Clinic, GMC = Glaucoma Management Clinic; WEI = Wilmer Eye Institute.

Table 2. The prerequisite skills of the non-medical staff working in the corresponding shared care scheme.

SC/ Recommendations	NMS	History Taking	IOP	VA	Slit-Lamp Examination	+Gonio	VF	Fundus Photographs	OCT	HRT	GDx	CCT
ANGIG& RANZCO	NS	x	x	x	x(a&p)	x	x	x	x*	x*	x*	x
SC-RVAC	Opto	NS°	NS°	NS°	NS°	NS°	NS°	NS°	NS°	NS°	NS°	NS°
CGSC	Opto	x	x	NS	x(a&p)	x	x	x	x**	x**	x**	0
SC-GFU	Opto OT	x	x	x	0	0	x	0	0	0	x	0
SC-MC	Opto	x	x	x	x(a&p)	0	x	x	x	0	0	0
SC-MEH	Opto	x	x	NS	x(a&p)	x	x	x***	x***	x***	x***	x***
SC-QMC	Opto	x	x	NS	x(a&p)	x	x	0	x	x	0	x
SC-SGC	Opto	x	x	NS	NS	NS	x	x	0	x	0	NS
SC-GMC	Opto	x	x	x	x(a&p)	x	x	NS	0	x	0	0

Abbreviations: x = task performed by the corresponding member of the non-medical staff; 0 = task not performed by any member of the non-medical staff; x* = preferable rather than mandatory; x** = automated imaging tests, not further specified; x*** = could decide on further assessment if indicated; NS = not specified; NS° = not specified, but based on the recommendations of the Australian and New Zealand Glaucoma Interest Group and the Royal Australian and New Zealand College of Ophthalmologists; Opto = optometrists; OT = Ophthalmic technician; (a&p) = anterior&posterior segment; SC = shared care clinic; NMS = non-medical staff; IOP = intra-ocular pressure; VA = visual acuity; Gonio = gonioscopy; VF = visual field; OCT = optical coherence tomography; HRT = Heidelberg retinal tomography; GDx = GDx ECC scanning laser polarimetry; CCT = central corneal thickness; ANGIG&RANZCO = recommendations of the Australian and New Zealand Glaucoma Interest Group and the Royal Australian and New Zealand College of Ophthalmologists; SC-RVAC = shared care clinic, established between the Royal Victorian Eye & Ear Hospital and the Australian College of Optometry; CGSC = recommendations from the Canadian Glaucoma Society Committee; GFU = Glaucoma Follow-up Unit; MC = Mayo Clinic's campus in Rochester; MEH = Moorfield Eye Hospital; QMC = Queen's medical centre; SGC = Stable Glaucoma Clinic in New Zealand; GMC = Glaucoma Management Clinic in Australia.

In all SC schemes/recommendations, the non-medical staff had to perform and interpret a patient's history, visual acuity (VA), IOP and visual field (VF). Depending on the SC scheme/recommendation, their required skill set also included optic disc assessment, slit-lamp examination of the posterior segment, assessment of GDx, OCT and HRT, measuring the central corneal thickness (CCT), gonioscopy and/or fundus photography.

3.3.3. Patient Characteristics

Table 3 provides an overview of the characteristics that render patients suitable or unsuitable for each SC clinic, along with a list of conditions requiring referral to a GE.

Table 3. The characteristics that render patients suitable or unsuitable for each shared care clinic, along with a list of conditions requiring referral to a Glaucoma Expert.

SC/Recommendations	NMS	Suitable	Unsuitable	Model-Specific Referral	Patient-Specific Referral
ANGIG& RANZCO	NS	OHT; GS; G: stable & low/moderate risk	High risk of visual loss, e.g., other ocular diseases; advanced glaucoma (both stable and unstable); closed angles	GS: every 3–4 y; G early/moderate stable: every 2 y	Recent diagnosis; start of therapy; unstable disease; acutely raised or very high IOP; narrow angles
SC-RVAC	Opto	NS°	NS°	NS°	NS°
CGSC	Opto	OHT; GS; G: stable & low risk; Other concurrent eye diseases related to G	G: unstable/moderate/advanced	GS: every 3–4 y; G early: every 2–3 y	Recent diagnosis; start of therapy; GS with high risk (suspected progression); unstable G; acutely raised or very high IOP

Table 3. Cont.

SC/Recommendations	NMS	Suitable	Unsuitable	Model-Specific Referral	Patient-Specific Referral
SC-GFU	Opto OT	OHT; GS; G: stable	Complex cases: other ocular diseases; H laser therapy for DRP	G and GS: every third visit	Recent diagnosis; suspected progression
SC-MC	Opto	G: stable (mild/moderate/advanced); Other concurrent eye diseases	G: unstable	Mild G: every 3 y; moderate G: every 2 y; advanced G: every 1 y	Recent diagnosis; suspected progression; significant cataract; intolerant of medications
SC-MEH	Opto	OHT; GS; G; Other concurrent eye diseases	Known clinical complication, H laser therapy/surgery	OHT: every 1 y; stable G: every 6 mo; after change in therapy: 1 mo	Recent diagnosis; changes in treatment
SC-QMC	Opto	OHT; GS; G; Other concurrent eye diseases	H laser therapy/surgery	NS	Recent diagnosis; changes in treatment
SC-GSC	Opto	OHT; GS; G: stable	Other ocular diseases; G: unstable; recent treatment changes	NS	Unstable G
SC-QMC	Opto	OHT; GS; G: stable	G: severe and complicated; other ocular diseases	NS	Narrow angles

Abbreviations: OHT = ocular hypertension patient; GS = glaucoma suspect patients; G = glaucoma patient; NS = not specified; NS° = not specified, but based on the recommendations of the Australian and New Zealand Glaucoma Interest Group and the Royal Australian and New Zealand College of Ophthalmologists; Opto = Optometrist; OT = Ophthalmic Technician; ONP: Ophthalmic Nurse Practitioner; H = history of; y = year(s); DRP = diabetic retinopathy; mo = month(s); IOP = intra-ocular pressure; PDS = pigment dispersion syndrome; PXF = pseudo exfoliation syndrome; SC = Shared Care clinic; NMS = Non-Medical Staff; ANGIG&RANZCO = recommendations of the Australian and New Zealand Glaucoma Interest Group and the Royal Australian and New Zealand College of Ophthalmologists; SC-RVAC = shared care clinic, established between the Royal Victorian Eye & Ear Hospital and the Australian College of Optometry; CGSC = recommendations from the Canadian Glaucoma Society Committee; GFU = Glaucoma Follow-up Unit; MC = Mayo Clinic's campus in Rochester; MEH = Moorfield Eye Hospital; QMC = Queen's medical centre; SGC = Stable Glaucoma Clinic in New Zealand; GMC = Glaucoma Management Clinic in Australia.

- Unsuitable

As a general rule, new patients were considered unsuitable and needed an initial assessment by a GE. According to Ho et al. [39], decision-making at a first appointment was more related to diagnosis rather than continuing management.

Except for the SC-MEH [40,42] and the SC-QMC [39], patients with unstable glaucoma were considered unsuitable. A patient was considered to be unstable, if the tIOP was exceeded, or if progression was detected using functional or structural testing.

Complicated cases were also excluded, due to the high risk of visual loss. Patients were deemed to fall into this category if they had other eye diseases, advanced glaucoma (definite optic disc pathology or repeatable visual field loss over 12 dB and/or within 10 degrees of fixation, with or without normal IOP [28]), clinical complications or (recently) underwent surgery or laser therapy.

- Suitable

Generally, a patient was considered suitable when being stable, a glaucoma suspect, or with a low-to-moderate risk of visual loss.

- Back-referral

A patient could be referred back to the GE, in case of patient-specific conditions or at regular intervals, regardless of the glaucoma status, as an internal quality check.

3.4. Impact on Glaucoma Care

3.4.1. Quality of Care (QoC)

Distinction is made between the QoC provided by the non-medical staff and the QoC provided by the SC clinic in general (see Table 4). Quality is measured by evaluating completeness, accuracy and management decisions.

Table 4. The quality of care provided by the non-medical staff and the quality of care provided by the shared care clinic in general.

SC/Hospital	First Author	Compliance with Protocol (GFU)/Guidelines	Results of Tests and Examinations	Glaucoma Status	Referral	MD: Clinical Management
SC-RVAC	Bentley et al. [41]	SC vs. AAO PPPg, ANGIG&RANZCO - >85%	Optic nerve assessment skills (% correct diagnosis): -mean increase of 14.0% *	NS	NS	NS
SC-GFU	Holtzer-Goor et al. [38]	NMS vs. protocol - >98.8% of the visits	NS	SC vs. StC - % visits stable: SC (17.0%) ≈ StC (16.0%) ** - % visits with shortening of FU-interval: SC (16.0%) ≈ StC (15.1%) **	NMS: correct referral to GE - 84.4% of the remarkable cases	SC vs. StC - Treatment changes: SC (14.0%) ≈ StC (15.0%) **
SC-GFU	Holtzer-Goor et al. [36]	NMS vs. protocol - IOP, VA, GDx: > 97.5% - VF: 25.4% SC/StC vs. protocol - IOP: SC ≈ StC ** - VA: SC > StC * - GDx: SC > StC * - VF: SC ≈ StC **	SC vs. StC - VA decline (% visits): SC (3.9%) < StC (6.3%) * - IOP: SC ≈ StC ** - VF: SC ≈ StC ** - GDx: SC ≈ StC **		NMS: correct referral to seek advice from GE - 100.0%: SOF on GDx/VA- 84.6%: IOP > tIOP - 68.2%: VA declined >2 lines	SC vs. StC -Treatment changes: SC (14.0%) ≈ StC (15.0%) ** -Reason for change: SC ≈ StC **
SC-GFU	Lemij et al. [37]	NMS vs. protocol - IOP, VA, GDx: > 97.5% - VF: 41.2% *** SC/StC vs. protocol - IOP: SC ≈ StC ** - VA: SC > StC * - GDx: SC > StC * - VF: SC ≈ StC ** -Slit-lamp exam: SC < StC *	SC vs. StC - IOP: SC ≈ StC ** - VA: SC ≈ StC ** - GDx: SC ≈ StC ** - VF: SC ≈ StC **		NMS: correct referral to GE (50.0%) - 92.0%: SOF on GDx - 75.0% SOF on VF - 66.7%: IOP > tIOP - 36.0%: VA declined >2 lines	SC vs. StC -Treatment changes: SC (14.1%) ≈ StC (15.4%) ** -Reason for change: SC ≈ StC **
SC-MC	Damento et al. [37]	SC/StC vs. AAO PPPg (mean number of diagnostic tests) - 13 mo: SC > StC * - 25 mo: SC > StC *	NS	SC vs. StC (number of patients visits) - 13 mo: SC > StC * - 25 mo: SC > StC *	NS	NS
SC-MC	Winkler et al. [35]	SC/StC vs. AAO PPPg (% of patient visits) - Combined compliance *: SC > StC * - VF: SC ≈ StC ** - Gonio: SC > StC * - Fundus photographs: SC > StC * - OCT: SC > StC * - CCT: SC ≈ StC **	NS	NS	NS	NS

Table 4. Cont.

SC/Hospital	First Author	Compliance with Protocol (GFU)/Guidelines	Results of Tests and Examinations	Glaucoma Status	Referral	MD: Clinical Management
SC-MC	Shah et al. [33]	Opto vs. GE (frequency of clinical test data used to assess progression) - IOP: opto > GE * - Disc hemorrhage: opto≈ GE ** -Fundus photographs: opto≈ GE ** - VF: opto < GE (p=0.07, tendency) - OCT: opto < GE *	Among all HCP (GEs and optos); among GEs only: - IOP: κ = 0.57; κ = 0.57 - Disc hemorrhage: κ = 0.65; κ = 0.59 -Fundus photographs: 77%; 89% - VF: κ = 0.45; κ = 0.47 - OCT: κ = 0.26; κ = 0.51	Among all HCP (GEs and optos); among GEs only: - κ = 0.37; κ = 0.39	NS	NS
SC-MEH	Banes et al. [40]	NS	Opto vs. GE - IOP: OD median difference = -0.25 mmHg, OS median difference = 0.00 mmH - Slit-lamp exam (cup/disc): median difference = 0, greatest difference = 0.15 - VF: κ = 0.80–0.81	Opto vs. GE - FU-interval: κ = 0.97	NS	Opto vs. GE - Medical and surgical treatment: κ = 0.93–1.00
	Banes et al. [42]		Opto vs. GE - Slit lamp exam: sensitivity and specificity ≈ 83% Opto vs. GE; GE vs. GE - VF: κ = 0.37–0.33; κ = 0.39	Opto vs. GE; GE vs. GE - FU-interval: κ = 0.35; κ = 0.41	Opto vs. GE; GE vs. GE - Correct referral to GE: 72.0% agreement; 72.0% agreement	Opto vs. GE; GE vs. GE - "eye drop" treatment: κ = 0.67; κ = 0.74 - cataract surgery: 94.0%; 93.0% - glaucoma surgery: 95.0%; 97.0%
SC-QMC	Ho et al. [39]	NS	Opto vs. GE - VF: κ = 0.81–0.93	Opto vs. GE - next appointment: κ = 0.88–0.97	Opto vs. GE - Correct referral to GE: κ = 0.96–1.00	Opto vs. GE - "eye drop" treatment: κ = 0.96–1.00
SC-SGC	Bhota et al. [43]	NS	NS	NS	Opto vs. GE - Correct referral to GE: 66.1% agreement	NS
SC-GMC	Phu et al. [44]	NS	Opto vs. GE - Gonio: 59.8% agreement on structures (fair to moderate), 93.4% exact agreement with final diagnosis	NS	NS	NS

Abbreviations: SC = shared care clinic; StC = standard care clinic; * = statistical significant difference ($p \leq 0.05$); ** = no statistical significant difference ($p > 0.05$); κ = kappa; IQR = interquartile range; GE = glaucoma expert; NMS = non-medical staff; Opto = optometrist; HCP = health care providers; IOP = intra-ocular pressure; VA = visual acuity; VF = visual field; Gonio = gonioscopy; OCT = optical coherence tomography; HRT = Heidelberg retinal tomography; GDx = GDx ECC scanning laser polarimetry; CCT = central corneal thickness; Combined compliance* = combined completion of visual field, gonioscopy, measurement of central corneal thickness, and imaging (OCT or fundus photographs); SOF = suspicion of progression; VF: 41.2% ***: Out of the 34 patients who required a visual field examination on a yearly basis, 20 patients did not receive it in the SC-GFU; mo = month(s); AAO PPPg = American Academy of Ophthalmology Preferred Practice Pattern guidelines; ANGIG&RANZCO = recommendations of the Australian and New Zealand Glaucoma Interest Group and the Royal Australian and New Zealand College of Ophthalmologists; SC-RVAC = shared care clinic, established between the Royal Victorian Eye & Ear Hospital and the Australian College of Optometry; GFU = glaucoma follow-up unit; MC = Mayo Clinic's campus in Rochester; MEH = Moorfield Eye Hospital; QMC = Queen's medical centre; GHGC = Greenwich hospital glaucoma clinic; SGC = Stable Glaucoma Clinic in New Zealand; GMC = Glaucoma Management Clinic in Australia.

Performance of the Non-Medical Staff

Performance of the non-medical staff was evaluated by comparison with the "gold standard", which was the performance of the GE or a working protocol of the corresponding SC clinic.

- Completeness of data collection:

The non-medical staff working at the SC-GFU performed the required tests as per protocol in almost all visits [36–38]. VF was the only test with a poor compliance, i.e., in only 25.4% of the visits that required VF according to the protocol, the test was actually performed. Of note, also in the StC-GFU run by the GE, VFs were only performed in 16.9% of the visits where a VF was required according to the protocol [36].

- Accuracy of data collection:

Agreement between GEs and optometrists on IOP was evaluated in two studies [33,40] and was found to be good. Banes et al. [40] noted that optometrists tended to record lower IOP, but differences were small.

Agreement on structural glaucomatous damage was evaluated in three studies [33,40,42]. When performing slit-lamp examination, the optometrist's cup/disc ratio was comparable to that of GEs [40] and the optometrist's ability to decide whether or not an optic disc was glaucomatous was also found to be good (sensitivity and specificity ~83.0%) [42]. When evaluating fundus photographs on stability, the agreement between all HCP (GEs and optometrists) of the SC-MC [33] was found to be good and comparable to the agreement between GEs alone. Banes et al. [40] demonstrated the (dis)agreement rate to be independent of the cup/disc ratio values. Only Shah et al. [33] examined the agreement on OCT interpretation between all HCPs, including GEs and optometrists, and found it to be "fair". The study of Phu et al. [44] evaluated the agreement between optometrists and ophthalmologists on gonioscopy. The agreement in the exact assessment of the angle was "fair to moderate". Consistency with a final diagnosis, whether the angle was open or closed, was 93.4% [44].

Agreement on functional glaucomatous damage was evaluated in four studies [33,39,40,42]. The agreement on VF-status was "fair" [42], "moderate" [33] and "almost perfect" [39,40]. Banes et al. [42] pointed out that optometrists were more cautious than GEs, by classifying more eyes as being "progressive".

- Management decisions:

Several studies examined the non-medical staff's ability to make management decisions based on their interpretation of tests and examinations [33,36,37,39,40,42].

As for glaucoma status, in the SC-GFU, the non-medical staff referred half of the cases which met one of the back-referral criteria in the protocol back to the GE. Out of the cases that met the GDx- or VF-criterion (indicating suspected progressive damage), 92.0% and 75.0% of the cases, respectively, were actually sent back. These values amounted to 66.7% for the IOP-criterium (IOP > tIOP) and 36.0% for the VA-criterium (declined $\geq$ 2 lines) [37]. In the SC-GFU, the non-medical staff could also opt to seek advice of the GE when one the above criteria was met. In 100% of the cases that met the GDx- or the VF-criterium, the non-medical staff asked for advice or referred back. This value amounted to 84.6% and 68.2% for the IOP- and VA-criterium, respectively [36].

In the SC-MC, disease progression was defined as IOP > tIOP, progression on optic nerve photographs, OCT or VF [33,34]. Shah et al. [33] showed a "fair" level of agreement on glaucoma progression diagnosis between all HCPs (optometrists and GEs) and between GEs alone. The level of agreement between all HCPs was higher when relying on IOP or disc hemorrhages compared with the agreement when relying on OCT or VF [33]. Of all the available test data, the OCT and VF data were considerably less used by the optometrists than by the GEs. This discrepancy in use was also reflected in the high discrepancy in interpreting OCT and VF between all HCPs (agreement of 36.0%, κ = 0.26, for OCT, and agreement of 53%, κ = 0.45, for VF) [33].

Two other articles evaluated the agreement between HCPs on whether a patient should be discussed with the GE [39,42]. Ho et al. [39] found this agreement to be "almost perfect" between the GE and the non-medical staff. Banes et al. [42] found this agreement to be slightly smaller (72.0%), but equal to the agreement between two GEs on whether a patient should be discussed with them. Three studies [39,40,42] evaluated the agreement on disease status by using the proposed follow-up interval as a measure. A shortened interval indicated that the disease status was judged to be worsening. Overall, the agreement was "almost perfect" [39,40]. Only Banes et al. [42] showed a "fair" agreement.

As for ordering tests, the non-medical staff of the SC-MH [40,42] and the SC-QMC [39] was allowed to do so. Ho et al. [39] showed a high agreement on ordering a VF at the next appointment between the optometrists and GE. Although Banes et al. [42] assessed lower values, the agreement was still good and similar to the agreement between two GEs. In both clinics, the optometrists tended to order more additional tests than the GEs [39,40,42].

The non-medical staff of the SC-MH [40,42] and the SC-QMC [39] were also able to decide on further treatment. In both clinics, agreement was high for both the medical and surgical treatments.

Performance of the SC Clinic

In this case, the "gold standard" corresponds to the StC or the guidelines used (Table 4).

- Completeness of data collection:

The Mayo Clinic showed an increase in compliance on initial testing to the American Academy of Ophthalmology Preferred Practice Pattern (AAO PPP) guidelines [45] after implementation of the SC-MC [35]. Similarly, the SC-RVAC [41] showed a high compliance to both the AAO PPP [45] and the ANGIG&RANZCO recommendations [28]. The compliance on rate of testing was weak, but similar, for VF in both SC-GFU and StC-GFU [36,37].

- Accuracy of data collection:

No difference was found between the results obtained by the SC-GFU [36,37] and the StC-GFU. One exception was VA, which declined in more visits of the StC-GFU than in the SC-GFU [36]. Holtzer-Goor et al. attributed this difference to the different protocols used in both clinics; the SC-GFU had to perform VA at every visit while the StC-GFU had to perform VA only when judged to be necessary (but at least once a year) [36]. In other words, the StC-GFU would mainly perform VA for those patients who mentioned having difficulties with their sight [36]. The implementation of SC-RVAC resulted in a 14.0% increase in correct diagnosis when assessing the optic nerve compared to the StC clinic [41].

- Management decisions:

No difference was found between the StC-GFU and the SC-GFU in the decision on the number of patients judged to be stable or progressive [36,38]. Holtzer-Goor et al. concluded that a SC scheme did not miss a significant number of cases of suspected progression [36]. Damento et al. assessed the decision on "disease status" in the Mayo Clinic by using the "number of patient visits" as a measure [34]. The rationale was that, if an HCP judged the disease status to be worsening, that HCP decided to shorten the follow-up interval, which resulted in more visits taking place in a certain amount of time. No difference was found in the number of patient visits between the SC-MC and the StC-MC [34].

Furthermore, the number of treatment changes was similar between the SC-GFU and the StC-GFU [36–38]. Moreover, no difference was found concerning the reason for change, i.e., IOP exceeding the tIOP, intolerance to the medication, structural or functional progression [36,37]. Likewise, the number of procedures carried out in the SC-MC and the StC-MC did not differ [34]. However, the number of procedures performed by the GE tended to increase after implementation of the SC scheme [34].

3.4.2. Acceptance

Patients

Patient satisfaction was about the same in the SC-GFU and the StC-GFU [36,37]. No difference was noted in the dimensions "overall mark", "knowledge", "waiting area", and "information received". Patients scored the SC-GFU higher on 'taking sufficient time" and "giving sufficient information".

When comparing HCPs, Holtzer-Goor et al. assessed a higher score on the "overall mark" for the non-medical staff [36]. The GE got a higher score on the dimension "information received". Patients gave both the GE and the non-medical staff similar scores on "knowledge" and "waiting area". Lemij et al. [37] found similar scores as Holtzer-Goor et al. [36], but assessed a higher score for the GE on "knowledge" and "information received". In the SC-RVAC, almost 95% of the responders opted to be treated in the SC-RVAC rather than remaining on the waiting list of the StC-RVAC [41].

Staff

All clinicians of the SC-RVAC found the SC clinic an excellent opportunity to exchange knowledge, and 82.0% wanted to stay working in the clinic [41]. Similarly, the GE and the ophthalmic technicians were very pleased to work in the SC-GFU [37,38]. The ophthalmic technicians indicated the patient contact and the increased responsibility to be the main reasons. However, the optometrists working in the SC-GFU found their work tedious, and thought the shared clinic was not working satisfactorily [37].

3.4.3. Productivity

In the SC-RVAC, the waiting list was reduced by 32.0% after 17 months and by 92.0% after 28 months [41]. Holtzer-Goor et al. hypothesized that the implementation of the GFU reduced the waiting list, because of the increased number of patients (+23.0%) and patient visits (+16.0%) [38]. Another article on the SC-GFU by Holtzer-Goor et al. showed that for each patient transferred to the SC-GFU, approximately 0.57 extra stable glaucoma patients could be managed in the hospital [36]. However, this seemed to be a short-term effect. In the long term, the patients' outflow would be limited because glaucoma is a chronic disease [36]. Moreover, the inflow would increase as the number of patients with glaucoma is predicted to increase as indicated above (cfr. Section 1). Damento et al. documented an increased access for complex patients to the GE after implementing the SC-MC [34]. Botha et al. demonstrated an improvement in IOP control and decreased progression rates since the implementation of SC-SGC, partly attributable to less delays in follow-up [43].

4. Results of Virtual Clinics' Studies

4.1. Literature Search

From the 445 articles identified, 14 were selected, complemented with one additional article obtained from the reference lists. The processes of identification, screening, duplicates removal and full-text assessment are shown in Figure 2.

4.2. Description of the Included Articles

Baseline characteristics of the included articles are shown in Table 5. Unlike SC clinics, VCs are not widespread. All VCs included in this review are located in the UK. A VC could be implemented in the initial assessment of a patient who had been referred from primary care, in which case these clinics served as a triaging service. These types of VCs included the glaucoma assessment clinic (GAC) [46–48] at the Singleton hospital and the Glaucoma Screening clinic (GSC) [49] as part of a broader service transformation program being established at the MEH. Gunn et al. did not focus on a specific VC but investigated the proportion, the characteristics and the acceptability of the Hospital Eye Service (HES)-units that implemented a VC for glaucoma care [50].

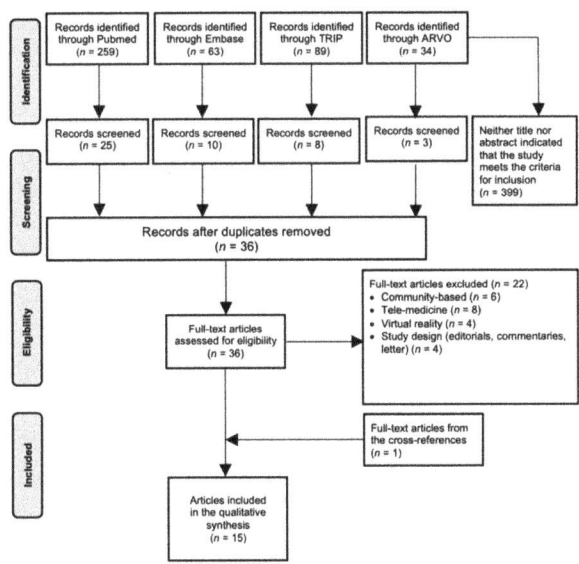

Figure 2. Study selection PRISMA flow chart on Virtual Clinics. Abbreviations: ARVO = Annual Meeting of the Association for Research in Vision and Ophthalmology; n = amount.

Table 5. Baseline Characteristics "Virtual Clinics".

First Author, Year	Country	Hospital	VC	Study Sample	NG/OSR vs. FU-Patients
Banes et al., 2018	UK	Units from the HES	/	/	NG/OSR and FU-patients
Wright and Diamond, 2014	UK	3 glaucoma clinics: Bristol, Nuneaton and Kingston	GCC	24,257 patients	FU-patients
Kotecha et al., 2017	UK	MEH	GSC (GSMS)	1380 patients	NG/OSR
Clarke et al., 2017	UK	MEH	SMS (GSMS)	204 patients	FU-patients
Kotecha et al., 2015	UK	MEH	SMS (GSMS)	1575 patients	FU-patients
Nikita et al., 2019	UK	MEH	SMS (GSMS)	2015 patients	FU-patients
Kotecha et al., 2005	UK	MEH	GSMS	43 patients	NG/OSR and FU-patients
Choong et al., 2003	UK	SH	GAC	100 patients	NG/OSR
Rathod et al., 2008	UK	SH	GAC	78 patients	NG/OSR
Court and Austin, 2015	UK	SH	GAC	170 patients (85 StC and 85 GAC)	NG/OSR
Tatham et al., 2021	UK	PAEP	VC-PAEP	105 patients (55 StC and 50 VC-PAEP)	FU-patients
Gunn et al., 2021	UK	MREH; BEH	VC-MREH; VC-BEH	148 patients	FU-patients
Mostafa et al., 2020	UK	PAEP	VC-PAEP	116 patients	FU-patients
Nikita et al., 2021	UK	MEH	VC-MEH	2017 patients	NG/OSR and FU-patients
Spackman et al., 2020	UK	REIP	VC-REIP	68 patients	FU-patients

Abbreviations: UK = United Kingdom; MEH = Moorfield Eye Hospital; HES = Hospital Eye Services; SH = Singleton Hospital; GCC = Glaucoma Classifying Clinic; GSC = Glaucoma Screening Clinic; SMS = Stable Monitoring Service; GSMS = Glaucoma Screening and Stable Monitoring Service; GAC = Glaucoma Assessment Clinic; VC = virtual clinic; StC = standard care clinic; NG/OSR = new glaucoma/ocular hypertension suspect referrals; FU = follow-up, PAEP = Princess Alexandra Eye Pavilion, MREH = Manchester Royal Eye Hospital, BEH = Bristol Eye Hospital, REIP = The Royal Eye Infirmary Plymouth.

A VC could also play a role in patient follow-up. These types of VCs included the virtual triaging clinic established in Bristol, Nuneaton and Kingston, referred to as the glaucoma classifying clinic (GCC) [51] in this paper, the virtual clinic in Princess Alexandra Eye Pavilion (VC-PAEP) [52,53], the virtual clinic in Manchester Royal Eye Hospital (VC-MREH) [54] and in Bristol Eye Hospital (VC-BREH) [54], the virtual clinic in The Royal Eye Infirmary Plymouth (VC-REIP) [55] and the Stable Monitoring Service [56–58] (SMS) which was the other part of the virtual service transformation implemented at the MEH [50]. The complete virtual service at MEH was named the Glaucoma Screening and Stable Monitoring Service (GSMS) [59], implementing both the GSC [49] for initial assessment and the SMS [56–58] for patient follow-up. Nikita at al studied expanded patient eligibility criteria at MEH (VC-MEH); both new and follow-up patients were included [60].

4.3. The Organization: Implementing a VC for Glaucoma

4.3.1. Role of the Staff

The prerequisite skills of the non-medical staff working in the corresponding VC are listed in Table 6.

Table 6. The prerequisite skills of the non-medical staff working in the corresponding virtual clinic.

VC	First Author	NMS	History Taking	IOP	VA	Slit-Lamp	Von Herick	OCT (Angle)	VF	Fundus Photographs	OCT	HRT	CCT
GCC	Wright and Diamond	Opto	x*	x*	x*	x*	x*	0	-	-	0	0	-
		OT	x*	x*	x*	x*	x*	0	x	x	0	0	x
GSC (GSMS)	Kotecha et al.	Clinician;	-	-	-	0	0	-	-	-	0	0	-
		OT	x*	x	x	0	0	x	x	x	0	0	x
SMS (GSMS)	Clarke et al. Kotecha et al. Nikita et al.	ONP	x*	-	-	x(a)	NS	0	-	-	0	-	0
		OT	-	x*	x	-	0	0	x	x	0	x	0
		OT	x*	x	x	0	0	0	x	x	0	0	0
		NS	NS	x	x	0	0	0	x	x	x	0	0
GSMS	Kotecha et al.	Clinician	-	-	-	-	-	-	-	-	-	-	-
		OT	NS	NS	NS	NS	NS	NS	NS	NS	NS	NS	NS
GAC	Choong et al. Rathod et al. Court and Austin	ONP	x	x	0	0	0	0	x	0	0	0	0
		ONP	x	x	0	x	x	0	x	x	0	x	0
		ONP	x	x	0	x	NS	0	x	x	0	x	0
VC-PAEP	Tatham et al. Mostafa et al.	OT	x	x	NS	x	NS	0	x	x	x	x	x
		OT	x	x	NS	x	NS	0	x	x	x	x	x
		ONP	x	x	NS	x	NS	0	x	x	x	x	x
VC-MREH; VC-BEH	Gunn et al.	OT	x	x	x	0	0	0	x	0	0	x	0
VC-MEH	Nikita et al.	OT	x	x	x	0	0	x*	x	x	0	x	0
VC-RAEP	Spackman et al.	NS	NS	NS	NS	NS	NS	NS	NS	NS	NS	NS	NS

Abbreviations: x = task performed by the corresponding member of the non-medical staff; - = task performed by the other member of the non-medical staff; 0 = task not performed by any member of the non-medical staff; x* = not specified which member of the non-medical staff performed the clinical assessment; Opto = optometrist; OT = ophthalmic technician; ONP: ophthalmic nurse practitioner; HCA = health care assistant; x(a) = anterior segment; NS = not specified; NMS = non-medical staff; IOP = intra-ocular pressure; VA = visual acuity; OCT(angle) = anterior segment optical coherence tomography for angle assessment; VF = visual field; OCT = optical coherence tomography; HRT = Heidelberg retinal tomography; CCT = central corneal thickness; VC = virtual clinic; GCC = Glaucoma Classifying Clinic; GSC = Glaucoma Screening Clinic; SMS = Stable Monitoring Service; GSMS = Glaucoma Screening and Stable Monitoring Service; GAC = Glaucoma Assessment Clinic, PAEP = Princess Alexandra Eye Pavilion, MREH = Manchester Royal Eye Hospital, BEH = Bristol Eye Hospital, REIP = The Royal Eye Infirmary Plymouth.

4.3.2. Initial Assessment

In the GSC, a new patient was evaluated by a clinician who decided if the patient was eligible for the VC, based on the referral letter from primary care [49]. If eligible, the patient underwent testing, performed by ophthalmic technicians. Patients were also given a questionnaire enquiring about their medical and family history. The GE reviewed the collected clinical data and decided on a follow-up at the hospital or a discharge. In the GAC, new patients were systematically seen by the ONP without prior triage [46–48]. The ONP took the patient's history, performed tests, clinically examined the patient and assessed the patient's risk profile. The article of Choong et al. could be considered as the pilot study of the GAC, which did not include a VC yet [47]. It was presented as a fast-track system, which allowed an ONP to triage patients, including defining the time-interval in which patients needed to have their face-to-face appointment with the GE. Rathod et al. built further on this system and added a virtual service [48]. The ONP would again triage these patients, but the GE would do the initial assessment by reviewing the GAC data instead of a face-to-face assessment [48].

4.3.3. Follow-Up

The non-medical staff working at SMS varied between articles [56–58]. In the pilot study, ophthalmic technicians performed VA, VF and optic disc imaging [56]. An ONP took the patient's history by reviewing a questionnaire and was in charge of the clinical examination, including tests that required more expertise (IOP, slit-lamp examination). Furthermore, they could offer advice on common eye complaints and drop delivery technique. The GE reviewed the notes of previous appointments and included these in the management decisions. In a later study, the ONP was removed from the SMS [57]. A slit-lamp examination was no longer performed, and the ophthalmic technicians took over IOP measurement. In the study of Nikita et al., the SMS also incorporated OCT for the virtual review [58]. However, the profession of the non-medical staff was not specified in this article [58]. Similar to the GSC [49], a follow-up patient was evaluated by a clinician who decided if the patient was eligible for the SMS [59]. In the GCC, an optometrist supported by ophthalmic technicians met the patient first and collected clinical data from the clinical history, clinical examination, VF and color optic disc images [51]. After data interpretation, the optometrist classified the patient into one of five risk categories, each associated with a required time interval for a face-to-face consultation with a GE. Subsequently, in the virtual review, the GE confirmed or changed the optometrist's classification, based on the same clinical data. If a patient was classified to have no strong evidence of glaucoma, the patient would be discharged, and would not be seen by a GE [51].

4.3.4. Patient Suitability

Table 7 provides an overview of new patients who are considered suitable and unsuitable for each VC.

Table 7. The characteristics that render patients suitable or unsuitable for each virtual clinic.

VC	First Author	NG/OSR vs. FU-Patients	Suitable	Unsuitable
GCC	Wright and Diamond	FU-patients	General FU-pool (all types and various stages of risk)	NS
GSC (GSMS)	Kotecha et al.	NG/OSR	First: low risk of developing G Later: up to three risk factors for G	Definitive signs of G; angle closure suspects; IOP > 32 mmHg
SMS (GSMS)	Clarke et al.	FU-patients	OHT; GS; G: stable and low risk; open angle inclusive PDS and PXF	Poor mobility: poor VF; poor disc imaging
	Kotecha et al.	FU-patients	OHT; GS; G: stable and low/moderate risk	Phakic angle closure/suspects; monocular; coexisting ocular comorbidity; best-corrected VA < Snellen 6/12; H glaucoma filtration surgery; concerns regarding adherence; requirement of hospital transport to attend; signs of cognitive impairment
	Nikita et al.	FU-patients	G: most types, various stages of risk	NS
GSMS	Kotecha et al.	NG/OSR;	Low/moderate risk of developing G	NS
		FU-patients	OHT; GS; G: stable and low/moderate risk, open-angle	NS
GAC	Choong et al.	NG/OSR	All NG/OSR *	NS
	Rathod et al.	NG/OSR	All NG/OSR *	NS
	Court and Austin	NG/OSR	All NG/OSR *	NS
VC-PAEP	Tatham et al.	FU-patients	G: mild to moderate stable	H glaucoma filtration surgery; phakic angle closure/suspects
	Mostafa et al.	FU-patients	GS; OHT	
VC-MREH; VC-BEH	Gunn et al.	FU-patients	G; GS; OHT	<18 years of age; unable to speak English
VC-MEH	Nikita et al.	NG/OSR and FU-patients	G (most types); GS; H ocular surgery/glaucoma laser/retinal laser	Unstable advanced G
VC-REIP	Spackman et al.	FU-patients	NS	NS

Abbreviations: FU = follow-up; NG/OSR = new glaucoma/OHT suspect referrals; G = glaucoma patient; OHT = ocular hypertension patient; GS = glaucoma suspect patient; PDS = pigment dispersion syndrome; PXF = pseudoexfoliation syndrome; All NG/OSR * = all risks of developing glaucoma; H = history of; IOP = intra-ocular pressure; VA = visual acuity; VF = visual field; NS = not specified; VC = virtual clinic; GCC = glaucoma classifying clinic; GSC = Glaucoma Screening Clinic; SMS = Stable Monitoring Service; GSMS = Glaucoma Screening and Stable Monitoring Service; GAC = Glaucoma Assessment Clinic; PAEP = Princess Alexandra Eye Pavilion; MREH = Manchester Royal Eye Hospital; BEH = Bristol Eye Hospital; REIP = The Royal Eye Infirmary Plymouth. PCAG = Primary closed-angle glaucoma.

New Patients
- Suitable:

At the start of the GSC, only "low risk" glaucoma suspects were considered to be suitable [49]. These patients only had one of the following risk factors: suspicious optic discs, suspicious VF or IOP >20 mm Hg. In a second stage, "low-to-moderate risk" glaucoma suspects (having up to two risk factors, including and a positive family history in a first-degree relative) were also eligible for the GSC [49]. Finally, at a later stage, patients could have up to three of those risk factors and still be eligible for the GSC [49]. A clinician decided if a patient would be included in the VC or would be sent to the GE immediately. In the GAC, all new glaucoma/OHT suspect referrals were included in the VC [46,48].

- Unsuitable:

The clinician excluded new glaucoma/OHT suspect referrals from the GSC if they did not meet the inclusion criteria [49]. Patients were also excluded if they showed definitive signs of glaucoma, were angle-closure suspects or were referred with an IOP >32 mm Hg [49]. If a patient showed an IOP >32 mm Hg at the initial assessment of the GSC, the patient would be sent to a GE on the same day [49].

Follow-Up Patients

- Suitable:

Only stable patients with a low risk of glaucomatous damage progression were suitable for the SMS [56–58]. In the "pilot" study by Clarke et al., patients were included if their planned follow-up frequency was more than six months [56]. This study concluded that patients were suitable if they had stable glaucoma and were at low risk of progression to significant visual loss over each follow-up interval [56]. Recent studies conducted by Nikita et al. expanded patient suitability from glaucoma suspects and low-risk glaucoma to most types of glaucoma and in various stages of disease progression, and provided firm evidence that expanded patient eligibility criteria are able to deliver high-quality glaucoma care that is safe and effective [58,60]. In the GCC, patients were taken from the general follow-up pool and could have any type of glaucoma at any stage [51]. In the VC-PAEP, patients with mild to moderate stable open-angle glaucoma or patients with mild to moderate stable primary closed-angle glaucoma who are bilaterally pseudophakic were suitable [52,53].

- Unsuitable:

In the "pilot" study of the SMS, patients were excluded if they had poor mobility or if the quality of their VF or fundus photographs was poor [56]. When the SMS was eventually established, other exclusion criteria were added, including monocular, concurrent eye diseases/morbidities, a low VA and if there were concerns about the patients' adherence to treatment [57]. The expanded monitoring service studied by Nikita et al. did not specify the exclusion criteria [58]. Both the SMS and the VC-PAEP excluded phakic angle-closure glaucoma/glaucoma suspects and patients who had a history of glaucoma filtration surgery [52,53,57].

4.4. Impact on Glaucoma Care
4.4.1. QoC
New Patients (GSC and GAC)

In the GSC, 20.0% of patients were discharged wrongly by the GE, but only a minority required medical intervention, leading to a "significant" false rate of 4.0% [49]. The GSC missed two narrow angles with one requiring surgery [49]. In the GAC, the similarity of a GE's virtual assessment was "substantial" ($\kappa = 0.72$) to those made through a face-to-face assessment [48].

Follow-Up Patients (GCC, SMS, VC-PAEP, VC-MREH and VC-BEH, VC-REIP)

In the GCC, a "substantial" ($\kappa = 0.69$) agreement on triaging was found between the optometrists and supervising GEs [51]. In general, optometrists tended to be overcautious by considering patients more at risk. Still, the optometrists discharged 15.0% of the cases having glaucoma according to the GE. Another concern was the 6.5% of cases considered as low-risk by the optometrist who were identified as unstable by the GE [51]. Kotecha et al. compared the face-to-face assessment by a GE in the SMS with a virtual assessment by a different GE (inter-GE agreement) or by the same GE (intra-GE agreement) [57]. The inter-GE agreement was found to be "fair" ($\kappa = 0.32$). In this analysis, seven out of 14 unstable cases were detected during the virtual review (sensitivity of 50.0%). The other seven patients (3.4% of all patients) had been "misclassified" as stable during the virtual clinic assessment, two of whom (1.9%) having advanced VF loss. The sensitivity increased to 75.0% when only considering consultants and excluding fellows from the GE population [57]. Regarding the analysis made by the same GE, the intra-GE agreement was "fair" ($\kappa = 0.26$–0.27). The disagreements would only pose a risk for six patients (3.1% of all patients), since these were deemed as stable during the virtual review, but unstable at the face-to-face review by the same GE. The sensitivity amounted to 75.0% for the consultant and 60.0% for the fellow [57]. The study of Mostafa et al. showed that Goldmann applanation tonometry measurements only have moderate agreement when performed by different operators and that repeat Ocular Response Analyzer (ORA) IOP measurements were more consistent [53].

4.4.2. Acceptance
Patients

According to Kotecha et al., patients with a low risk of progression were more open to a VC [59]. Patients were pleased with the reduced waiting time, the expertise of the staff and the productivity of the VC [57,59]. Court and Austin found that patients in the VC did not consider they were receiving inferior quality care compared to patients in StC [46]. However, some patients were disappointed by not receiving immediate feedback and not seeing a doctor on the same day [57]. Tatham et al. found no significant difference in knowledge of glaucoma between patients of VC-PAEP and StC-PAEP, suggesting that patients' knowledge is not disadvantaged by virtual clinics [52]. Study patients of Gunn et al. reported reduced waiting times as a key aspect of positive experiences [54]. These patients demonstrated high levels of trust in the staff performing tests in the glaucoma VC [53]. Spackman et al. evaluated patient satisfaction with the glaucoma VC in comparison with StC in The Royal Eye Infirmary Plymouth [55]. Overall, 98% of patients felt that the VC was the same or better than the StC [55].

Staff

Gunn et al. [50] investigated the perspective of the GE; 92.9% of the respondents considered the VC as safe and efficient as StC, with 31.0% rating the efficiency as very good. The authors also identified the main reasons for not implementing a VC: insufficient staff, inadequate space, insufficient time or funding to train the non-medical staff, the risk of missing pathology and the lack of face-to-face discussion [50]. Later, Gunn et al. [54] investigated the perceptions of the technicians working in the glaucoma SC clinic. The technicians reported satisfaction in working within the glaucoma service. However, they commonly felt they would benefit from more detailed training, particularly around knowledge of the conditions and medications [54].

4.4.3. Productivity

In the GSC, the GE discharged 62.0% of new glaucoma/OHT suspect referrals, sent 1.0% for an urgent same-day assessment with a GE, referred 6.0% to SMS and booked 31.0% for the consultant-led outpatient clinic [49]. In the GAC, 20.5% were discharged, after being diagnosed virtually as "normal" [48]. In the GCC, the GE discharged 3.7% of new glaucoma/OHT suspect referrals, which is 1.2% more than the number of patients that would have been discharged by the optometrists [51]. The virtual supervision by the GE also reduced the number of additional visits, e.g., the follow-up appointments, by 2.4% of the total number of visits [51]. The implementation of the SMS led to 13.0% of the patients being discharged, 57.0% of the patients being rebooked in the SMS and 30.0% being sent to a GE for a face-to-face appointment [58].

5. Discussion

5.1. Application of SC/VC

All the studies regarding SC clinics in this review concentrated on patient follow-up, while the studies regarding VCs were done with a follow up setting—GCC [51], SMS [56,57,59], VC-PAEP [52,53], VC-MREH [54], VC-BEH [54] and VC-REIP [55] or for an initial assessment only—GAC [46–48] and GSC [49].

5.2. Generalizability to Other Hospitals/Countries

The guidelines for the management of glaucoma are mainly country-specific: the AAO PPP [45] in the USA, the Royal College of Ophthalmologists' (RCO) guidelines [61] in the UK, the COSgcpg [31] in Canada and the NHMRC guidelines [30] in Australia. The guidelines from the RCO [61] and guidelines from NICE [62] are commonly used in the UK, however not in other countries. Furthermore, in the VCs of the UK-based articles, the non-medical staff entrusted with a particular task probably followed the same UK-based required training. Hence, one should be careful in extrapolating to other countries, e.g., the non-medical staff from the REH are not trained to perform slit-lamp examination to assess the optic disc [36].

5.3. Skills of the Non-Medical Staff

In all SC clinics and VCs operating during follow-up, the non-medical staff had to take a clinical history, measure IOP and perform a functional (VF) and a structural (fundus photographs, OCT, HRT or GDx) evaluation. In all SC clinics [33–44], at least one non-medical staff member had to interpret the results from these examinations to decide on the glaucoma status and the (possible) presence of progression. In the VCs [46–51,56–59] the non-medical staff had to perform all examinations a GE would normally do without making any treatment decisions. In only two VCs (GCC and GAC), a non-medical staff member had to be able to interpret these examinations to triage patients [46,48,51]. In the other virtual services, (GSMS, VC-PAEP, VC-MREH, VC-BEH, VC-MEH and VC-REIP), the non-medical staff had only to collect and to deliver data to the GE.

5.4. Suitable Patients

In all clinics, patients who were stable and were at low risk of progression were considered suitable. Patients with narrow angles, with or without glaucoma, were found suitable, if the non-medical staff was able to assess the angle of the anterior chamber; hence, such patients were only accepted in the GCC, GAC, SC-MEH and the SC-QMC [41–43,48,51].

5.5. Pathway of a High-Risk Patient

In the GSMS, a clinician triaged both new patients and follow-up patients, whereby high-risk patients were sent directly to the GE for a face-to-face appointment [49,56–59]. The GAC and the GCC, however, did not foresee such triage system, in that the non-medical staff assessed all new patients [48,51]. However, high-risk patients were sent to a GE immediately.

In all implemented SC schemes, a GE assessed all new patients to decide on their eligibility. The ANGIG&RANZCO [28] and the Canadian Glaucoma Society [29] recommendations on SC were an exception in that the initial assessment by a GE was not mandatory if the non-medical staff considered a new patient to be low-to-moderate risk [29], without significant ocular risk factors [28].

5.6. Compliance to Guidelines

An increase in compliance with guidelines was noted when implementing a SC clinic due to the combined examination efforts of the non-medical staff and the GE [35,41,47].

Compliance was also higher when following a standardized protocol [35,36,47]. Moreover, by delegating some tasks to the non-medical staff, the GE would have more time and would not have to give up examinations [40]. Banes et al. showed that the lack of time in the often very busy StC clinic caused the GE to skip some examinations [40]. Such was also the case in the GFU, where a low compliance rate was noted in the SC-GFU as well as in the StC-GFU [36,62]. This clinic admitted only low risk patients with no proven glaucoma (but with positive family history, OHT and/or suspicious looking discs) or early glaucoma damage. In such cases, structural measurements were deemed to be more important, for being more informative and also quicker to perform than VFs [36,62]. None of the VC-articles examined the effect on compliance.

5.7. Data Interpretation: Importance of Training

The accuracy of the data interpretation increased with the level of experience/training of the non-medical staff. As the optometrists from the SC-MEH [40,42] and SC-QMC [39] got extra training in these tasks, their interpretation of the fundus photographs and VF was more accurate than in the SC-MC. The lack of training could also explain why the agreement on evaluating OCT between optometrists from the SC-MC and GEs was less good, and worse than the agreement between GEs [33]. The optometrists from the SC-MEH and SC-QMC assessed the optic disc through slit-lamp examination and showed a high agreement with the GE because they were trained to use these devices [39,40,42]. None of the VC-articles investigated the accuracy of the non-medical staff.

5.8. Quality of Management Decisions

In their decisions on progression/referral, the non-medical staff of the SC-GFU followed the referral criteria strictly [36,37]. More importantly, adherence to these criteria increased when, besides referring patients to the GE directly [37], they could also ask for the GE's advice [36]. The level of agreement on progression between optometrists and the GEs from the SC-MC was only "fair", but similar to the level of agreement between two GEs. A point of concern was that almost 1/3 of the glaucoma cases being progressive would not be referred to the GE. Possible reasons were an incorrect interpretation of data (see above) and not using all data when making decisions. However, optometrists tended to be overcautious in general. In both the SC-MEH and GCC, the optometrists classified more patients as progressive or at higher risk than the GE [42,51]. Most likely, the reason was to make a safer decision. As a consequence, the optometrists tended to order more additional tests than the GEs [39,40,42].

Decisions on discharge/follow-up were also safeguarded. In the GCC, decisions of the non-medical staff in this respect were supervised virtually by the GE [51]. In the GFU, the non-medical staff could not discharge and could only decide to keep or shorten the interval as planned [36–38]. Similarly, in the GAC the non-medical staff could not discharge, and the GE would (virtually) assess the patient within a maximum time interval of three months [48]. The agreement with the face-to-face diagnosis was also high. In the GSC out of the 16 patients for whom the diagnosis differed between the face-to-face and virtual review, only three patients required medical intervention [49]. Two of these patients were diagnosed as having OHT, one of whom had an IOP at the face-to-face consultation which was twice as high as what had been found in the virtual review and in the referral letter. The third patient had narrow, occludable angles requiring prophylactic laser iridotomy [49]. In the SMS, the sensitivity of detecting unstable cases was dependent on the expertise of the GE; a higher sensitivity was noted for the consultant than for the fellow, both in the inter- and intra-observer agreement analyses [56]. The arbitrary stable/unstable classification, which was used in the SMS for deciding on the time to the next FU appointment, was explained as a possible reason for the low sensitivity [56]. However, since only stable and low-to-moderate risk patients could enter the clinic, the actual number of missed unstable patients was low, and even lower with advanced VF loss [56]. Due to the wide confidence intervals, it was suggested to perform more extensive studies to provide a more accurate answer on the virtual clinic's sensitivity [56]. In the SC-MEH studies, the optometrist(s) and the GE independently decided on the follow-up interval and the further treatment [40,42]. The agreement was high and comparable to the agreement between two GEs. In SC-QMC study, where the GE had to state (dis)approval with the optometrists' decisions, the agreement was even higher [39].

5.9. Acceptance

All findings showed that the acceptance of care provided by a SC clinic or a VC was at least as good as in the StC clinic. In the SC-GFU, the GE scored higher on "knowledge" and "information received"; however, the difference was too small to be relevant [37]. In the study of Spackman et al., 98% of patients felt that the glaucoma VC was the same or better than the StC [55].

Acceptance of SC and VCs by the GEs was overall good; some medical staff however found their work in SC to be tedious [37].

5.10. Productivity

The waiting list for new glaucoma/OHT suspect referrals to the GE decreased; most of the follow-up appointments of stable, low risk glaucoma suspects/patients were given to the non-medical staff, thereby saving the GE time [36,41]. Also, the non-medical staff could ensure these patients got their appointments on time.

The access of complex patients and unstable patients to the GE increased [34]. The non-medical staff was made responsible for monitoring stable glaucoma, thereby saving time for the GE to accept more complex patients and to see all patients on time and detect progression quickly. Holtzer-Goor et al. found a significantly lower VA in the StC-GFU; this could indicate that more complex patients were directed to the StC-GFU, thereby achieving one of the main goals of SC [36]. Likewise, the number of procedures performed by the GE tended to increase when cooperating with the non-medical staff in the SC-MC suggesting better access of complex patients to care provided by the GE [34].

By delegating triaging, GEs were also less busy with the initial assessment. The GAC and the GSC respectively sent only 79.5% and 32.0% to the GE for a face-to-face assessment [48,49]. The GSC sent less people to the StC outpatient clinic because they could refer stable OHT/glaucoma suspects/glaucoma patients with low-to-moderate risk to the SMS [49,56,57].

5.11. Directions for Future Research

Since hospitals do not always employ all non-medical staff professions, the effect of replacing one profession by another should be studied. Furthermore, the impact of VCs on compliance to guidelines/protocol should be investigated. Decisions made through virtual review were not completely similar to those made through face-to-face assessment, which could be caused by not assessing the patient face-to-face, or by the non-medical staff not providing accurate data. A deeper analysis is needed to improve our knowledge regarding these findings. An economic analysis of SC/VCs versus StC, the long-term effect of SC/VCs on the disease itself and possible synergetic effects when combining SC and VCs are other interesting topics for future studies. Furthermore, since all the VCs in this review are located in the UK, the conclusions drawn may not apply in other countries, especially outside the Anglo-Saxon world. Therefore, future studies conducted outside the UK/Anglo-Saxon world can be an added value.

6. Conclusions

This literature review examines different implementations of SC and VCs in a hospital-based setting and compares them with the conventional ophthalmologist-led outpatient service in terms of the QoC delivered, the acceptance and the productivity.

A high acceptance seems to be linked to the reduced waiting time in the clinic and the social skills of some non-medical staff members having contact with the patient. Furthermore, by dividing the workload among the ophthalmologists and the non-medical staff, more patients could enter the glaucoma care pathway and be seen on time. Due to their reduced workload, ophthalmologists could assess new and high-risk patients more rapidly and with access to more auxiliary tests. Progressive glaucoma could be detected earlier, the treatment could be adjusted faster and further damage could be prevented.

In summary, SC and VCs are two promising approaches to tackle the upcoming capacity problems of glaucoma care within a hospital-based setting, without compromising the acceptance and the QoC delivered.

Author Contributions: Conceptualization, J.B.-B. and I.S.; methodology, A.-S.S., J.V., J.B.-B. and I.S.; validation, J.B.-B. and I.S.; formal analysis, A.-S.S. and J.V.; investigation, A.-S.S., J.V. and J.B.-B.; resources, I.S.; data curation, A.-S.S. and J.V.; writing—original draft preparation, A.-S.S. and J.V.; writing—review and editing, J.B.-B. and I.S.; visualization, J.B.-B.; supervision, J.B.-B. and I.S.; project administration, J.B.-B.; funding acquisition, I.S. All authors have read and agreed to the published version of the manuscript.

Funding: This research received no external funding.

Institutional Review Board Statement: Not applicable.

Informed Consent Statement: Not applicable.

Conflicts of Interest: The authors declare no conflict of interest.

References

1. Conlon, R.; Saheb, H.; Ahmed, I.I. Glaucoma treatment trends: A review. *Can. J. Ophthalmol.* **2017**, *52*, 114–124. [CrossRef]
2. Hitchings, R. Shared care for glaucoma. *Br. J. Ophthalmol.* **1995**, *79*, 626. [CrossRef] [PubMed]
3. Klein, B.E.; Klein, R.; Sponsel, W.E.; Franke, T.; Cantor, L.B.; Martone, J.; Menage, M.J. Prevalence of glaucoma. The Beaver Dam Eye Study. *Ophthalmology* **1992**, *99*, 1499–1504. [CrossRef]
4. Constable, I.J.; Yogesan, K.; Eikelboom, R.; Barry, C.; Cuypers, M. Fred Hollows lecture: Digital screening for eye disease. *Clin. Exp. Ophthalmol.* **2000**, *28*, 129–132. [CrossRef] [PubMed]
5. Wollstein, G.; Garway-Heath, D.F.; Fontana, L.; Hitchings, R.A. Identifying early glaucomatous changes. Comparison between expert clinical assessment of optic disc photographs and confocal scanning ophthalmoscopy. *Ophthalmology* **2000**, *107*, 2272–2277. [CrossRef]
6. De Silva, S.R.; Riaz, Y.; Purbrick, R.M.; Salmon, J.F. There is a trend for the diagnosis of glaucoma to be made at an earlier stage in 2010 compared to 2008 in Oxford, United Kingdom. *Ophthalmic Physiol. Opt.* **2013**, *33*, 179–182. [CrossRef]
7. National Collaborating Centre for Acute Care; National Institute for Health and Clinical Excellence. *Guidance. Glaucoma: Diagnosis and Management of Chronic Open Angle Glaucoma and Ocular Hypertension*; National Collaborating Centre for Acute Care: London, UK, 2009.
8. Ratnarajan, G.; Newsom, W.; Vernon, S.A.; Fenerty, C.; Henson, D.; Spencer, F.; Wang, Y.; Harper, R.; McNaught, A.; Collins, L.; et al. The effectiveness of schemes that refine referrals between primary and secondary care-the UK experience with glaucoma referrals: The Health Innovation & Education Cluster (HIEC) Glaucoma Pathways Project. *BMJ Open* **2013**, *3*, e002715.
9. Ratnarajan, G.; Newsom, W.; French, K.; Kean, J.; Chang, L.; Parker, M.; Garway-Heath, D.F.; Bourne, R.R. The impact of glaucoma referral refinement criteria on referral to, and first-visit discharge rates from, the hospital eye service: The Health Innovation & Education Cluster (HIEC) Glaucoma Pathways project. *Ophthalmic Physiol. Opt.* **2013**, *33*, 183–189.
10. Chalk, D.; Smith, M. Guidelines on glaucoma and the demand for services. *Br. J. Health Care Manag.* **2013**, *19*, 476–481. [CrossRef]
11. Smith, R. Our Ophthalmology Service is 'Failing', Please Help! Available online: https://www.rcophth.ac.uk/2013/08/our-ophthalmology-service-is-failingplease-help/ (accessed on 30 July 2021).
12. Resnikoff, S.; Felch, W.; Gauthier, T.M.; Spivey, B. The number of ophthalmologists in practice and training worldwide: A growing gap despite more than 200,000 practitioners. *Br. J. Ophthalmol.* **2012**, *96*, 783–787. [CrossRef]
13. NPSA. *Rapid Response Report NPSA/2009/RRR004: Preventing Delay to Follow Up for Patients with Glaucoma*; National Patient Safety Agency: London, UK, 2009.
14. Tuck, M.W.; Crick, R.P. Efficiency of referral for suspected glaucoma. *BMJ* **1991**, *302*, 998–1000. [CrossRef]
15. OECD. *OECD Health Policy Studies Value for Money in Health Spending*; OECD Publishing: Paris, France, 2010.
16. Morley, A.M.; Murdoch, I. The future of glaucoma clinics. *Br. J. Ophthalmol.* **2006**, *90*, 640–645. [CrossRef] [PubMed]
17. Integrated care for asthma: A clinical, social, and economic evaluation. Grampian Asthma Study of Integrated Care (GRASSIC). *BMJ* **1994**, *308*, 559–564.
18. Serrano, V.; Rodriguez-Gutierrez, R.; Hargraves, I.; Gionfriddo, M.R.; Tamhane, S.; Montori, V.M. Shared decision-making in the care of individuals with diabetes. *Diabet. Med.* **2016**, *33*, 742–751. [CrossRef]

19. Congalton, A.T.; Oakley, A.M.; Rademaker, M.; Bramley, D.; Martin, R.C. Successful melanoma triage by a virtual lesion clinic (teledermatoscopy). *J. Eur. Acad. Dermatol. Venereol.* **2015**, *29*, 2423–2428. [CrossRef]
20. Harnett, P.; Jones, M.; Almond, M.; Ballasubramaniam, G.; Kunnath, V. A virtual clinic to improve long-term outcomes in chronic kidney disease. *Clin. Med.* **2018**, *18*, 356–363. [CrossRef]
21. Khouri, A.S.; Fechtner, R.D.; Shaarawy, T.M.; Sherwood, M.B.; Hitchings, R.A.; Crowston, J.G. *Primary Open-Angle Glaucoma*, 2nd ed.; Elsevier/Saunders: London, UK, 2015; Volume 29, pp. 333–345.
22. Quigley, H.A.; Broman, A.T. The number of people with glaucoma worldwide in 2010 and 2020. *Br. J. Ophthalmol.* **2006**, *90*, 262–267. [CrossRef]
23. Van Melkebeke, L.; Barbosa-Breda, J.; Huygens, M.; Stalmans, I. Optical coherence tomography angiography in glaucoma: A review. *Ophthalmic Res.* **2018**, *60*, 139–151. [CrossRef] [PubMed]
24. Pitha, I.F.; Kass, M.A. Ocular Hypertension. In *Glaucoma*; Elsevier/Saunders: Philadelphia, PA, USA, 2015; Volume 28, pp. 325–332. Available online: https://www.sciencedirect.com/science/article/pii/B9780702051937000285?via%3Dihub (accessed on 30 July 2021).
25. Sunaric-Mégevand, G.; Aclimandos, W.; Creuzot-Garcher, C.; Traverso, C.E.; Tuulonen, A.; Hitchings, R.; Mathysen, D.G. Can 'Fellow of the European Board of ophthalmology Subspecialty Diploma in Glaucoma', a subspecialty examination on glaucoma induce the qualification standard of glaucoma clinical practice in Europe? *J. Educ. Eval. Health Prof.* **2016**, *13*, 28. [CrossRef] [PubMed]
26. The Royal College of Ophthalmologists. So You Want to Be an Ophthalmologist? A Short Guide in Ophthalmology in the UK. Available online: https://www.rcophth.ac.uk/wp-content/uploads/2014/07/RCOphth-Ophthalmology-Career-Feb2017.pdf (accessed on 30 July 2021).
27. Landis, J.R.; Koch, G.G. The measurement of observer agreement for categorical data. *Biometrics* **1977**, *33*, 159–174. [CrossRef] [PubMed]
28. White, A.; Goldberg, I.; Australian and New Zealand Glaucoma Interest Group and the Royal Australian and New Zealand College of Ophthalmologists. Guidelines for the collaborative care of glaucoma patients and suspects by ophthalmologists and optometrists in Australia. *Clin. Exp. Ophthalmol.* **2014**, *42*, 107–117. [CrossRef] [PubMed]
29. Canadian Glaucoma Society Committee on Interprofessional Collaboration in Glaucoma Care. Model of interprofessional collaboration in the care of glaucoma patients and glaucoma suspects. *Can. J. Ophthalmol.* **2011**, *46*, S1–S10. [CrossRef] [PubMed]
30. NHMRC Guidelines for the screening, prognosis, diagnosis, management and prevention of glaucoma. Available online: https://www.nhmrc.gov.au/sites/default/files/2018-10/cp113_glaucoma_120404.pdf (accessed on 30 July 2021).
31. Canadian Ophthalmological Society Glaucoma Clinical Practice Guideline Expert Committee; Canadian Ophthalmological Society. Canadian Ophthalmological Society evidence-based clinical practice guidelines for the management of glaucoma in the adult eye. *Can. J. Ophthalmol.* **2009**, *44*, S7–S93. [CrossRef]
32. Damji, K.F.; Behki, R.; Wang, L.; Target IOP Workshop participants. Canadian perspectives in glaucoma management: Setting target intraocular pressure range. *Can. J. Ophthalmol.* **2003**, *38*, 189–197. [CrossRef]
33. Shah, S.M.; Choo, C.; Odden, J.; Zhao, B.; Fang, C.; Schornack, M.; Stalboerger, G.; Bennett, J.R.; Khanna, C.L. Provider agreement in the assessment of glaucoma progression within a team model. *J. Glaucoma* **2018**, *27*, 691–698. [CrossRef] [PubMed]
34. Damento, G.M.; Winkler, N.S.; Hodge, D.O.; Khanna, S.S.; Khanna, C.L. Healthcare utilization by glaucoma patients in a team care model. *Semin. Ophthalmol.* **2018**, *33*, 829–837. [CrossRef] [PubMed]
35. Winkler, N.S.; Damento, G.M.; Khanna, S.S.; Hodge, D.O.; Khanna, C.L. Analysis of a physician-led, team-based care model for the treatment of glaucoma. *J. Glaucoma* **2017**, *26*, 702–707. [CrossRef]
36. Holtzer-Goor, K.M.; Van Vliet, E.J.; Van Sprundel, E.; Plochg, T.; Koopmanschap, M.A.; Klazinga, N.S.; Lemij, H.G. Shared care in monitoring stable glaucoma patients: A randomized controlled trial. *J. Glaucoma* **2016**, *25*, e392–e400. [CrossRef]
37. Holtzer-Goor, K.M.; Klazinga, N.S.; Koopmanschap, M.A.; Lemij, H.G.; Plochg, T.; Van Sprundel, E. *Monitoring of Stable Glaucoma Patients: Evaluation of the Effectiveness and Efficiency of a Glaucoma Follow-up Unit, Staffed by Nonphysician Health Care Professionals, as an Intermediate Step Towards Glaucoma Monitoring in Primary Care*; Erasmus University Rotterdam: Rotterdam, The Netherlands, 2010.
38. Holtzer-Goor, K.M.; van Sprundel, E.; Lemij, H.G.; Plochg, T.; Klazinga, N.S.; Koopmanschap, M.A. Cost-effectiveness of monitoring glaucoma patients in shared care: An economic evaluation alongside a randomized controlled trial. *BMC Health Serv. Res.* **2010**, *10*, 312. [CrossRef]
39. Ho, S.; Vernon, S.A. Decision making in chronic glaucoma-optometrists vs ophthalmologists in a shared care service. *Ophthalmic Physiol. Opt.* **2011**, *31*, 168–173. [CrossRef]
40. Banes, M.J.; Culham, L.E.; Crowston, J.G.; Bunce, C.; Khaw, P.T. An optometrist's role of co-management in a hospital glaucoma clinic. *Ophthalmic Physiol. Opt.* **2000**, *20*, 351–359. [CrossRef]
41. Bentley, S.A.; Green, C.; Malesic, L.; Siggins, T.; Escott, C.; O'Keefe, M.; Clarke, C. Establishing a collaborative model of glaucoma care in an Australian public hospital setting. *Invest. Ophthalmol. Vis. Sci.* **2019**, *60*, 1020.
42. Banes, M.J.; Culham, L.E.; Bunce, C.; Xing, W.; Viswanathan, A.; Garway-Heath, D. Agreement between optometrists and ophthalmologists on clinical management decisions for patients with glaucoma. *Br. J. Ophthalmol.* **2006**, *90*, 579–585. [CrossRef]
43. Bhota, V.; Taylor, S.; Benefield, J.; Ah-Cha, J. Approach to collaborative glaucoma care in New Zealand: An update. *Clin. Exp. Ophthalmol.* **2019**, *47*, 798–799.

44. Phu, J.; Wang, H.; Khuu, S.; Zangerl, B.; Hennessy, M.; Masselos, K.; Kalloniatis, M. Anterior Chamber Angle Evaluation: Consistency and Agreement between Optometrists and Ophthalmologists. *Optom. Vis. Sci.* **2019**, *96*, 751–760. [CrossRef]
45. Prum, B.E., Jr.; Rosenberg, L.F.; Gedde, S.J.; Mansberger, S.L.; Stein, J.D.; Moroi, S.E.; Herndon, L.W.; Lim, M.C.; Williams, R.D. Primary open-angle glaucoma preferred practice pattern® guidelines. *Ophthalmology* **2016**, *123*, P41–P111. [CrossRef]
46. Court, J.H.; Austin, M.W. Virtual glaucoma clinics: Patient acceptance and quality of patient education compared to standard clinics. *Clin. Ophthalmol.* **2015**, *9*, 745–749. [CrossRef]
47. Choong, Y.F.; Devarajan, N.; Pickering, A.; Pickering, S.; Austin, M.W. Initial management of ocular hypertension and primary open-angle glaucoma: An evaluation of the royal college of ophthalmologists' guidelines. *Eye* **2003**, *17*, 685–690. [CrossRef] [PubMed]
48. Rathod, D.; Win, T.; Pickering, S.; Austin, M.W. Incorporation of a virtual assessment into a care pathway for initial glaucoma management: Feasibility study. *Clin. Exp. Ophthalmol.* **2008**, *36*, 543–546. [CrossRef] [PubMed]
49. Kotecha, A.; Brookes, J.; Foster, P.J. A technician-delivered 'virtual clinic' for triaging low-risk glaucoma referrals. *Eye* **2017**, *31*, 899–905. [CrossRef] [PubMed]
50. Gunn, P.J.G.; Marks, J.R.; Au, L.; Waterman, H.; Spry, P.G.D.; Harper, R.A. Acceptability and use of glaucoma virtual clinics in the UK: A national survey of clinical leads. *BMJ Open Ophthalmol.* **2018**, *3*, e000127. [CrossRef]
51. Wright, H.R.; Diamond, J.P. Service innovation in glaucoma management: Using a Web-based electronic patient record to facilitate virtual specialist supervision of a shared care glaucoma programme. *Br. J. Ophthalmol.* **2015**, *99*, 313–317. [CrossRef]
52. Tatham, J.; Ali, A.; Hillier, N. Knowledge of Glaucoma Among Patients Attending Virtual and Face-to Face Glaucoma Clinics. *J. Glaucoma* **2021**, *30*, 325–331. [CrossRef]
53. Mostafa, I.; Bianchi, E.; Brown, L.; Tatham, A. What is the best way to measure intraocular pressure in a virtual clinic? *Eye* **2020**, *35*, 448–454. [CrossRef] [PubMed]
54. Gunn, P.; Marks, R.; Au, L.; Read, S.; Waterman, H.; Spry, P.; Harper, R. Virtual Clinics for glaucoma care–Patients' and clinicians' experiences and perceptions: A qualitative evaluation. *Eye* **2021**, 1–10.
55. Spackman, W.; Waqar, S.; Booth, A. Patient satisfaction with the virtual glaucoma clinic. *Eye* **2021**, *35*, 1017–1018. [CrossRef] [PubMed]
56. Clarke, J.; Puertas, R.; Kotecha, A.; Foster, P.J.; Barton, K. Virtual clinics in glaucoma care: Face-to-face versus remote decision-making. *Br. J. Ophthalmol.* **2017**, *101*, 892–895. [CrossRef] [PubMed]
57. Kotecha, A.; Baldwin, A.; Brookes, J.; Foster, P.J. Experiences with developing and implementing a virtual clinic for glaucoma care in an NHS setting. *Clin. Ophthalmol.* **2015**, *9*, 1915–1923. [CrossRef] [PubMed]
58. Nikita, E.; Kortuem, K.; Fasolo, S.; Tsoukanas, D.; Sim, D. Expanded teleglaucoma clinics. An opportunity to manage the increasing demand for glaucoma care with safety and efficiency. *Invest. Ophthalmol. Vis. Sci.* **2019**, *60*, 5480.
59. Kotecha, A.; Bonstein, K.; Cable, R.; Cammack, J.; Clipston, J.; Foster, P. Qualitative investigation of patients' experience of a glaucoma virtual clinic in a specialist Ophthalmic Hospital in London, UK. *BMJ Open* **2015**, *5*, e009463. [CrossRef] [PubMed]
60. Nikita, E.; Gazzard, G.; Sim, D.; Fasolo, S.; Kortum, K.; Jayaram, H. Expansion of patient eligibility for virtual glaucoma clinics: A long-term strategy to increase the capacity of high-quality glaucoma care. *Br. J. Ophthalmol.* **2021**, 1–6. [CrossRef]
61. The Royal College of Ophthalmologists. Commissioning Guide. Glaucoma (Long Version). Available online: https://www.college-optometrists.org/uploads/assets/97a30d3e-f6ba-4504-875d6a91d73ba5e3/Commissioning-Guide-Glaucoma-Full-report.pdf (accessed on 30 July 2021).
62. National Institute for Health and Care Excellence. *National Institute for Health and Care Excellence: Clinical Guidelines. Glaucoma: Diagnosis and Management*; National Institute for Health and Care Excellence: London, UK, 2017.

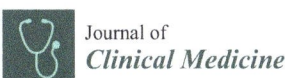

Article

Macular Pigment and Open-Angle Glaucoma in the Elderly: The Montrachet Population-Based Study

Louis Arnould [1,2,3,*], Alassane Seydou [3], Christine Binquet [2], Pierre-Henry Gabrielle [1,3], Chloé Chamard [4,5], Lionel Bretillon [3], Alain M. Bron [1,3], Niyazi Acar [3] and Catherine Creuzot-Garcher [1,3]

1. Department of Ophthalmology, Dijon University Hospital, 21000 Dijon, France; phgabrielle@gmail.com (P.-H.G.); alain.bron@chu-dijon.fr (A.M.B.); catherine.creuzot-garcher@chu-dijon.fr (C.C.-G.)
2. Clinical Epidemiology/Clinical Trials Unit, Clinical Investigation Center, INSERM, CIC 1432, Dijon University Hospital, 21000 Dijon, France; christine.binquet@u-bourgogne.fr
3. Centre des Sciences du Goût et de l'Alimentation, AgroSup Dijon, CNRS, INRAE, Université Bourgogne Franche-Comté, 21000 Dijon, France; alassanemaiga7@yahoo.fr (A.S.); lionel.bretillon@inrae.fr (L.B.); niyazi.acar@inrae.fr (N.A.)
4. Department of Ophthalmology, Gui de Chauliac Hospital, 34000 Montpellier, France; chloe.chamard@gmail.com
5. Neuropsychiatry—Epidemiological and Clinical Research, Inserm, PSNREC, Montpellier University, 34000 Montpellier, France
* Correspondence: louis.arnould@chu-dijon.fr; Tel.: +33-380293536

Abstract: (1) Background: To compare macular pigment optical density (MPOD) and its spatial distribution between eyes with primary open-angle glaucoma (POAG) and control eyes in an elderly population. (2) Methods: The Montrachet study (Maculopathy Optic Nerve and nutrition neurovAs-Cular and HEarT) is a population-based study including participants aged 75 years and over. All participants had a slit lamp examination, fundus photographs, and a questionnaire about their medical past history and smoking status. Optic disc spectral domain optical coherence tomography was also performed. All glaucoma-suspected patients were convocated to have a new full examination. We only retained one eye with POAG for analysis in the glaucoma group and one eye without optic neuropathy in the control participants group. MPOD measurements were performed with the two-wavelength autofluorescence method (488 and 514 nm). (3) Results: Overall, 601 eyes had MPOD measurements among 1153 participants. Among the 601 eyes, 48 had POAG. The mean age for the glaucoma and control participants was 84.01 ± 4.22 years and 81.94 ± 3.61 years, respectively ($p < 0.001$). In the multivariable analysis, we could not find any association between POAG and MPOD at 0.5° ($p = 0.336$). We found no significant difference regarding MP spatial distribution between the two groups ($p = 0.408$). (4) Conclusion: In this elderly population-based study, eyes with POAG and control eyes without optic neuropathy did not differ in terms of MPOD and MP spatial distribution.

Keywords: mcular pigment optical density; glaucoma; two-wavelength autofluorescence; elderly; population-based study

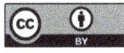

1. Introduction

Macular pigment (MP) plays an important role in visual function [1] and in the protection of the retina against oxidative damage [2,3]. It is located in the inner layers of the retina [4] and composed of three carotenoids. Two of them are exclusively from dietary origin (lutein and zeaxanthin) while the third one (meso-zeaxanthin) is synthetized from lutein. The highest MP concentration is located in the Henle's fiber layer of the fovea and rapidly decreases to be undetectable outside the macula. In the literature, three MP patterns have been reported: the no-ring profile, ring-like profile, and an intermediate profile [5–8].

MP and oral dietary carotenoid supplementation have been extensively studied in macular disorders, especially in age-related macular degeneration (AMD). Numerous studies suggested the role of carotenoid in the prevention of AMD [9,10].

Glaucoma is the most common optic neuropathy in adulthood, leading to irreversible damages of the structure and function of the optic nerve [11]. It is defined as a multifactorial progressive optic neuropathy with a typically acquired loss of optic nerve fibers (death of the retinal ganglion cell axons) [12,13]. Primary open-angle glaucoma (POAG) is the most common form of this disease [14]. In 2020, it was estimated that nearly 52 million people are affected by POAG worldwide and that this number would increase to 79 million by 2040 [15].

To date, the relationship between MPOD and POAG is conflicting and the association between neurodegenerative disease and MP is less straightforward. MP and glaucoma could be linked based on two major hypotheses: microvascular and oxidative stress processes [16]. According to several research teams, MP could absorb vision blue light, hence decreasing light energy in the inner retina and photo-oxidative injury [17]. Some studies found that lower densities of MP were found in glaucoma patients, [18] whereas other studies could not support this assumption [19]. The primary objective of this study was to compare MPOD between eyes with POAG and control eyes in an elderly population. The secondary objective was to compare the MP spatial distribution between both groups.

2. Materials and Methods

2.1. Population Study

The Montrachet study (Maculopathy Optic Nerve and nutrition neurovAsCular and HEarT) was an ancillary study of the population-based Three Cities (3C) study, which had been previously reported [20]. In the 3C cohort study, 9294 persons were randomly selected from the electoral rolls of three French urban cities (Bordeaux, Dijon, and Montpellier) and aged 65 years. Ten years later, the subgroup of participants from Dijon was invited to participate in the Montrachet study.

The methodology of the Montrachet study and baseline characteristics of volunteers have already been described [21]. From October 2009 to March 2013, 1153 volunteers underwent complete eye examination in the Department of Ophthalmology of the Dijon University Hospital, France. All participants were asked to complete a questionnaire about their lifestyle (alcohol consumption and smoking status) and environment (sun exposure). This examination included the collection of self-reported eye disease and treatment history, visual acuity measurement, intraocular pressure measurement (Tonoref II, Nidek, Gamagori, Japan), central corneal thickness measurement with an ultrasonic contact pachymeter (DGH 500, DGH Technology, Exton, PA, USA), visual field examination with a screening program (Frequency-Doubling Technology, Carl Zeiss Meditec, Dublin, CA, USA), and spectral-domain optical coherence tomography (SD-OCT; software version 5.4.7.0; Spectralis, Heidelberg Engineering Co., Heidelberg, Germany) for both the macula and the optic nerve head after pupil dilation. The high-speed resolution mode and the eye-tracking system were activated to acquire the images. For the optic disc, the retinal nerve fiber layer (RNFL) thickness acquisition was obtained with a circle diameter of 3.5 mm. Moreover, each participant benefited from two retinal photographs: one centered on the macula and one on the optic nerve (TRC NW6S, Topcon, Tokyo, Japan). In addition, fasting blood samples were drawn to measure plasma carotenoids and fatty acids. We also used a semiquantitative food frequency questionnaire to quantify the dietary intake of lutein and zeaxanthin among participants. The study was approved by the regional ethics committee and was registered as 2009-A00448-49. All participants gave their informed consent. This study adhered to the tenets of the Declaration of Helsinki and we followed the STROBE policy according to the EQUATOR guidelines [22].

2.2. Glaucoma Diagnosis

Glaucoma diagnosis in the Montrachet study has already been reported [23,24]. Briefly, optic disc photographs were reviewed by two trained ophthalmologists (LA and PHG) masked for clinical and RNFL thickness information. In case of discrepancy, a senior glaucoma specialist (AMB) made an adjudication. Suspected-glaucoma eyes benefited from a new examination with gonioscopy and a Humphrey Swedish Interactive Thresholding Algorithm 24-2 visual field (Carl Zeiss Meditec, Dublin, CA, USA). Glaucoma was defined by the glaucoma classification of the International Society of Geographical and Epidemiological Ophthalmology (ISGEO) [25]. In case of bilateral disease, the eye with the most severe presentation was kept for analysis. Only cases of primary open-angle glaucoma (POAG) were considered for the present analysis. Secondary glaucoma, angle-closure glaucoma, and non-glaucomatous optic neuropathy were excluded from the analysis.

2.3. MPOD Measurements

The MPOD was measured with the two-wavelength autofluorescence method using a modified Heidelberg Retina Angiograph (HRA; Heidelberg Engineering, Heidelberg, Germany). After pupil dilation with tropicamide 0.5% (Thea, Clermont-Ferrand, France), two acquisitions were performed at a 30 s interval and captured at 488 and 514 nm excitation wavelengths by a trained technician for both eyes (Figure S1). Glaucomatous status was masked to the operator. MPOD maps were generated by digital subtraction of the log autofluorescence images. We recorded MPOD at $0°$, $0.5°$, $1°$, $2°$, and $6°$ eccentricities using the software provided by the manufacturer of the device. MPOD was expressed in optical density units (DU). In the control participants group without optic neuropathy, the eye with the best image quality was retained for analysis. The right eye was chosen when image quality was similar in both eyes. We excluded participants with poor image quality in both eyes and those who suffered from late age-related macular degeneration (AMD). Classification of late AMD was based on both color fundus and OCT images [26]. From the graphs generated by the software of the modified HRA, we divided the different MP spatial distribution profiles into three groups (ring-like, no ring, and intermediate). A second investigator (PHG) analyzed fifty eyes of our population randomly chosen independently from the first investigator (LA).

2.4. Blood Sampling

Blood samples were collected from fasted volunteers for plasma lipids and fatty acids analysis [27]. Lipids extracted from plasma were stored under inert gas and then transmethylated with boron trifluoride in methanol [28]. Finally, fatty acid methyl esters were isolated with hexane and analyzed by gas chromatography using the Hewlett Packard Model 5890 (Palo Alto, CA, USA) with a CPSIL-88 column (100 m × 0.25 mm i.d., fim thickness 0.20 µm; Varian, Les Ulis, France) equipped with a flame ionization detector. The carrier gas used was hydrogen.

2.5. Statistical Analysis

Categorical variables were expressed as a number (n, percentage) and continuous variables as mean ± standard deviation (SD) or median (interquartile range (Q1–Q3)) according to their distribution. We performed our analysis with one eye per individual as the unit of analysis. We displayed two groups: control eyes and eye with POAG. Bivariate analysis was performed with Pearson's chi-square or Fisher exact tests for percentage comparisons as appropriate. Student test or analyses of variance, or the Kruskal–Wallis test was used for comparison of mean or median when appropriate. Cohen's kappa coefficient was used to measure the concordance between the two eyes for MPOD and for MP spatial distribution profiles between the two investigators. For multivariable analysis between MPOD at $0.5°$ and the presence of POAG as a dependent variable, all variables associated with glaucoma in the bivariate analysis with a p-value < 0.20 were included in the model. The smoking status variable was forced in the model. Then, a final model adjusted for age, sex, smoking status, lens status, plasma alpha-linoleic acid (ALA), and eicosapentaenoic acid (EPA) n-3 polyunsaturated fatty acids (PUFAs) was obtained by manual backward selection. For all analyses, the tests were two-tailed and the results were considered significant when p-values were less than 0.05. Analyses were performed using SAS software (version 9.4; SAS Institute, Inc., Cary, NC, USA).

3. Results

3.1. Demographics and Baseline Characteristics

A total of 702 participants had MPOD measurements among the 1153 from the Montrachet study (Figure 1).

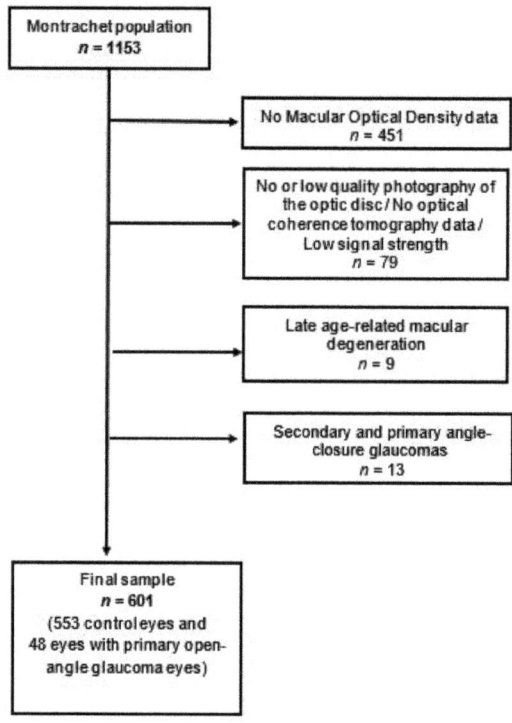

Figure 1. Eyes (553 eyes without optic neuropathy and 48 eyes with POAG). The baseline demographics and clinical characteristics of participants and non-participants are shown in Table 1.

Table 1. Baseline characteristics between participants and non-participants in the Montrachet study.

	Total (n = 1153)	Participants (n = 601)	Non-Participants (n = 552)	p-Value
Age, years	82.25 ± 3.75	82.11 ± 3.70	82.41 ± 3.76	0.165
Gender				
Men	430 (37.29)	232 (38.60)	190 (35.87)	0.339
Smoking status	390 (34.42)	208 (35.25)	182 (33.52)	0.539
Alcohol consumption	64 (6.29)	31 (5.87)	33 (6.75)	0.565
Body mass index, kg/m^2				
<25	598 (51.86)	315 (52.41)	283 (51.27)	0.698
≥25	555 (48.14)	286 (47.59)	269 (48.73)	
Central retinal thickness, μm	292.51 ± 49.56	293.60 ± 44.55	293.40 ± 54.59	0.942
Cup-to-disc ratio	0.34 ± 0.21	0.34 ± 0.22	0.33 ± 0.21	0.407

Table 1. Cont.

	Total (n = 1153)	Participants (n = 601)	Non-Participants (n = 552)	p-Value
Spherical equivalent, diopters	0.06 ± 2.11	0.13 ± 2.06	−0.03 ± 2.18	0.241
Lens status				
Phakic	583 (50.70)	274 (45.59)	309 (56.28)	<0.001
Pseudophakic	567 (49.30)	327 (54.41)	240 (43.72)	
Sun protection				
Never	115 (10.02)	60 (10.02)	55 (10.02)	
Occasionally	258 (22.47)	130 (21.70)	128 (23.32)	0.799
Often	775 (67.51)	409 (68.28)	366 (66.67)	
Iris color				
Blue/gray	465 (40.33)	244 (40.60)	221 (40.04)	
Green/hazel	360 (31.22)	202 (33.61)	158 (28.62)	0.067
Dark brown/black	328 (28.45)	155 (25.79)	173 (31.34)	
AMD stages				
No AMD	587 (54.96)	322 (54.95)	265 (54.98)	
Early AMD stage 1	337 (31.55)	198 (33.79)	139 (28.84)	
Early AMD stage 2	100 (9.36)	53 (9.04)	47 (9.75)	<0.0001
Early AMD stage 3	22 (2.06)	13 (2.22)	9 (1.87)	
Late AMD	22 (2.06)	0 (0.00)	22 (4.56)	
Plasma xanthophylls, μg/L				
L	271.41 (178.07–453.91)	277.87 (177.89–448.29)	266.59 (179.10–454.84)	0.863
Z	17.81 (11.28–26.00)	17.39 (11.49–26.32)	18.17 (10.65–25.63)	0.946
L/Z supplementation, yes	65 (5.64)	34 (5.56)	31 (5.72)	0.909
Plasma n-3 PUFAs				
ALA	0.63 ± 0.21	0.63 ± 0.21	0.63 ± 0.22	0.859
EPA	1.29 ± 0.62	1.32 ± 0.65	1.25 ± 0.58	0.084
DHA	2.22 ± 0.65	2.27 ± 0.67	2.16 ± 0.62	0.022
Plasma lipids, mmol/L				
Total cholesterol	5.83 ± 0.93	5.83 ± 0.93	5.77 ± 0.97	0.324
LDL cholesterol	3.60 ± 0.83	3.62 ± 0.83	3.58 ± 0.84	0.511
HDL cholesterol	1.66 ± 0.40	1.66 ± 0.40	1.67 ± 0.41	0.869
Triglycerides	1.17 ± 0.52	1.20 ± 0.54	1.14 ± 0.49	0.055

p-value was calculated between participants and non-participants. The results are displayed as n (%) for categorical variables and as mean ± standard deviation or as median (interquartile range (IQR)) depending on their distribution for continuous variables. AMD = age-related macular degeneration; L = lutein; Z = zeaxanthin; PUFA = polyunsaturated fatty acids; ALA = alpha-linoleic acid; EPA = eicosapentaenoic acid; DHA = docosahexaenoic acid; LDL = low-density lipoprotein; and HDL = high-density lipoprotein. Missing data for smoking status (current or past, n = 20), alcohol consumption (current or past n = 136), central retinal thickness (n = 8), cup-to-disc ratio (n = 105), spherical equivalent (n = 103), lens status (n = 3), sun protection (n = 5), AMD stages (n = 85), L/Z (n = 358), plasma n-3 PUFAs (n = 339), LDL cholesterol (n = 14), HDL cholesterol (n = 14), and triglycerides (n = 15).

Non-participants were more likely to be phakic and to present late AMD. Participants' mean age was 82.11 ± 3.70 years.

The characteristics of the study population are displayed in Table 2.

Table 2. Baseline characteristics of eyes without optic neuropathy and eyes with primary open-angle glaucoma in the Montrachet study, n = 601.

	Eyes without Optic Neuropathy (n = 553)	Eyes with POAG (n = 48)	p-Value
Age, years	81.94 ± 3.61	84.01 ± 4.22	<0.001
Gender			
Men	206 (37.25)	26 (54.17)	0.021
Smoking status	191 (35.11)	17 (36.96)	0.801
Alcohol consumption	29 (5.97)	2 (4.76)	0.749

Table 2. *Cont.*

	Eyes without Optic Neuropathy (n = 553)	Eyes with POAG (n = 48)	p-Value
BMI, kg/m^2			
<25	291 (52.62)	24 (50.00)	0.727
≥25	262 (47.38)	24 (50.00)	
Central retinal thickness, µm	292.90 ± 43.29	302.30 ± 56.92	0.158
Global RNFL thickness, µm	95.3±11.7	79.6±19.0	<0.001
Cup-to-disc ratio	0.31 ± 0.19	0.73 ± 0.10	<0.001
Intraocular pressure, mmHg	15.49 ± 3.32	15.46 ± 3.32	0.407
Mean deviation of visual field, dB	NA	−11.69 ± 8.12	NA
Spherical equivalent, diopters	0.20 ± 2.04	−0.76 ± 2.09	0.002
Best-corrected visual acuity, <20/60	12 (2.2)	2 (4.2)	0.428
Lens status			
Phakic	264 (47.74)	10 (20.83)	<0.001
Pseudophakic	289 (52.26)	38 (79.17)	
Sun protection			
Never	58 (10.51)	2 (4.26)	
Occasionally	118 (21.38)	12 (25.53)	0.357
Often	376 (68.11)	33 (70.21)	
Macular pigment distribution			
No ring	395 (71.43)	38 (80.85)	
Intermediate	59 (10.67)	4 (8.51)	0.408
Ring-like	99 (17.90)	5 (10.64)	
Iris color			
Blue/gray	224 (40.51)	20 (41.67)	
Green/hazel	191 (34.54)	11 (22.92)	0.158
Dark brown/black	138 (24.95)	17 (35.41)	
AMD stages			
No AMD	296 (54.82)	26 (56.53)	
Early AMD stage 1	184 (34.07)	14 (30.43)	0.625
Early AMD stage 2	47 (8.70)	6 (13.04)	
Early AMD stage 3	13 (2.41)	0 (0.00)	
Plasma xanthophylls, µg/L			
L	269.58 (176.846–443.43)	316.38 (180.00–435.20)	0.625
Z	17.44 (11.49–26.32)	15.78 (11.49–27.48)	0.905
L/Z supplementation, yes	31 (5.61)	0 (0.00)	NA
Plasma n-3 PUFAs			
ALA	0.63 ± 0.21	0.70 ± 0.26	0.057
EPA	1.34 ± 0.66	1.14 ± 0.35	0.068
DHA	2.27 ± 0.69	2.22 ± 0.45	0.628
Plasma lipids, mmol/L			
Total cholesterol	5.84 ± 0.94	5.69 ± 0.80	0.311
LDL cholesterol	3.62 ± 0.84	3.59 ± 0.77	0.836
HDL cholesterol	1.67 ± 0.39	1.58 ± 0.45	0.134
Triglycerides	1.21 ± 0.55	1.15 ± 0.40	0.468

p-value was calculated between participants and non-participants. The results are displayed as n (%) for categorical variables and as mean ± standard deviation or as median (interquartile range (IQR)) depending on their distribution for continuous variables. POAG = primary open-angle glaucoma; RNFL = retinal nerve fiber layer; AMD = age-related macular degeneration; L = lutein; Z = zeaxanthin; NA = not applicable; PUFA = polyunsaturated fatty acids; ALA = alpha-linoleic acid; EPA = eicosapentaenoic acid; DHA = docosahexaenoic acid; LDL = low-density lipoprotein; and HDL = high-density lipoprotein. Missing data for smoking status (n = 11), alcohol consumption (n = 73), sun protection (n = 2), central retinal thickness (n = 1), cup-to-disc ratio (n = 7), macular pigment distribution (n = 1), AMD stages (n = 15), plasma L/Z (n = 164), plasma n-3 PUFAs (n = 154), LDL cholesterol (n = 6), HDL cholesterol (n = 6), and triglycerides (n = 6).

The POAG patients were more likely to be men and they were significantly older. The eyes with POAG were more likely to be pseudophakic, to present with a larger cup-to-disc ratio and a thinner global RNFL thickness, and with a negative spherical equivalent.

3.2. MPOD and Primary Open-Angle Glaucoma

The concordance between the two eyes for MPOD among 50 randomly chosen subjects found an agreement with kappa 0.79 (confidence interval = 0.64–0.95). The MPOD means at the 0°, 0.5°, 1°, 2°, and 6° eccentricities for the two groups are presented in Table 3.

Table 3. Macular pigment optic density at several degree eccentricities from the fovea in control and primary open-angle glaucoma eyes in the Montrachet study.

	Total ($n = 601$)	Eyes without Optic Neuropathy ($n = 553$)	Eyes with POAG ($n = 48$)	p-Value
MPOD at 0°	0.73 ± 0.32	0.72 ± 0.32	0.77 ± 0.30	0.308
MPOD at 0.5°	0.56 ± 0.26	0.55 ± 0.26	0.61 ± 0.25	0.165
MPOD at 1°	0.48 ± 0.22	0.47 ± 0.22	0.51 ± 0.21	0.345
MPOD at 2°	0.30 ± 0.14	0.30 ± 0.14	0.32 ± 0.13	0.427
MPOD at 6°	0.07 ± 0.04	0.07 ± 0.04	0.08 ± 0.04	0.505

p-value was calculated between control and primary open-angle glaucoma eyes. The results are displayed as mean ± standard deviation. POAG = primary open-angle glaucoma and MPOD = macular pigment optical density. MPOD was measured in optical density units.

In this univariate analysis, there was no statistically significant difference at each eccentricity degree between the two groups. After adjustment for age, gender, smoking and lens status, and plasma PUFAs, we compared the MPOD at 0.5° eccentricity between eyes without optic neuropathy and eyes with POAG. We could not find a statistically significant difference (p = 0.336; Table 4).

Table 4. Multivariable analysis of association between MPOD at 0.5° and the presence of primary open-angle glaucoma in the Montrachet study.

	OR (95% CI)	p-Value
Age, years	1.10 (1.01–1.20)	0.041
Sex, male	2.73 (1.19–6.25)	0.017
Smoking status, yes	0.60 (0.25–1.43)	0.251
Lens status, pseudophakic	2.49 (1.01–6.16)	0.044
Plasma PUFAs		
ALA	7.16 (1.42–36.16)	0.017
EPA	0.47 (0.21–1.04)	0.063
MPOD at 0.5°	2.08 (0.47–9.23)	0.336

PUFA = polyunsaturated fatty acids; ALA = alpha-linoleic acid; EPA = eicosapentaenoic acid; MPOD = macular pigment optical density; OR = odds ratio; and CI = Confidence interval. In total, 162 observations were deleted due to missing values from smoking status, lens status, and plasma PUFAs. MPOD was measured in optical density units.

Similarly, we did not find a statistical difference for MPOD at 1°, 2°, and 6° eccentricity (data not shown). In the multivariable analysis, older age (p = 0.041), male sex (p = 0.017), pseudophakic status (p = 0.044), and the elevated plasma level of ALA (p = 0.017) were significantly associated with the presence of POAG. The agreement for MP spatial distribution profiles between the two investigators was 0.71 (confidence interval = 0.48–0.93). MP spatial distribution was classified into three patterns, namely ring-like (10.64%), intermediate (8.51%), and no ring-like (80.85%) in eyes with POAG as well as 17.90%, 10.67%, and 71.43% in the control eyes. There was no significant difference regarding the MP spatial distribution between eyes with POAG and eyes without optic neuropathy (p = 0.408; Table 2).

4. Discussion

Our study was designed to compare MPOD in an elderly population between POAG and control eyes using the two-wavelength autofluorescence method. Additionally, we aimed to investigate the MP spatial distribution between these two groups. We found no difference of MPOD and MP spatial distribution between eyes with POAG and eyes without optic neuropathy. These results are not in agreement with previous studies [16,29,30]. Igras E. et al. found a statistically significant difference for MPOD between glaucoma patients and controls with a MPOD median of 0.23 (−0.19; 0.65) and 0.36 (−0.08; 0.80) at 0.5° eccentricity, respectively [16]. Ji Y. et al. found MPOD significantly reduced in the glaucoma group compared to the control group, with 0.116 ± 0.033 UD and 0.137 ± 0.026 UD, respectively [30]. Recently, Siah WF. et al. [29] found that MPOD was lower in glaucomatous eyes with foveal ganglion cell complex involvement. We should note that these three case-control studies focused on smaller samples of selected patients ($n = 40$, $n = 30$, and $n = 88$, respectively). Nevertheless, our results could be difficult to compare to other studies as the MP measurement procedures were different. We measured MP with a two-wavelength autofluorescence method whereas Siah WF. et al. [29], Igras E. et al. [16], and Ji Y. et al. [30] used customized heterochromatic flicker photometry (cHFP) and a fundus reflectance method. On one hand, the reflectance method has some limitations because it uses only one wavelength, which is problematic in the case of lens opacification [31]. On the other hand, cHFP results should be interpreted with caution as it is influenced by the operator's execution and participants' cooperation [32]. Moreover, cHFP is a time-consuming technique (approximately 30 min), which is difficult to realize in elderly participants. The two-wavelength autofluorescence method for MPOD measurement is faster (2 to 3 min for each participant) and objective, and can be performed by trained technicians. Nevertheless, MP values obtained by means of the Heidelberg Spectralis (HRA) with the two-wavelength autofluorescence method were comparable to MP values obtained using the densitometer (cHFP) [33].

In contrast to the three previous research groups, our results are in line with Daga FB and Bruns Y et al. [19,34]. Daga FB et al. found that patients diagnosed with glaucoma (mean age of 72.5 years) had comparable MP levels to control subjects (mean age of 70.0 years) with the same two-wavelength autofluorescence method. Moreover, they also demonstrated no significant relationship between MP, standard automated perimetry, and retinal nerve fiber layer thickness measurements [19]. Bruns Y et al. presented that there was no evidence for lower MPOD in their 43 glaucomatous-patient (mean age of 70.0 years) case-control study [34]. These conflicting results could also be found in epidemiology studies. Jae H. Kang et al. presented in a large population-based study (Nurses' Health Study and Health Professionals Follow-up Study) that increased dietary levels of carotenoid were associated with a lower risk of POAG [35]. On the other hand, in the Rotterdam study, no protective effect was found between carotenoids and POAG [36].

A negative correlation has been demonstrated between BMI and MPOD but in our study, we did not show any significant difference between the controls and POAG participants regarding their BMI [37].

In our study, the eyes with POAG were more likely to be pseudophakic, which could have influenced the MPOD measurement as mentioned by Sasamoto et al. [38]. Nevertheless, the difference between the phakic and pseudophakic eyes found in the literature is mainly due to the absorption of blue light by the cataractous lens. Thus, we took into account the lens status in the multivariable analysis in order to limit misinterpretation of the MPOD measurement secondary to blurred media due to cataract.

Carotenoids supplementation is a confounding factor for MPOD because it has been reported that supplementation increased the concentration of carotenoids in plasmatic serum and MPOD [39,40]. Unfortunately, we were not able to evaluate this point as there was no lutein/zeaxanthin supplementation in the POAG group. We used a semiquantitative food frequency questionnaire to quantify the dietary intake in terms of carotenoid among participants in order to control for any disparity in MPOD caused by diet. In our study, there was no significant difference between the two groups in term of carotenoids intake (data not shown).

One school of thought suggests from preclinical studies of the glaucoma model that MP could operate as a neuroprotective agent. MP could regulate the production of pro-oxidant stressors in the early ischemic retinal injury and protect the inner retina from the neurodegenerative process [41,42]. Another school of thought strengthened by the results of the present study found no association between MP and glaucoma [19,34,36]. Hence, positive results could be explained by many confounders (healthy diet and lifetime exposure) and not independently by carotenoids and MP.

We found a significant difference between glaucomatous and control participants for age, gender, and lens status. These results are in agreement with previous studies which showed that POAG prevalence increased with age and men were more likely to present with POAG compared to women [43–45]. Regarding lens status and POAG prevalence, results in the literature are not clear as in some situations, cataract surgery is part of the treatment of POAG. Significative association between an elevated plasma level of ALA and POAG is conflicting. It was previously presented that there was no significant difference regarding isolated plasma FAs between participants with POAG and participants without optic neuropathy in elderly [46]. Considering the dispersion of the results for elevated plasma levels of ALA and POAG in this study, this association should be confirmed by further clinical studies.

We acknowledge several limitations of this study. First, we analyzed only 611 eyes of 1153 participants in the Montrachet study due to imaging quality and availability of MP evaluation. Thus, missing data could decrease the power of our analysis even though there was no difference between participants and non-participants. Second, these findings are based on a Caucasian European population and cannot be extrapolated to other parts of the world and other ethnicities. Third, this exploratory cross-sectional study only enhanced a potential absence of association between MPOD, MP spatial distribution, and glaucomatous optic neuropathy. This should be confirmed by a longitudinal study to validate our findings. Fourth, it is also important to acknowledge that our two groups are unequal ($n = 48$ versus $n = 553$) with a small sample size of glaucomatous patients, which could lead to statistical bias and lower statistical power. Fifth, we did not collect ganglion cell layer thickness measurements, which could have given us the opportunity to focus the analysis on glaucomatous eyes with foveal ganglion cell complex loss.

We thought that the strengths of a population-based study could help to clarify the debate on the relationship of MP and glaucoma. In contrast to control-case studies, participants were enrolled in the Montrachet study regardless of their glaucomatous status.

5. Conclusions

In conclusion, our study investigated the difference of MPOD and MP spatial distribution between POAG eyes and control eyes in the elderly in the frame of a population-based study. We found no significant difference between these two groups. The clinical relevance of the relationship between POAG and macular pigment warrants further studies.

Supplementary Materials: The following supporting information can be downloaded at: https://www.mdpi.com/article/10.3390/jcm11071830/s1, Figure S1: A digital subtraction image with intensity corresponding to MPOD (right) and their measurements plotted from center to periphery of fovea corresponding to the mean MPOD at each eccentricity (left).

Author Contributions: Conceptualization, C.C.-G. and A.M.B.; methodology, C.B.; software, A.S.; validation, N.A., C.C.-G. and A.M.B.; formal analysis, A.S.; investigation, L.A. and P.-H.G.; resources, C.C.-G.; data curation, A.S.; writing—original draft preparation, L.A., P.-H.G. and C.C.; writing—review and editing, L.A., P.-H.G., C.C. and L.B.; supervision, C.C.-G., A.M.B., C.B., L.B. and N.A.; project administration, C.B.; funding acquisition, C.C.-G. and N.A. All authors have read and agreed to the published version of the manuscript.

Funding: National Research Institute for Agriculture, Food and Environment (INRAE); Regional Council of Burgundy (PARI Grant); European Regional Development Fund (FEDER); Agence Nationale de la Recherche (ANR-11-LABX-0021-01).

Institutional Review Board Statement: The study was conducted in accordance with the Declaration of Helsinki and approved by the Institutional Review Board (or Ethics Committee) of the Three Cities Study Group (protocol code 2009-A00448).

Informed Consent Statement: Informed consent was obtained from all subjects involved in the study. Written informed consent has been obtained from the patient(s) to publish this paper.

Data Availability Statement: Data are available upon reasonable request. A Three Cities data request form has to be sent to louis.arnould@chu-dijon.fr.

Acknowledgments: We thank Sandrine Daniel for her data management support.

Conflicts of Interest: The authors declare no conflict of interest.

References

1. Loughman, J.; Akkali, M.C.; Beatty, S.; Scanlon, G.; Davison, P.A.; O'Dwyer, V.; Cantwell, T.; Major, P.; Stack, J.; Nolan, J.M. The relationship between macular pigment and visual performance. *Vis. Res.* **2010**, *50*, 1249–1256. [CrossRef] [PubMed]
2. Wu, J.; Seregard, S.; Algvere, P.V. Photochemical damage of the retina. *Surv. Ophthalmol.* **2006**, *51*, 461–481. [CrossRef]
3. Junghans, A.; Sies, H.; Stahl, W. Macular pigments lutein and zeaxanthin as blue light filters studied in liposomes. *Arch. Biochem. Biophys.* **2001**, *391*, 160–164. [CrossRef]
4. Trieschmann, M.; van Kuijk, F.J.G.M.; Alexander, R.; Hermans, P.; Luthert, P.; Bird, A.C.; Pauleikhoff, D. Macular pigment in the human retina: Histological evaluation of localization and distribution. *Eye Lond. Engl.* **2008**, *22*, 132–137. [CrossRef] [PubMed]
5. Alassane, S.; Binquet, C.; Arnould, L.; Fleck, O.; Acar, N.; Delcourt, C.; Bretillon, L.; Bron, A.M.; Creuzot-Garcher, C. Spatial Distribution of Macular Pigment in an Elderly French Population: The Montrachet Study. *Investig. Ophthalmol. Vis. Sci.* **2016**, *57*, 4469–4475. [CrossRef] [PubMed]
6. Meyer zu Westrup, V.; Dietzel, M.; Pauleikhoff, D.; Hense, H.-W. The association of retinal structure and macular pigment distribution. *Investig. Ophthalmol. Vis. Sci.* **2014**, *55*, 1169–1175. [CrossRef] [PubMed]
7. Delori, F.C.; Goger, D.G.; Keilhauer, C.; Salvetti, P.; Staurenghi, G. Bimodal spatial distribution of macular pigment: Evidence of a gender relationship. *J. Opt. Soc. Am. A Opt. Image Sci. Vis.* **2006**, *23*, 521–538. [CrossRef] [PubMed]
8. Berendschot, T.T.J.M.; van Norren, D. Macular pigment shows ringlike structures. *Investig. Ophthalmol. Vis. Sci.* **2006**, *47*, 709–714. [CrossRef]
9. Delcourt, C.; Carrière, I.; Delage, M.; Barberger-Gateau, P.; Schalch, W.; The POLA Study Group. Plasma Lutein and Zeaxanthin and Other Carotenoids as Modifiable Risk Factors for Age-Related Maculopathy and Cataract: The POLA Study. *Investig. Ophthalmol. Vis. Sci.* **2006**, *47*, 2329–2335. [CrossRef]
10. Meyers, K.J.; Mares, J.A.; Igo, R.P., Jr.; Truitt, B.; Liu, Z.; Millen, A.E.; Klein, M.; Johnson, E.J.; Engelman, C.D.; Karki, C.K.; et al. Genetic Evidence for Role of Carotenoids in Age-Related Macular Degeneration in the Carotenoids in Age-Related Eye Disease Study (CAREDS). *Investig. Ophthalmol. Vis. Sci.* **2014**, *55*, 587–599. [CrossRef]
11. Jonas, J.B.; Aung, T.; Bourne, R.R.; Bron, A.M.; Ritch, R.; Panda-Jonas, S. Glaucoma. *Lancet Lond. Engl.* **2017**, *390*, 2183–2193. [CrossRef]
12. Nork, T.M.; Ver Hoeve, J.N.; Poulsen, G.L.; Nickells, R.W.; Davis, M.D.; Weber, A.J.; Sarks, S.H.; Lemley, H.L.; Millecchia, L.L. Swelling and loss of photoreceptors in chronic human and experimental glaucomas. *Arch. Ophthalmol.* **2000**, *118*, 235–245. [CrossRef] [PubMed]
13. Kanis, M.J.; Lemij, H.G.; Berendschot, T.T.J.M.; van de Kraats, J.; van Norren, D. Foveal cone photoreceptor involvement in primary open-angle glaucoma. *Graefes Arch. Clin. Exp. Ophthalmol.* **2010**, *248*, 999–1006. [CrossRef] [PubMed]
14. Kapetanakis, V.V.; Chan, M.P.Y.; Foster, P.J.; Cook, D.G.; Owen, C.G.; Rudnicka, A.R. Global variations and time trends in the prevalence of primary open angle glaucoma (POAG): A systematic review and meta-analysis. *Br. J. Ophthalmol.* **2016**, *100*, 86–93. [CrossRef]
15. Tham, Y.-C.; Li, X.; Wong, T.Y.; Quigley, H.A.; Aung, T.; Cheng, C.-Y. Global prevalence of glaucoma and projections of glaucoma burden through 2040: A systematic review and meta-analysis. *Ophthalmology* **2014**, *121*, 2081–2090. [CrossRef] [PubMed]
16. Igras, E.; Loughman, J.; Ratzlaff, M.; O'Caoimh, R.; O'Brien, C. Evidence of lower macular pigment optical density in chronic open angle glaucoma. *Br. J. Ophthalmol.* **2013**, *97*, 994–998. [CrossRef] [PubMed]
17. Kijlstra, A.; Tian, Y.; Kelly, E.R.; Berendschot, T.T.J.M. Lutein: More than just a filter for blue light. *Prog. Retin. Eye Res.* **2012**, *31*, 303–315. [CrossRef] [PubMed]
18. Siah, W.F.; O'Brien, C.; Loughman, J.J. Macular pigment is associated with glare-affected visual function and central visual field loss in glaucoma. *Br. J. Ophthalmol.* **2018**, *102*, 929–935. [CrossRef]

19. Daga, F.B.; Ogata, N.G.; Medeiros, F.A.; Moran, R.; Morris, J.; Zangwill, L.M.; Weinreb, R.N.; Nolan, J.M. Macular Pigment and Visual Function in Patients With Glaucoma: The San Diego Macular Pigment Study. *Investig. Ophthalmol. Vis. Sci.* **2018**, *59*, 4471–4476. [CrossRef]
20. 3C Study Group. Vascular factors and risk of dementia: Design of the Three-City Study and baseline characteristics of the study population. *Neuroepidemiology* **2003**, *22*, 316–325. [CrossRef]
21. Creuzot-Garcher, C.; Binquet, C.; Daniel, S.; Bretillon, L.; Acar, N.; de Lazzer, A.; Arnould, L.; Tzourio, C.; Bron, A.M.; Delcourt, C. The Montrachet Study: Study design, methodology and analysis of visual acuity and refractive errors in an elderly population. *Acta Ophthalmol.* **2016**, *94*, e90–e97. [CrossRef] [PubMed]
22. Von Elm, E.; Altman, D.G.; Egger, M.; Pocock, S.J.; Gøtzsche, P.C.; Vandenbroucke, J.P. STROBE Initiative The Strengthening the Reporting of Observational Studies in Epidemiology (STROBE) statement: Guidelines for reporting observational studies. *J. Clin. Epidemiol.* **2008**, *61*, 344–349. [CrossRef]
23. Maupin, E.; Baudin, F.; Arnould, L.; Seydou, A.; Binquet, C.; Bron, A.M.; Creuzot-Garcher, C.P. Accuracy of the ISNT rule and its variants for differentiating glaucomatous from normal eyes in a population-based study. *Br. J. Ophthalmol.* **2020**, *104*, 1412–1417. [CrossRef] [PubMed]
24. Arnould, L.; Lazzer, A.D.; Seydou, A.; Binquet, C.; Bron, A.M.; Creuzot-Garcher, C. Diagnostic ability of spectral-domain optical coherence tomography peripapillary retinal nerve fiber layer thickness to discriminate glaucoma patients from controls in an elderly population (The MONTRACHET study). *Acta Ophthalmol.* **2020**, *98*, e1009–e1016. [CrossRef] [PubMed]
25. Foster, P.J.; Buhrmann, R.; Quigley, H.A.; Johnson, G.J. The definition and classification of glaucoma in prevalence surveys. *Br. J. Ophthalmol.* **2002**, *86*, 238–242. [CrossRef] [PubMed]
26. Gabrielle, P.-H.; Seydou, A.; Arnould, L.; Acar, N.; Devilliers, H.; Baudin, F.; Ghezala, I.B.; Binquet, C.; Bron, A.M.; Creuzot-Garcher, C. Subretinal Drusenoid Deposits in the Elderly in a Population-Based Study (the Montrachet Study). *Investig. Ophthalmol. Vis. Sci.* **2019**, *60*, 4838–4848. [CrossRef] [PubMed]
27. Moilanen, T.; Nikkari, T. The effect of storage on the fatty acid composition of human serum. *Clin. Chim. Acta Int. J. Clin. Chem.* **1981**, *114*, 111–116. [CrossRef]
28. Morrison, W.R.; Smith, L.M. Preparation of fatty acid methyl esters and dimethylacetals from lipids with boron fluoride–methanol. *J. Lipid Res.* **1964**, *5*, 600–608. [CrossRef]
29. Siah, W.F.; Loughman, J.; O'Brien, C. Lower Macular Pigment Optical Density in Foveal-Involved Glaucoma. *Ophthalmology* **2015**, *122*, 2029–2037. [CrossRef]
30. Ji, Y.; Zuo, C.; Lin, M.; Zhang, X.; Li, M.; Mi, L.; Liu, B.; Wen, F. Macular Pigment Optical Density in Chinese Primary Open Angle Glaucoma Using the One-Wavelength Reflectometry Method. *J. Ophthalmol.* **2016**, *2016*, 2792103. [CrossRef]
31. Berendschot, T.T.J.M.; van Norren, D. Objective determination of the macular pigment optical density using fundus reflectance spectroscopy. *Arch. Biochem. Biophys.* **2004**, *430*, 149–155. [CrossRef] [PubMed]
32. Stringham, J.M.; Hammond, B.R.; Nolan, J.M.; Wooten, B.R.; Mammen, A.; Smollon, W.; Snodderly, D.M. The utility of using customized heterochromatic flicker photometry (cHFP) to measure macular pigment in patients with age-related macular degeneration. *Exp. Eye Res.* **2008**, *87*, 445–453. [CrossRef] [PubMed]
33. Dennison, J.L.; Stack, J.; Beatty, S.; Nolan, J.M. Concordance of macular pigment measurements obtained using customized heterochromatic flicker photometry, dual-wavelength autofluorescence, and single-wavelength reflectance. *Exp. Eye Res.* **2013**, *116*, 190–198. [CrossRef] [PubMed]
34. Bruns, Y.; Junker, B.; Boehringer, D.; Framme, C.; Pielen, A. Comparison of Macular Pigment Optical Density in Glaucoma Patients and Healthy Subjects—A Prospective Diagnostic Study. *Clin. Ophthalmol.* **2020**, *14*, 1011–1017. [CrossRef]
35. Kang, J.H.; Willett, W.C.; Rosner, B.A.; Buys, E.; Wiggs, J.L.; Pasquale, L.R. Association of Dietary Nitrate Intake with Primary Open-Angle Glaucoma: A Prospective Analysis from the Nurses' Health Study and Health Professionals Follow-up Study. *JAMA Ophthalmol.* **2016**, *134*, 294–303. [CrossRef]
36. Ramdas, W.D.; Wolfs, R.C.W.; Kiefte-de Jong, J.C.; Hofman, A.; de Jong, P.T.V.M.; Vingerling, J.R.; Jansonius, N.M. Nutrient intake and risk of open-angle glaucoma: The Rotterdam Study. *Eur. J. Epidemiol.* **2012**, *27*, 385–393. [CrossRef]
37. Nolan, J.; O'Donovan, O.; Kavanagh, H.; Stack, J.; Harrison, M.; Muldoon, A.; Mellerio, J.; Beatty, S. Macular pigment and percentage of body fat. *Investig. Ophthalmol. Vis. Sci.* **2004**, *45*, 3940–3950. [CrossRef]
38. Sasamoto, Y.; Gomi, F.; Sawa, M.; Sakaguchi, H.; Tsujikawa, M.; Nishida, K. Effect of cataract in evaluation of macular pigment optical density by autofluorescence spectrometry. *Investig. Ophthalmol. Vis. Sci.* **2011**, *52*, 927–932. [CrossRef] [PubMed]
39. Alassane, S.; Binquet, C.; Cottet, V.; Fleck, O.; Acar, N.; Daniel, S.; Delcourt, C.; Bretillon, L.; Bron, A.M.; Creuzot-Garcher, C. Relationships of Macular Pigment Optical Density with Plasma Lutein, Zeaxanthin, and Diet in an Elderly Population: The Montrachet Study. *Investig. Ophthalmol. Vis. Sci.* **2016**, *57*, 1160–1167. [CrossRef]
40. Connolly, E.E.; Beatty, S.; Thurnham, D.I.; Loughman, J.; Howard, A.N.; Stack, J.; Nolan, J.M. Augmentation of macular pigment following supplementation with all three macular carotenoids: An exploratory study. *Curr. Eye Res.* **2010**, *35*, 335–351. [CrossRef]
41. Dilsiz, N.; Sahaboglu, A.; Yildiz, M.Z.; Reichenbach, A. Protective effects of various antioxidants during ischemia-reperfusion in the rat retina. *Graefes Arch. Clin. Exp. Ophthalmol.* **2006**, *244*, 627–633. [CrossRef] [PubMed]
42. Li, S.-Y.; Fu, Z.-J.; Ma, H.; Jang, W.-C.; So, K.-F.; Wong, D.; Lo, A.C.Y. Effect of lutein on retinal neurons and oxidative stress in a model of acute retinal ischemia/reperfusion. *Investig. Ophthalmol. Vis. Sci.* **2009**, *50*, 836–843. [CrossRef] [PubMed]

43. Rudnicka, A.R.; Mt-Isa, S.; Owen, C.G.; Cook, D.G.; Ashby, D. Variations in primary open-angle glaucoma prevalence by age, gender, and race: A Bayesian meta-analysis. *Investig. Ophthalmol. Vis. Sci.* **2006**, *47*, 4254–4261. [CrossRef] [PubMed]
44. Grzybowski, A.; Och, M.; Kanclerz, P.; Leffler, C.; De Moraes, C.G. Primary Open Angle Glaucoma and Vascular Risk Factors: A Review of Population Based Studies from 1990 to 2019. *J. Clin. Med.* **2020**, *9*, 761. [CrossRef]
45. Gordon, M.O.; Beiser, J.A.; Brandt, J.D.; Heuer, D.K.; Higginbotham, E.J.; Johnson, C.A.; Keltner, J.L.; Miller, J.P.; Parrish, R.K.; Wilson, M.R.; et al. The Ocular Hypertension Treatment Study: Baseline factors that predict the onset of primary open-angle glaucoma. *Arch. Ophthalmol.* **2002**, *120*, 714–720; discussion 829–830. [CrossRef] [PubMed]
46. Chemaly, A.; Arnould, L.; Seydou, A.; Gabrielle, P.-H.; Baudin, F.; Acar, N.; Creuzot-Garcher, C. Plasma fatty acids and primary open-angle glaucoma in the elderly: The Montrachet population-based study. *BMC Ophthalmol.* **2021**, *21*, 146. [CrossRef] [PubMed]

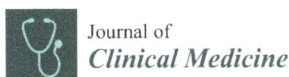

Review

Psychopharmacological Treatment, Intraocular Pressure and the Risk of Glaucoma: A Review of Literature

Adela Magdalena Ciobanu [1,2,*], Vlad Dionisie [2,3,*], Cristina Neagu [2], Otilia Maria Bolog [4], Sorin Riga [5,6] and Ovidiu Popa-Velea [7]

[1] Neuroscience Department, Discipline of Psychiatry, Faculty of Medicine, 'Carol Davila' University of Medicine and Pharmacy, 020021 Bucharest, Romania
[2] Department of Psychiatry, 'Prof. Dr. Alexandru Obregia' Clinical Hospital of Psychiatry, 041914 Bucharest, Romania; romcrys@yahoo.com
[3] Department of Psychiatry and Psychology, 'Carol Davila' University of Medicine and Pharmacy, 020021 Bucharest, Romania
[4] Service d'Ophtalmologie, Centre Hospitalier 'Rene Dubos', 95300 Pontoise, France; bologotilia@gmail.com
[5] Department of Stress Research and Prophylaxis, 'Prof. Dr. Alexandru Obregia' Clinical Hospital of Psychiatry, 041914 Bucharest, Romania; D_S_Riga@yahoo.com
[6] Romanian Academy of Medical Sciences, 927180 Bucharest, Romania
[7] Department of Medical Psychology, Faculty of Medicine, 'Carol Davila' University of Medicine and Pharmacy, 020021 Bucharest, Romania; ovidiu.popa-velea@umfcd.ro
* Correspondence: adela.ciobanu@yahoo.com (A.M.C.); vlad.dionisie@gmail.com (V.D.)

Abstract: Through the years, the available psychopharmacological treatments have expanded with numerous new drugs. Besides weight gain, gastro-intestinal problems or Parkinson-like symptoms, ocular adverse effects of psychiatric drugs have been reported. These adverse effects are not common, but can be dangerous for the patient. This review summarises the current knowledge on the risk of raised intraocular pressure and glaucoma entailed by psychopharmacological treatment. Also, it provides updated data for clinicians involved in the treatment of patients with glaucoma or glaucoma risk factors. For this purpose, we performed an extensive literature search in the PubMed database using specific terms. Selective serotonin and noradrenaline reuptake inhibitors are the best evidenced as having no association with glaucoma. Antipsychotics, and especially first generation, seem to have no correlation with an increased intraocular pressure and therefore possibly with a risk of glaucoma, although a special attention should be paid when using ziprasidone. Tricyclic antidepressants, benzodiazepines and topiramate should be avoided in patients diagnosed with glaucoma or at risk. Clinicians should be aware of the possible psychotropic drug induced glaucoma and monitor at risk patients closely in order to prevent this condition. Irrespective of the psychopharmacological regimen taken into consideration, the glaucoma patient should be under the strict supervision of the ophthalmologist.

Keywords: glaucoma; intraocular pressure; antidepressant; antipsychotic; benzodiazepine; topiramate; SSRI; SNRI

1. Introduction

Glaucoma represents a heterogeneous group of chronically progressive neurodegenerative bilateral diseases of the optic nerve, clinically characterized by optical neuropathy, resulting in retinal ganglion cell death, optic nerve head cupping, and associated specific loss of the visual field [1–3]. The aetiology of the disease is considered to be multifactorial [4], while the clinical picture can differ, with a substantial risk of associated blindness, especially in adults over the age of 60 [5].

Studies have shown that in Europe glaucoma occurs in 2.93% of people aged 40 to 80, reaching 10% at the age of over 90 [6]. Several types of glaucoma are described, which form a group of eye diseases and are the main cause of permanent blindness worldwide. [7,8].

Based on the mechanism by which aqueous outflow is impaired with respect to the anterior chamber configuration, the disease is typically divided into 2 basic subtypes: open angle and angle closure [9,10]. Clinical presentation of open-angle glaucoma (OAG) includes mainly chronic, slow and irreversible loss of peripheral vision, ultimately leading to blindness. Because of the gradual and insidious development, more than 50% of patients are unaware of their condition (known as 'the sneak thief of sight'), especially due to the pattern of visual field loss that spares the central vision until advanced stages [9]; therefore, periodic ophthalmologic evaluation is important [11,12]. On the other hand, acute angle-closure glaucoma (AACG) represents a dramatic urgent event that is caused by the sudden increase in the intraocular pressure (IOP) due to occlusion of the trabecular meshwork by the peripheral iris (in predisposed eyes with a narrow iridocorneal angle), obstructing aqueous outflow, that can lead to a potential risk of rapid blinding. ACG patients usually present more acute symptoms such as hyperaemia, teary, and painful eyes, sudden blurring of vision, or halos around lights secondary to corneal oedema from a sudden rise in IOP. Increased IOP is responsible for additional symptoms such as headache, nausea, and vomiting [9]. It must also be kept in mind that a narrow angle can be asymptomatic in the absence of a predisposing factor for angle-closure (e.g., pupillary dilatation) or that there are cited cases of insidious angle-closure glaucoma, which tends to be more visually destructive subtypes [9].

Above all, we have to make a firm distinction between acute angle-closure and angle-closure glaucoma. The major difference between the two entities is the absence and presence of optic nerve damage and visual field defects, respectively, especially when a specific treatment is rapidly received by the patient. The notion of glaucoma is under discussion when an optic neuropathy with elements specific to glaucoma damage occurs.

The scientific literature identifies several local and systemic risk factors associated with the development and progression of glaucoma [13]. In the case of OAG the local risk factors are represented by IOP (the key modifiable factor), family history of primary OAG, intraocular anti-VEGF (vascular endothelial growth factor) therapy, decreased thickness of the central region of the cornea, pre-existing myopia (low–moderate and high), low intraocular vascular pressure, optic nerve pathology, visual field changes, disc haemorrhage, and pseudo-exfoliation. Systemic risk factors include cardiovascular diseases, diabetes mellitus, dyslipidaemia, cerebral stroke, steroid treatment, arterial hypertension, with old age and male gender acting as additional risks [8,10,14]. Concerning the rapid progression of glaucoma, the most important favouring factors are considered to be high IOP and cardiovascular diseases [15].

On the other hand, the risk factors for developing ACG mentioned in the literature are the following: age (62 years being the average age at presentation), gender (more commonly female), race (Asian descent), family history, hyperopic eyes, short eyes. Those at risk for ACG with packed angle configuration can develop an attack exacerbated by mydriasis either spontaneously (primary) or pharmacologically (secondary) [9,10].

Medication represents a distinct risk for glaucoma. Corticosteroids are the most common cause of open-angle glaucoma (OAG), but several non-steroidal anti-inflammatory agents can also lead to OAG [16]. Regarding ACG, the list of potentially risky drugs includes antidepressants, such as selective serotonin reuptake inhibitors (SSRIs), tricyclic antidepressants and monoamine oxidase inhibitors, antipsychotic drugs, antihistaminic medication, antiparkinsonian agents, anticonvulsants (e.g., topiramate), mydriatic agents, sympathomimetic drops, antispasmodic drugs, and botulinum toxin.

Among the two types of glaucoma, ACG represents a pathology of interest concerning psychiatric treatment. Medications with anticholinergic effects could induce a precipitation of iridocorneal angle closure in patients with predisposition via mydriasis which is the primary pathogenic mechanism in the appearance of glaucoma in psychiatric patients [17,18] This rapid onset of the angle obstruction produces an imbalance between the production and drainage of aqueous humour in the anterior chamber, thus an accumulation of liquid and the increase of IOP. Other presumed involved mechanisms in the development of glaucoma are the anterior dislocation of the iris and lens or the inflammation of the ciliary body [7].

The challenges presented by glaucoma in psychiatry are bidirectional: on the one hand, patients with risk factor for angle-closure may develop clinical symptoms (eye pain, visual changes, headache) as a direct side effect of the psychiatric treatment. In case of patients with non-diagnosed OAG the raise in IOP can lead to severe aggravation of the disease, which can pass unnoticed until advanced stages [19]. On the other hand, glaucoma patients may exhibit a wide array of psychiatric symptoms, as a consequence of progression of vision loss, such as depression [20], anxiety [21] and insomnia [22].

Therefore, a minimal and specific screening before initiating a psychiatric treatment should be kept in mind, at least for the patients who have risk factors to develop OAG (IOP measure, fundus examination, +/− optic coherence tomography—OCT of the optic nerve head) or ACG (IOP measure, gonioscopy, +/− OCT of the optic nerve head) depending on the mechanism of action of the class of drugs used. Nevertheless, a good multidisciplinary collaboration between the psychiatrist and the ophthalmologist is strongly recommended, especially in complex cases.

Given the importance of glaucoma in influencing the choice of psychiatric drugs, we propose to review the main psychiatric therapeutic agents and their potential effects on glaucoma occurrence. Secondly, our aim is to provide a useful review of current data for clinicians facing dilemmas regarding the pharmacology treatment of psychiatric disorders in patients with glaucoma or glaucoma risk factors.

2. Methodology

We conducted an extensive literature search in the PubMed database from 1977 until 2021. The search was performed during March-May 2021 using the following terms: 'psychotropic medication', 'SSRI', 'citalopram', 'escitalopram', 'paroxetine', 'fluvoxamine', 'fluoxetine', 'sertraline', 'SNRI', 'duloxetine', 'venlafaxine', 'tricyclic antidepressants', 'clomipramine', 'amitriptyline', 'imipramine', 'doxepin', 'desipramine', 'nortriptyline' 'NDRI', 'bupropion', 'benzodiazepine', 'alprazolam', 'diazepam' 'antipsychotics', 'haloperidol', 'ziprasidone', 'risperidone', 'olanzapine', 'quetiapine', 'clozapine', 'topiramate' cross-referenced with 'glaucoma' and 'intraocular pressure'. We selected only articles written in English and based on clinical reports. After review of title, keywords and abstract, we retrieved 128 articles. Following removal of duplicates, full text assessment and then screening of the remaining articles for relevant studies that could be included in our paper, we finally included 90 articles divided as it follows: SSRI-7, citalopram-2, escitalopram-2, paroxetine-5, fluvoxamine-1, sertraline-1, SNRI-2, duloxetine-2, venlafaxine-5, tricyclic antidepressants-1, clomipramine-1, amitriptyline-1, imipramine-1, bupropion-4, benzodiazepine-2, diazepam-1, antipsychotics-8, haloperidol-3, risperidone-1, topiramate-40.

3. Antidepressants

3.1. Selective Serotonin Reuptake Inhibitors (SSRIs) and Serotonin and Noradrenaline Reuptake Inhibitors (SNRIs)

SSRIs and SNRIs are currently the first line drugs for the treatment of depression according to international guidelines [23,24]. SSRIs and SNRIs are the most prescribed drugs for depression and have the best overall tolerability and safety among all antidepressants. Also, these drugs are indicated as first choice for the treatment of anxiety, post-traumatic and obsessive compulsive disorders [25–27].

Since the discovery in 1974 of the first member of SSRI class, namely fluoxetine, continuing with sertraline, paroxetine, fluvoxamine, citalopram and escitalopram, these drugs have revolutionised the pharmacological therapy of depression. SSRIs mechanism of action implies a selective blockage of the reuptake of serotonin in the synaptic gap, therefore increasing the availability of the neurotransmitter and normalising the function of synapses. Until now seven families of serotonin receptors (5HT1-5HT7) have been described as having a diffuse localisation, including eye structures. Experimental studies have determined that 5HT1A, 5HT2A/2C and 5HT7 are located in the iris-ciliary body complex. Stimulation of 5HT1A receptor reduces the IOP through the reduction of aqueous humour, while 5HT2A/2C receptors increase IOP by stimulation of the ciliary body blood flow, therefore they enhance the production of aqueous humour. 5HT7 receptors are responsible for mydriasis through the relaxation of the sphincter muscle and for rising IOP by increasing the production of aqueous humour [28,29]. In addition, mydriatic effects might appear due to their weak anticholinergic and noradrenergic actions [30]. These contrary possible effects of stimulating serotonin receptors have determined researchers to study the possible real relationship between glaucoma and SSRIs and SNRIs in order to shed some light on the field (Table 1, Figure 1).

The SNRI class has similar indications in psychiatry to SSRI, although they have been later on introduced, in the twentieth century. The SNRI class comprises venlafaxine (the first drug discovered from this class) and duloxetine. Their main mechanism is the inhibition of serotonin and norepinephrine reuptake, with weak dopamine transporter blockage. Noradrenaline is suggested to cause mydriasis and lid retraction through stimulation of α1 receptors; α2 inhibitory receptors from the ciliary epithelium can cause an increase in outflow facility of the aqueous humour while the blockage of these receptors by SNRI could reverse these effects leading to increased IOP [31]. The noradrenergic effect of SNRI is more dominant than the one of SSRI, suggesting a possible high risk of ACG. However, current data suggest that the systemic usage of SNRI could lead in long-term treatment to a decrease in the IOP. Another possible cause of mydriasis due to SNRI treatment would be the stimulation of serotoninergic receptors, mainly 5HT7, which in turn could lead to relaxation of the sphincter muscle [29,32].

Table 1. Mechanisms of ction of psychopharmacological drugs and their possible effect on intraocular pressure, pupil size and glaucoma risk.

Effector	Receptors	Location	Drugs	Possible Induced Effect	Effect on IOP
Adrenaline	α1	Iris dilator muscle	Citalopram Escitalopram Paroxetine Fluvoxamine Fluoxetine Sertraline Ziprasidone Other atypical antipsychotics	Mydriasis (Hypertension, lid retraction) [33–35]	-
	α2	Ciliary epithelium	Escitalopram, Paroxetine, Sertraline Atypical antipsychotics	Increased outflow of aqueous humour	↓IOP [33,35]
	β2	Ciliary epithelium	Paroxetine	Increase production of aqueous humour	↑IOP [36]

Table 1. Cont.

Effector	Receptors	Location	Drugs	Possible Induced Effect	Effect on IOP
Serotonin	5HT7	sphincter of the pupil, iris ciliary body	Paroxetine, Ziprasidone	Mydriasis	↑IOP [28,33,37]
	5HT1A	Iris-ciliary body	Escitalopram, Paroxetine, Fluvoxamine, Sertraline, Ziprasidone Other atypical antipsychotics	-	↓IOP [28,33–35,37]
	5HT2A	Iris-ciliary body	Escitalopram Paroxetine, Fluoxetine Sertraline, Venlafaxine, Ziprasidone Other atypical antipsychotics	-	↓IOP [28,33,37]
	5HT2C	Iris-ciliary body	Citalopram Escitalopram, Fluvoxamine Fluoxetine, Paroxetine, Sertraline, Venlafaxine Ziprasidone, Other atypical antipsychotics	-	↑IOP [28,33,35,37]
Dopamine	DA1	The ciliary body, trabecular meshwork, and uveoscleral tissue	Paroxetine	Increased production of aqueous humour	↑IOP [33,35,38]
	DA2	Anterior segment	Escitalopram Paroxetine, Sertraline, Ziprasidone Typical and other atypical antipsychotics	Suppression of the production of aqueous humour	↓IOP [33,35,38]
Acetylcholine (miotic effect)	Muscarinic (Blockade)	Smooth muscle around the pupil	Citalopram, Paroxetine Escitalopram, Fluoxetine. Sertraline Tricyclic antidepressants Typical and atypical antipsychotics	Mydriasis	↑IOP [36]
TNF	TNF-R1	Aqueous humour outflow channels	Bupropion	Increased caspase activity, mitochondrial dysfunction	↑IOP [39]
Sulpha based drugs	-	-	Topiramate	Allergic reaction (myopia, swelling of the ciliary body, forward displacement of the lens-iris diaphragm)	↑IOP [40]

↑, increased; ↓, decreased; IOP, intraocular pressure; 5HT, 5-hydroxytryptamine (serotonin); DA, dopamine; TNF, tumour necrosis factor; R, receptor.

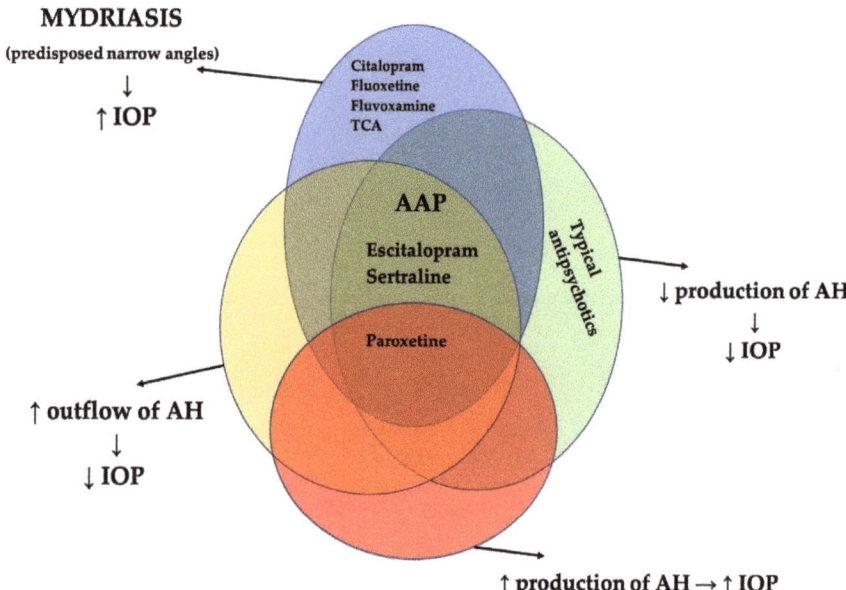

Figure 1. Schematic representation of the relationship between antidepressant and antipsychotic drugs and the various ocular side effects related to glaucoma pathogenic mechanisms. AAP, atypical antipsychotics; IOP, intraocular pressure; AH, aqueous humour; TCA, tricyclic antidepressants; ↑, increased; ↓, decreased.

3.1.1. OAG

Zheng et al. (2018) documented a potential negative association between SSRIs with primary open angle glaucoma (POAG). More precisely, Zheng et al. (2018) showed that POAG patients treated with systemic medication and under SSRI therapy have a significant lower risk of developing POAG that would require a procedure (patients undergoing treatment with SSRI were at an averagely 30% lower risk for the development of OAG than non-SSRIs users). An approximately 30% reduced risk was also associated with the SNRI class, although less significantly. Also, it has been suggested that there is a dose-response relationship with lower odds of POAG with greater days of treatment [41].

These findings are similar to another cross-sectional study in which three groups of patients with open angle eyes were compared (patients receiving SSRI for 1 week to 6 months, longer than 6 months, or patients under no treatment). IOP was lower in patients under SSRI treatment for less 6 month or more than 6 months in comparison with controls, but the pupil diameter was higher in the abovementioned groups [30].

In contrast, a rise in IOP was documented in the case of a patient with chronic OAG during the initiation of treatment with venlafaxine (a SNRI). After the patient complained of headaches, the starting dose of 225 mg was reduced to 75 mg. No symptoms were reported after the dosage was lowered. Although asymptomatic at 3 months, the IOP increased and the retinal nerve suffered damages [42].

3.1.2. ACG

Regarding ACG, in a large population-based study it was associated with a recent exposure to antidepressants in older adults [43], whereas long exposure to SSRIs did not influence the risk of ACG [44]. Another study conducted by Chen et al. (2017) concluded that individuals under SSRIs therapy had a greater risk of glaucoma (OAG, PACG, glaucoma state, glaucoma suspicion, other forms of glaucoma) incidence. Also, long-term use (>365 days) and/or high dosage were associated with a greater risk of developing glaucoma with an additive effect when both variables were included [37]. In a case-control study that included 1456 ACG patients, immediate SSRI users had 5.80 higher chances to develop ACG as compared to nonusers [45].

Conversely, a recent meta-analysis outlined that treatment with SSRIs was not associated with a higher risk of POAG or PACG and that IOP seemed to be lower in patients exposed to SSRIs. Also, Wang et al. (2018) concluded that pupillary diameter was higher in subjects under this type of antidepressant treatment [46].

Regarding the individual risk of each drug from the SSRIs class to cause glaucoma, current research is scarce and only a few case reports are available in the literature.

Citalopram-induced glaucoma (unilateral ACG) was reported in the literature in a case of drug overdose where the patient presented with blurred vision, pain and corneal oedema, in association with a high IOP. This patient was noted to have shallow anterior chambers in both eyes. After initial ophthalmologic treatment her IOP maintained normal without anti-glaucoma maintenance treatment [47]. Another case of citalopram induced bilateral symptomatic acute angle closure was reported in a patient with a history of 5 months of treatment with a normal dosage (the patient presented with blurred vision and headache) [48].

A case report of escitalopram-induced bilateral ACG described ciliochoroidal effusions after 4 weeks of treatment with a daily dose of 20 mg in a patient that presented with blurred vision. Ophthalmic examination revealed: high IOP, bilateral shallow anterior chamber, best corrected visual acuity was 20/40 bilaterally and a myopic shift of 4 dioptres over the current spectacle prescription. The condition was resistant to medical and surgical treatment but the patient recovered completely after escitalopram was discontinued [49]. Another article reported headache, blurred vision, vomiting, and photophobia (typical symptoms of AACG) in a patient that suddenly stopped escitalopram 1 month before the debut of symptoms. The risk factors identified in this case included hypertension (under control with beta-blockers) and escitalopram use for 1 year [50].

Patients under paroxetine therapy have reported ACG specific symptoms (i.e., loss of visual acuity or blurred vision) between 1 day and 4 months of treatment [51–55]. Interestingly, Sierra-Rodriguez et al. (2013) presented a case report of a unilateral visual loss due to chronic ACG under paroxetine treatment for 4 months. After discontinuation of paroxetine and laser iridotomy, the IOP normalised. Unfortunately, the patient resumed treatment on her own with consequent IOP rise despite patent iridotomies [53].

Regarding fluvoxamine, a patient with a previous history of narrow angle glaucoma (with no iridectomy) presented with daily headaches for 3 months and depressive symptoms (for anxiety the patient was taking lorazepam 2mg/day) and was prescribed fluvoxamine. After two months treatment the patient reported severe orbital pain and blurred vision (increased IOP and mydriasis). Despite specific therapy, IOP decreased only after the withdraw of the antidepressant [56].

Similar ACG symptoms were reported after three days of sertraline treatment, in a 64 year old Chinese woman with hypermetropia. It is worth to mention that Chinese ethnicity, old age, female gender and hypermetropia are risk factors for AACG [57].

Concerning SNRIs, the current literature describes only two and four ACG case reports involving duloxetine and venlafaxine, respectively.

The possible association of duloxetine with the appearance of ACG symptoms was reported in two female patients (46 and 81 years old, respectively). It is important to mention that the 81 years old patient was suffering from other comorbidities, hypermetropia and cataract [33,58].

Regarding venlafaxine, literature reports 4 possible cases of AACG after recent administration of this antidepressant, with the onset of symptoms ranging between 4 h and 10 days. In all reported cases, the patients were females of different age (between 35 and 70 years old) and had blurred vision as a common symptom [59–62].

Taking into account all the described current literature data, SSRIs and SNRIs have in general no association with either types of glaucoma or increased IOP. Moreover, it is worth emphasizing that long term treatment with SSRIs or SNRIs is associated with a decrease in the IOP, which suggests a possible protective effect of these drugs that needs further investigation. Of course, studies that assess the relationship between specific SSRIs or SNRIs and the risk of raised IOP and glaucoma are necessary in order to better characterise each drug regarding this possible side effect. The current case reports that describe a possible relationship between a specific SSRI or SNRI and ACG should warn the prescribers to closely monitor patients during treatment, especially the individuals with associated risk factors.

3.2. Bupropion

Bupropion is a noradrenaline and dopamine reuptake inhibitor (NDRI) and has been used since 1985 mainly as an antidepressant and more recently as adjuvant for smoking cessation. Bupropion is known to have anti-tumour necrosis factor (TNF) effects and a decreased activity on acetylcholine receptors that result in less anticholinergic side effects [63]. Studies hypothesised that IOP might be raised by TNF through increased caspase activity or mitochondrial dysfunction in the aqueous humour outflow channels. TNF synthesis is decreased by noradrenaline (β2 receptor) and dopamine (D1 receptor) activation [39,64]. All these effects led to the possible conclusion that bupropion could have some protective proprieties regarding IOP and glaucoma (Table 1).

A cross-sectional study that included patients over 40 years old investigated the relationship between self-reported glaucoma and self-reported bupropion use for at least 1 year. Masis et al. (2017) concluded that the usage of bupropion for longer than one year may be associated with a lower risk of self-reported glaucoma. Other covariates associated with high risk included Hispanic/Black ethnicity, increased age, cataract extraction, and diabetic neuropathy. One important limitation of this study is the lack of specificity in glaucoma type (ACG or OAG) [64].

3.2.1. OAG

A cohort-type study regarding the risk of OAG coupled with bupropion treatment, reported a reduced hazard of developing this type of glaucoma. More precisely, the percentage of bupropion users that developed OAG was 1.8% and the percentage of non-users who developed OAG was 2.4%. Moreover, usage of this drug for 24–48 months has been associated with a 21% reduced chance of OAG [39].

3.2.2. ACG

A case-control study conducted on patients under 50 years old reported bupropion treatment to be associated with an increased risk of ACG. No new prescriptions were issued afterwards, which could imply that predisposed eyes with narrow angles and pupillary dilation were not likely since iridotomy would have allowed continuation of treatment. Although the manufacturer's information references the occurrence of ACG secondary to a pharmacological pupillary dilation, there is a possibility that choroidal effusion can occur [36].

Also, 2 weeks bupropion treatment (300 mg/day) was incriminated as a cause ACG in a 40 years old woman, with complains of blurred vision. Ultrasound bio microscopy revealed bilateral choroidal effusions that caused shallow angles [65].

3.3. Tricyclic Antidepressants (TCAs)

TCAs are the first generation of antidepressants and have been used in the psychopharmacological treatment of depression since around 1950. TCAs inhibit, through action on specific transporters, the reuptake of serotonin and noradrenaline in the synapse cleft. Also, TCAs block the postsynaptic histamine, acetylcholine and alpha-adrenergic receptors. Unfortunately, due to the cardiovascular and gastrointestinal serious adverse effects and their lethality in overdose quantities, TCAs have been replaced over time by SSRIs and SNRIs in the management of depression [66].

According current literature data, tricyclic antidepressants (clomipramine, amitriptyline, imipramine, doxepin, desipramine, nortriptyline etc.) are reported to be involved only in ACG and to precipitate AACG. The pupillary block via pupil dilatation that occurs during treatment with TCAs is attributed to the significant anticholinergic and serotonergic effects of these antidepressants [67]. The most frequent anticholinergic effects on the eye are mydriasis and cycloplegia, which in turn may cause the blockage of the trabecular meshwork. These effects result in blurred vision due to loss of accommodation and in precipitation of ACG [67–70] (Figure 1).

A relative large body of case reports that linked different TCAs treatment to the raise of IOP and glaucoma occurrence is present in the literature. Schlingemann et al. (1996) described the case of a 59-year-old woman with developed monocular vision loss, increased IOP and narrowed anterior chambers supposing due to treatment with clomipramine (75 mg/day) [71]. Lowe et al. (1966) also reported the cases of 4 patients on small dosage amitriptyline therapy that developed ACG [72]. In addition, Ritch et al. (1994) documented 4 cases of narrow angled patients who developed ACG related to imipramine treatment. Ritch et al. stated that uveal tract problems could be associated with TCA, mydriasis being often transient, without major consequences. Moreover, ACG can be promoted in susceptible patients (e.g., narrow angle individuals) [73].

All things considered, current data point out the risk of using drugs with potent anticholinergics proprieties, such as TCAs. The development of the new classes of antidepressants (i.e., SSRI and SNRI) provides important alternatives. In the case that TCAs must be used, the drugs with the less anticholinergic effects, such as desipramine and nortriptyline, should be taken into consideration [74]. No doubt, further cohort studies that assess the potential risk of angle closure glaucoma associated with TCAs are necessary in order to make conclusive recommendations.

4. Benzodiazepines (BZD)

Benzodiazepines are among the most commonly prescribed drug class in psychiatry and exhibit sedative, hypnotic, anxiolytic and muscle-relaxing properties by enhancing the effect of gamma aminobutyric acid (GABA). Due to this effect, benzodiazepines are incriminated to influence the sphincter pupillae and to determine the narrowing of iridocorneal angle [75]. Current literature documents only the relationship of BZD with ACG and AACG.

Until recently, few cases have been reported about the association of AACG with BZD treatment. The conclusions were rather ambiguous, given the fact that other psychotropic agents have been concomitantly used during the time AACG was reported to occur [75]. Park et al. (2019) tried to reveal the clear relationship between benzodiazepine usage and the risk of glaucoma. In this population-based case-control study on elderly patients, who are more susceptible to the adverse effects to BZD, the authors demonstrated a significant correlation between immediate new use of BZD (within 7 days of AACG diagnosis) and the occurrence of AACG. Oppositely, no significant change in AACG incidence in the non-immediate new users was reported. In addition, there was no significant difference between short half-life (<24 h) vs. long half-life (>24 h) benzodiazepine agents [76]. These findings are similar to the ones of Kim et al. (2020), who outlined an association between BZD therapy and AACG in a cohort of 6709 patients [75]. In the study group the most frequent prescribed BZD were Diazepam and Alprazolam. These drugs were also associated with the highest risk of AACG occurrence [75]. However, a different study concluded that diazepam reduced the IOP and would actually be safe in procedures where lowered IOP is desirable [77].

Therefore, we conclude that benzodiazepines could precipitate ACG in predisposed eyes and clinicians should be aware of these possible side effects.

5. Antipsychotics

Antipsychotic drugs are the cornerstone in the management of schizophrenia. Other indications for this category include schizoaffective disorder, bipolar disorder, delusional disorder, severe agitation, delirium, or psychotic features of major depressive disorder. They can be divided in two categories: typical or first generation (Haloperidol and Chlorpromazine as most known) and atypical or second generation (clozapine, asenapine, olanzapine, quetiapine, paliperidone, risperidone, sertindole, ziprasidone, zotepine, and aripiprazole). Typical antipsychotics manage the symptoms of psychosis through the blockage of the dopaminergic postsynaptic receptors, with additional histaminergic, α1 adrenergic and cholinergic blockade. Atypical antipsychotics are serotonin and dopamine antagonists with affinities for serotonin (5HT1A, 5HT2C, 5HT6, 5HT7), dopamine (D1, D3, D4) receptors, but also histamine (H1), muscarinic (M1, M2, M3, M4, M5) and adrenergic (α1, α2) receptors [78]. Most AAPs have in common a more potent 5HT2A action than dopamine (D2) antagonism. They are also partial agonists of 5HT1A. All these features contribute to the low extrapyramidal effects. Some other actions include the inhibition of muscarinic receptors (anticholinergic activity). A possible explanation for the association between antipsychotic drugs and glaucoma might be the cholinergic receptor blockade (muscarinic) [34,79] (Table 1, Figure 1).

Unfortunately, current research reports only the possible effects of antipsychotics on IOP and does not scrutinise the relationship between these drugs and OAG or ACG.

A cross-sectional study including 28 patients with schizophrenia showed that individuals under typical antipsychotics treatment had normal IOP [79]. This result is similar to the one reported by Reid et al. (1976). Moreover, Reid et al. (1976) study concluded that there was no IOP raise despite high dosage of typical antipsychotics [80]. Actually, not only haloperidol was found to lower IOP in glaucomatous eyes, but also it was proposed as a possible treatment for glaucoma [81–83].

Atypical antipsychotics (AAP) have cardiovascular side effects through the vasoconstriction determined by α1 adrenoreceptors blockage. Risperidone, clozapine, iloperidone and quetiapine may lead to hypotension via this mechanism [34]. Animal studies showed instilled APP into the eye determined a significant reduction of IOP observed after 1 h. Also, reduction of blood pressure occurred within 10 min after administration [84].

Reactive oxygen species (ROS) production is involved in the pathogenic mechanism of glaucoma. Risperidone was demonstrated to have the ability to decrease oxidative stress (OS) in schizophrenic patients by controlling the inflammatory response [85]. Other AAP that have been shown to decrease OS are clozapine and olanzapine [86]. However, the relationship between AAP, OS and glaucoma has been incompletely investigated. Therefore, future studies are necessary to elucidate this possible mechanism.

Several studies described that IOP elevation may lead to the inhibition of brain-derived-neurotrophic factor (BDNF) which could have in turn a contributing effect to the visual loss. Risperidone and clozapine have been found to increase levels of BDNF [87–89].

There is some evidence that AAPs could enhance glaucoma through anti-muscarinic action. For example, clozapine and olanzapine have high affinity for muscarinic receptors (inhibition) and anticholinergic activity, which could possibly exacerbate glaucoma [90]. Thus, the actions of AAP by downregulating OS and neurotrophins may be unbalanced because of their anti- muscarinic receptor action. This observation could explain that, in general, AAPs are not associated with a glaucoma risk [66].

A cross-sectional analysis of 28 patients with schizophrenia and under antipsychotic therapy (4 on typical antipsychotics, 16 on AAP, and 8 on both types) provided interesting conclusions. More precisely, a raise of IOP has been found only in patients under AAP therapy, particularly all on ziprasidone. Ziprasidone is known to exert a potent serotoninergic (5HT2A) and dopaminergic (D2) affinity [79].

In conclusion, clinicians should be aware that second generation antipsychotics could have some implication in the variations of IOP, therefore a special attention should be paid to patients at risk and also when prescribing ziprasidone. Increased IOP could have no clinical significance in certain situations (e.g., minor increase or lower basal IOP) or could lead to the development or progression of glaucoma (OAG or ACG) depending on the characteristics of the patient. Typical antipsychotics are suggested to be safer in relation to a possible rise of IOP.

6. Topiramate

Topiramate is a sulpha-derivative monosaccharide and it is commonly prescribed for treatment of epilepsy and migraine prevention. Off label indications include eating disorders, obesity and tobacco dependence. Regarding psychiatric recommendations, the current literature describes the benefits of topiramate in weight gain prevention and metabolic dysfunction in schizophrenic patients as a result of treatment with certain antipsychotics (i.e., olanzapine, clozapine) [91].

Topiramate's mechanism of action involves inhibition of carbonic anhydrase, calcium channels, and glutamate receptors, as well as blockage of the sodium channels and stimulation of gamma-aminobutyric acid receptors. Topiramate is suggested to cause or worsen glaucoma due to an acute hypersensitivity reaction and alteration of osmotic status. The mechanism is suggested to involve ciliochoroidal effusion which leads to anterior rotation of the swelled ciliary body with anterior shifting of lens-iris diaphragm and consequently shallowing of the anterior chamber and narrowing of the angle [92,93]. All these changes may also occur in normal eyes. Given this fact, clinicians should be more vigilant and it is advisable to adopt a watchful waiting approach for all patients treated with topiramate.

In a retrospective study, Ho JD et al. (2013) reported a greater risk of developing ACG after topiramate therapy in the first month of treatment (hazard ratio 7.41 times higher than control subjects) [93]. Other data showed an increased risk of ACG, myopia, suprachoroidal effusion, and abnormal vision, all reversible with the discontinuation of treatment [94,95].

Numerous case reports found in the current literature described the association of topiramate treatment with the development of ACG. In 38 reported cases [96–130], patients under topiramate treatment developed ACG after a short time from the treatment initiation (the majority between 1 day and 14 days), most of them being adult women (27 women/38 patients) with an age ranging from 23 to 59 years. Table 2 presents a summary of current topiramate induced acute angle closure or AACG case reports (Table 2).

Table 2. A summary of currently reported topiramate-induced acute (primary) angle-closure or acute (primary) angle-closure glaucoma cases (in adult patients).

Case Report	Patient's Gender, Age and Other Comorbidities	Onset after Drug Initiation
Alzendi et al. (2020) [96]	Female, 24 yo, migraines	13 days
Agarwal et al. (2019) [97]	Female, 25 yo, morbid obesity, obstructive sleep apnoea	11 days
Mahendradas et al. (2018) [98]	Female, 36 yo, hypothyroidism	5 days
Sierra-Rodríguez et al. (2018) [99]	Female, 29 yo, epilepsy	9 days
Lan et al. (2017) [100]	Female, 43 yo, arrhythmia	4 weeks
Czyz et al. (2014) [101]	Female, 40 yo, arterial hypertension, degenerative disk disease, fibromyalgia, migraines, chronic obstructive pulmonary disease	262 days
Pikkel et al. (2014) [102]	Male, 54 yo	7 days
Katsimpris et al. (2014) [103]	Female, 36 yo, migraines	14 days
Quagliato et al. (2013) [104]	Female, 55 yo, migraines, spasmodic torticollis, essential tremor	7 days
Caglar et al. (2012) [105]	Female, 36 yo, migraine	1 day
Cole et al. (2012) [106]	Female, 56 yo, depression treated with venlafaxine	2 days

Table 2. Cont.

Case Report	Patient's Gender, Age and Other Comorbidities	Onset after Drug Initiation
van Issum et al. (2011) [107]	Male, 34 yo, epilepsy	14 days
Willett et al. (2011) [108]	Male, 39 yo, arterial hypertension, migraines	7 days
Natesh et al. (2010) [109]	Male, 23 yo	5 days
Acharya et al. (2010) [110]	Male, 49 yo	14 days
Spaccapelo et al. (2009) [111]	Male, 34 yo, anxious-depressive syndrome treated with citalopram	7 days
Sbeity et al. (2009) [112]	Female, 59 yo, keratomileusis surgery, myopia	11 days
Chalam et al. (2008) [113]	Female, 34 yo, arterial hypertension, hypothyroidism	7 days
Boonyaleephan et al. (2008) [114]	Female, 23 yo	7 days
Aminlari et al. (2008) [115]	Female, 48 yo, bipolar disorder, depression, hypothyroidism, chronic pain	14 days
Aminlari et al. (2008)	Male, 53 yo, cluster headaches, hyperlipidaemia	6 weeks
Singh et al. (2007) [116]	Female, 33 yo, headaches	7 days
Parikh et al. (2007) [117]	Male, 51 yo, epilepsy	14 days
Viet et al. (2006) [118]	Male, 57 yo, bipolar disorder	7 days
Sachi et al. (2006) [119]	Female, 33 yo, migraines	3 weeks
Rhee et al. (2006) [120]	Female, 35 yo, migraines	2 months
Levy et al. (2006) [121]	Female, 35 yo, depression	7 days
Desai et al. (2006) [122]	Female, 36 yo, migraines	10 days
Mansoor et al. (2005) [123]	Female, 51 yo, surgery for hypermetropia, migraines	7 days
Craig et al. (2004) [124]	Female, 25 yo, epilepsy, depression treated with Venlafaxine	7 days
Boentert et al. (2003) [125]	Female, 23 yo, congenital hydrocephalus, Arnold-Chiari formation I, partial atrophy of the right optic nerve, astigmatism, vertical strabismus.	6 days
Medeiros et al. (2003) [126]	Male, 44 yo	5 days
Medeiros et al. (2003) [126]	Female, 42 yo, myopia	10 days
Chen et al. (2003) [127]	Female, 42 yo, hypertension, seizures	2.5 weeks
Banta et al. (2001) [128]	Male, 51 yo, bipolar disorder	14 days
Sankar et al. (2001) [129]	Female, 34 yo, depression	14 days
Sankar et al. (2001) [129]	Female, 53 yo, depression treated with venlafaxine, high cholesterol.	10 days
Rhee et al. (2001) [130]	Female, 43 yo, depression treated with paroxetine	1 day

yo, years old.

7. Conclusions

Based on the presented data, clinicians should be aware of the glaucoma-related risk-benefit profile of psychotropic medication and tailor their recommendations. The selective serotonin and noradrenaline reuptake inhibitors class is the medication group with the most solid results regarding a minimal possible risk of glaucoma. More precisely, SSRI and SNRI treatment seems to have even a protective role regarding OAG and no effect in relationship with ACG. Therefore, practitioners could use these drugs safely since there is no risk of a glaucoma induced effect. On the other hand, tricyclic antidepressants should be avoided in patients at risk to develop angle closure glaucoma or in angle closure glaucoma diagnosed individuals due to their strong anticholinergic and antimuscarinic proprieties. Regarding all antipsychotics, there is an important gap in the knowledge of their relationship with the risk of glaucoma. Based on the herein reviewed data, first generation antipsychotics do not seem to affect the intraocular pressure, but for the second generation antipsychotics, and especially ziprasidone, further studies are needed in order to bring some light to the current data. Also, topiramate is another drug that we advise not be used in the treatment of patients with possible risk factors or diagnosed with angle closure glaucoma, since current data point to an increased risk of trabecular obstruction and consequently a raise in intraocular pressure. Benzodiazepines should be prescribed carefully, especially in older patients. Whether or not it is identified as a contraindication, physicians should be aware of the possibility of psychotropic drug-induced glaucoma, especially angle closure type, and if the suspicion of glaucoma arises, ophthalmological assessment is recommended. Early recognition of this possible side effect and discontinuation of the drug in question are measures that should be immediately employed by the psychiatrist concomitantly with referring the patient to an ophthalmologist for a thorough evaluation. Due to the vast psychotropic medication and possible mechanisms and their interactions, future studies are needed to fill the literature gaps and enrich current knowledge on this subject.

Author Contributions: Conceptualization, A.M.C. and C.N.; methodology, A.M.C., V.D. and O.P.-V.; software, C.N.; validation, A.M.C., O.P.-V. and S.R.; formal analysis, C.N.; investigation, A.M.C., V.D., C.N.; resources, V.D., C.N., O.M.B.; data curation, V.D., O.M.B.; writing—original draft preparation, A.M.C., V.D., C.N.; writing—review and editing, A.M.C., O.P.-V., S.R., O.M.B.; visualization, O.P.-V.; supervision, S.R.; project administration, A.M.C.; funding acquisition, V.D., C.N. All authors have read and agreed to the published version of the manuscript.

Funding: This research received no external funding.

Institutional Review Board Statement: Not applicable.

Informed Consent Statement: Not applicable.

Data Availability Statement: All data relevant to this paper are included in the article.

Acknowledgments: We would like to thank Ioana Robu for the professional language assistance.

Conflicts of Interest: The authors declare no conflict of interest.

References

1. Balendra, S.I.; Shah, P.A.; Jain, M.; Grzybowski, A.; Cordeiro, M.F. Glaucoma: Hot Topics in Pharmacology. *Curr. Pharm. Des.* **2017**, *23*, 596–607.
2. Flaxman, S.R.; Bourne, R.R.A.; Resnikoff, S.; Ackland, P.; Braithwaite, T.; Cicinelli, M.V.; Das, A.; Jonas, J.B.; Keeffe, J.; Kempen, J.H.; et al. Global Causes of Blindness and Distance Vision Impairment 1990–2020: A Systematic Review and Meta-Analysis. *Lancet Glob. Health* **2017**, *5*, e1221–e1234. [CrossRef]
3. Bertaud, S.; Aragno, V.; Baudouin, C.; Labbé, A. Le glaucome primitif à angle ouvert. *Rev. Med. Interne* **2019**, *40*, 445–452. [CrossRef]
4. Casson, R.J.; Chidlow, G.; Wood, J.P.M.; Crowston, J.G.; Goldberg, I. Definition of Glaucoma: Clinical and Experimental Concepts: Definition of Glaucoma. *Clin. Exp. Ophthalmol.* **2012**, *40*, 341–349. [CrossRef]
5. Kingman, S. Glaucoma Is Second Leading Cause of Blindness Globally. *Bull. World Health Organ.* **2004**, *82*, 887–888.
6. Schuster, A.K.; Erb, C.; Hoffmann, E.M.; Dietlein, T.; Pfeiffer, N. The Diagnosis and Treatment of Glaucoma. *Dtsch. Arztebl. Int.* **2020**, *117*, 225–234.
7. Weinreb, R.N.; Aung, T.; Medeiros, F.A. The Pathophysiology and Treatment of Glaucoma: A Review. *JAMA* **2014**, *311*, 1901–1911. [CrossRef]
8. McMonnies, C.W. Glaucoma History and Risk Factors. *J. Optom.* **2017**, *10*, 71–78. [CrossRef] [PubMed]
9. Mantravadi, A.V.; Vadhar, N. Glaucoma. *Prim. Care* **2015**, *42*, 437–449. [CrossRef] [PubMed]
10. Salmon, J. *Kanski's Clinical Ophthalmology: A Systematic Approach*, 9th ed.; Elsevier Health Sciences: London, UK, 2019; pp. 349, 370–374.
11. Quigley, H.A. Number of People with Glaucoma Worldwide. *Br. J. Ophthalmol.* **1996**, *80*, 389–393. [CrossRef] [PubMed]
12. Friedman, D.S.; Wolfs, R.C.W.; O'Colmain, B.J.; Klein, B.E.; Taylor, H.R.; West, S.; Leske, M.C.; Mitchell, P.; Congdon, N.; Kempen, J.; et al. Prevalence of Open-Angle Glaucoma among Adults in the United States. *Arch. Ophthalmol.* **2004**, *122*, 532–538. [PubMed]
13. Pantalon, A.D.; Feraru, C.; Chiseliță, D. Risk Factors and Long Term Progression in Open Angle Glaucoma Patients. *Rom. J. Ophthalmol.* **2016**, *60*, 174–180. [PubMed]

14. Kim, K.E.; Kim, M.J.; Park, K.H.; Jeoung, J.W.; Kim, S.H.; Kim, C.Y.; Kang, S.W.; Epidemiologic Survey Committee of the Korean Ophthalmological Society. Prevalence, Awareness, and Risk Factors of Primary Open-Angle Glaucoma: Korea National Health and Nutrition Examination Survey 2008–2011. *Ophthalmology* **2016**, *123*, 532–541. [CrossRef]
15. Chan, T.C.W.; Bala, C.; Siu, A.; Wan, F.; White, A. Risk Factors for Rapid Glaucoma Disease Progression. *Am. J. Ophthalmol.* **2017**, *180*, 151–157. [CrossRef] [PubMed]
16. Phulke, S.; Kaushik, S.; Kaur, S.; Pandav, S.S. Steroid-Induced Glaucoma: An Avoidable Irreversible Blindness. *J. Curr. Glaucoma Pract.* **2017**, *11*, 67–72. [PubMed]
17. Flores-Sánchez, B.C.; Tatham, A.J. Acute Angle Closure Glaucoma. *Br. J. Hosp. Med.* **2019**, *80*, C174–C179. [CrossRef]
18. Boonyaleephan, S. Drug-Induced Secondary Glaucoma. *J. Med. Assoc. Thai* **2010**, *93*, S118–S122.
19. Distelhorst, J.S.; Hughes, G.M. Open-Angle Glaucoma. *Am. Fam. Physician* **2003**, *67*, 1937–1944.
20. Pelčić, G.; Ljubičić, R.; Barać, J.; Biuk, D.; Rogoić, V. Glaucoma, Depression and Quality of Life: Multiple Comorbidities, Multiple Assessments and Multidisciplinary Plan Treatment. *Psychiatr. Danub.* **2017**, *29*, 351–359. [CrossRef]
21. Zhang, D.; Fan, Z.; Gao, X.; Huang, W.; Yang, Q.; Li, Z.; Lin, M.; Xiao, H.; Ge, J. Illness Uncertainty, Anxiety and Depression in Chinese Patients with Glaucoma or Cataract. *Sci. Rep.* **2018**, *8*, 11671. [CrossRef]
22. Akhilesh, J. Associating Factors of Insomnia and Depression in Glaucoma: A Descriptive Analysis. *Int. Multispec. J. Health IMJH* **2018**, *4*, 41–49.
23. Kennedy, S.H.; Lam, R.W.; McIntyre, R.S.; Tourjman, S.V.; Bhat, V.; Blier, P.; Hasnain, M.; Jollant, F.; Levitt, A.J.; MacQueen, G.M.; et al. Canadian Network for Mood and Anxiety Treatments (CANMAT) 2016 Clinical Guidelines for the Management of Adults with Major Depressive Disorder: Section 3. Pharmacological Treatments: Section 3. Pharmacological Treatments. *Can. J. Psychiatry* **2016**, *61*, 540–560. [CrossRef]
24. Bauer, M.; Pfennig, A.; Severus, E.; Whybrow, P.C.; Angst, J.; Möller, H.-J.; World Federation of Societies of Biological Psychiatry. Task Force on Unipolar Depressive Disorders. World Federation of Societies of Biological Psychiatry (WFSBP) Guidelines for Biological Treatment of Unipolar Depressive Disorders, Part 1: Update 2013 on the Acute and Continuation Treatment of Unipolar Depressive Disorders. *World J. Biol. Psychiatry* **2013**, *14*, 334–385.
25. Kellner, M. Drug Treatment of Obsessive-Compulsive Disorder. *Dialogues Clin. Neurosci.* **2010**, *12*, 187–197.
26. Strawn, J.R.; Geracioti, L.; Rajdev, N.; Clemenza, K.; Levine, A. Pharmacotherapy for Generalized Anxiety Disorder in Adult and Pediatric Patients: An Evidence-Based Treatment Review. *Expert Opin. Pharmacother.* **2018**, *19*, 1057–1070. [CrossRef] [PubMed]
27. Asnis, G.M.; Kohn, S.R.; Henderson, M.; Brown, N.L. SSRIs versus Non-SSRIs in Post-Traumatic Stress Disorder: An Update with Recommendations. *Drugs* **2004**, *64*, 383–404. [CrossRef] [PubMed]
28. Costagliola, C.; Parmeggiani, F.; Sebastiani, A. SSRIs and Intraocular Pressure Modifications: Evidence, Therapeutic Implications and Possible Mechanisms. *CNS Drugs* **2004**, *18*, 475–484. [CrossRef]
29. Wiciński, M.; Kaluzny, B.J.; Liberski, S.; Marczak, D.; Seredyka-Burduk, M.; Pawlak-Osińska, K. Association between Serotonin-Norepinephrine Reuptake Inhibitors and Acute Angle Closure: What Is Known? *Surv. Ophthalmol.* **2019**, *64*, 185–194. [CrossRef] [PubMed]
30. Gündüz, G.U.; Parmak-Yener, N.; Kılınçel, O.; Gündüz, C. Effects of Selective Serotonin Reuptake Inhibitors on Intraocular Pressure and Anterior Segment Parameters in Open Angle Eyes. *Cutan. Ocul. Toxicol.* **2018**, *37*, 36–40. [CrossRef]
31. Loma, P.; Guzman-Aranguez, A.; de Lara, M.J.P.; Pintor, J. Beta2 Adrenergic Receptor Silencing Change Intraocular Pressure in New Zealand Rabbits. *J. Optom.* **2018**, *11*, 69–74. [CrossRef] [PubMed]
32. Uçan Gündüz, G.; Parmak Yener, N.; Kılınçel, O.; Gündüz, C. How Does Usage of Serotonin Noradrenaline Reuptake Inhibitors Affect Intraocular Pressure in Depression Patients? *J. Ocul. Pharmacol. Ther.* **2018**, *34*, 354–359. [CrossRef] [PubMed]
33. Mahmut, A.; Tunc, V.; Demiryurek, E.; Gursoy, A. Bilateral Acute Angle-Closure Glaucoma Induced by Duloxetine. *Ideggyogy. Sz.* **2017**, *70*, 358–360. [CrossRef] [PubMed]
34. Vallée, A.; Vallée, J.-N.; Lecarpentier, Y. Lithium and Atypical Antipsychotics: The Possible WNT/β Pathway Target in Glaucoma. *Biomedicines* **2021**, *9*, 473. [CrossRef]
35. Stahl, S.M. *Essential Psychopharmacology Series: Stahl's Essential Psychopharmacology: Neuroscientific Basis and Practical Applications*, 3rd ed.; Cambridge University Press: Cambridge, UK, 2008; pp. 284–369.
36. Symes, R.J.; Etminan, M.; Mikelberg, F.S. Risk of Angle-Closure Glaucoma with Bupropion and Topiramate. *JAMA Ophthalmol.* **2015**, *133*, 1187–1189. [CrossRef]
37. Chen, V.C.-H.; Ng, M.-H.; Chiu, W.-C.; McIntyre, R.S.; Lee, Y.; Lin, T.-Y.; Weng, J.-C.; Chen, P.-C.; Hsu, C.-Y. Effects of Selective Serotonin Reuptake Inhibitors on Glaucoma: A Nationwide Population-Based Study. *PLoS ONE* **2017**, *12*, e0173005.
38. Richelson, E. Pharmacology of antidepressants. *Mayo Clin. Proc.* **2001**, *76*, 511–527. [CrossRef]
39. Stein, J.D.; Talwar, N.; Kang, J.H.; Okereke, O.I.; Wiggs, J.L.; Pasquale, L.R. Bupropion Use and Risk of Open-Angle Glaucoma among Enrollees in a Large U.S. Managed Care Network. *PLoS ONE* **2015**, *10*, e0123682. [CrossRef] [PubMed]
40. Tripathi, R.; Tripathi, B.; Haggerty, C. Drug-Induced Glaucomas. *Drug Saf.* **2003**, *26*, 749–767. [CrossRef] [PubMed]
41. Zheng, W.; Dryja, T.P.; Wei, Z.; Song, D.; Tian, H.; Kahler, K.H.; Khawaja, A.P. Systemic Medication Associations with Presumed Advanced or Uncontrolled Primary Open-Angle Glaucoma. *Ophthalmology* **2018**, *125*, 984–993. [CrossRef]
42. Botha, V.E.; Bhikoo, R.; Merriman, M. Venlafaxine-Induced Intraocular Pressure Rise in a Patient with Open Angle Glaucoma: Venlafaxine Induced Intraocular Pressure Rise. *Clin. Exp. Ophthalmol.* **2016**, *44*, 734–735. [CrossRef]

43. Seitz, D.P.; Campbell, R.J.; Bell, C.M.; Gill, S.S.; Gruneir, A.; Herrmann, N.; Newman, A.M.; Anderson, G.; Rochon, P.A. Short-Term Exposure to Antidepressant Drugs and Risk of Acute Angle-Closure Glaucoma among Older Adults. *J. Clin. Psychopharmacol.* **2012**, *32*, 403–407. [CrossRef] [PubMed]
44. Chen, H.-Y.; Lin, C.-L.; Kao, C.-H. Long-Term Use of Selective Serotonin Reuptake Inhibitors and Risk of Glaucoma in Depression Patients. *Medicine* **2015**, *94*, e2041. [CrossRef] [PubMed]
45. Chen, H.-Y.; Lin, C.-L.; Lai, S.-W.; Kao, C.-H. Association of Selective Serotonin Reuptake Inhibitor Use and Acute Angle–Closure Glaucoma. *J. Clin. Psychiatry* **2016**, *77*, e692–e696. [CrossRef]
46. Wang, H.-Y.; Tseng, P.-T.; Stubbs, B.; Carvalho, A.F.; Li, D.-J.; Chen, T.-Y.; Lin, P.-Y.; Hsueh, Y.-T.; Chen, Y.-Z.; Chen, Y.-W.; et al. The Risk of Glaucoma and Serotonergic Antidepressants: A Systematic Review and Meta-Analysis. *J. Affect. Disord.* **2018**, *241*, 63–70. [CrossRef]
47. Croos, R.; Thirumalai, S.; Hassan, S.; Davis, J.D.R. Citalopram Associated with Acute Angle-Closure Glaucoma: Case Report. *BMC Ophthalmol.* **2005**, *5*, 23. [CrossRef]
48. Massaoutis, P.; Goh, D.; Foster, P.J. Bilateral Symptomatic Angle Closure Associated with a Regular Dose of Citalopram, an SSRI Antidepressant. *Br. J. Ophthalmol.* **2007**, *91*, 1086–1087. [CrossRef]
49. Zelefsky, J.R.; Fine, H.F.; Rubinstein, V.J.; Hsu, I.S.; Finger, P.T. Escitalopram-Induced Uveal Effusions and Bilateral Angle Closure Glaucoma. *Am. J. Ophthalmol.* **2006**, *141*, 1144–1147. [CrossRef] [PubMed]
50. AlQuorain, S.; Alfaraj, S.; Alshahrani, M. Bilateral Acute Closed Angle Glaucoma Associated with the Discontinuation of Escitalopram: A Case Report. *Open Access Emerg. Med.* **2016**, *8*, 61–65. [PubMed]
51. Eke, T.; Bates, A.K. Acute Angle Closure Glaucoma Associated with Paroxetine. *BMJ* **1997**, *314*, 1387. [CrossRef] [PubMed]
52. Kirwan, J.F.; Subak-Sharpe, I.; Teimory, M. Bilateral Acute Angle Closure Glaucoma after Administration of Paroxetine. *Br. J. Ophthalmol.* **1997**, *81*, 252. [CrossRef]
53. Sierra-Rodriguez, M.A.; Saenz-Frances, F.; Santos-Bueso, E.; Garcia-Feijoo, J.; Gonzelez-Romero, J.C. Chronic Angle-Closure Glaucoma Related to Paroxetine Treatment. *Semin. Ophthalmol.* **2013**, *28*, 244–246. [CrossRef] [PubMed]
54. Browning, A.C.; Reck, A.C.; Chisholm, I.H.; Nischal, K.K. Acute Angle Closure Glaucoma Presenting in a Young Patient after Administration of Paroxetine. *EYE* **2000**, *14*, 406–408. [CrossRef] [PubMed]
55. Levy, J.; Tessler, Z.; Klemperer, I.; Shneck, M.; Lifshitz, T. Late Bilateral Acute Angle-Closure Glaucoma after Administration of Paroxetine in a Patient with Plateau Iris Configuration. *Can. J. Ophthalmol.* **2004**, *39*, 780–781. [CrossRef]
56. Jiménez-Jiménez, F.J.; Ortí-Pareja, M.; Zurdo, J.M. Aggravation of Glaucoma with Fluvoxamine. *Ann. Pharmacother.* **2001**, *35*, 1565–1566. [CrossRef]
57. Ho, H.Y.; Kam, K.-W.A.; Young, A.L.; Chan, L.K.; Yu, E.C.-S. Acute Angle Closure Glaucoma after Sertraline. *Gen. Hosp. Psychiatry* **2013**, *35*, 575. [CrossRef] [PubMed]
58. Shifera, A.S.; Leoncavallo, A.; Sherwood, M. Probable Association of an Attack of Bilateral Acute Angle-Closure Glaucoma with Duloxetine. *Ann. Pharmacother.* **2014**, *48*, 936–939. [CrossRef]
59. de Guzman, M.H.P.; Thiagalingam, S.; Ong, P.Y.; Goldberg, I. Bilateral Acute Angle Closure Caused by Supraciliary Effusions Associated with Venlafaxine Intake. *Med. J. Aust.* **2005**, *182*, 121–123. [CrossRef]
60. Ezra, D.G.; Storoni, M.; Whitefield, L.A. Simultaneous Bilateral Acute Angle Closure Glaucoma Following Venlafaxine Treatment. *EYE* **2006**, *20*, 128–129. [CrossRef]
61. Ng, B.; Sanbrook, G.M.C.; Malouf, A.J.; Agarwal, S.A. Venlafaxine and Bilateral Acute Angle Closure Glaucoma. *Med. J. Aust.* **2002**, *176*, 241. [CrossRef] [PubMed]
62. Zhou, N.; Zhao, J.-X.; Zhu, Y.-N.; Zhang, P.; Zuo, Y. Acute Angle-Closure Glaucoma Caused by Venlafaxine. *Chin. Med. J. Engl.* **2018**, *131*, 1502–1503. [CrossRef]
63. Rudorfer, M.V.; Manji, H.K.; Potter, W.Z. Comparative Tolerability Profiles of the Newer versus Older Antidepressants. *Drug Saf.* **1994**, *10*, 18–46. [CrossRef]
64. Masís, M.; Kakigi, C.; Singh, K.; Lin, S. Association between Self-Reported Bupropion Use and Glaucoma: A Population-Based Study. *Br. J. Ophthalmol.* **2017**, *101*, 525–529. [CrossRef]
65. Takusagawa, H.L.; Hunter, R.S.; Jue, A.; Pasquale, L.R.; Chen, T.C. Bilateral Uveal Effusion and Angle-Closure Glaucoma Associated with Bupropion Use. *Arch. Ophthalmol.* **2012**, *130*, 120–122. [CrossRef]
66. Richa, S.; Yazbek, J.-C. Ocular Adverse Effects of Common Psychotropic Agents: A Review: A Review. *CNS Drugs* **2010**, *24*, 501–526. [CrossRef] [PubMed]
67. Ah-Kee, E.Y.; Egong, E.; Shafi, A.; Lim, L.T.; Yim, J.L. A Review of Drug-Induced Acute Angle Closure Glaucoma for Non-Ophthalmologists. *Qatar Med. J.* **2015**, *2015*, 6. [CrossRef] [PubMed]
68. Lieberman, E.; Stoudemire, A. Use of Tricyclic Antidepressants in Patients with Glaucoma. Assessment and Appropriate Precautions. *Psychosomatics* **1987**, *28*, 145–148. [CrossRef]
69. Sönmez, İ.; Aykan, Ü. Psychotropic Drugs and Ocular Side Effects. *Turk. J. Ophthalmol.* **2014**, *44*, 144–150. [CrossRef]
70. Razeghinejad, M.R.; Myers, J.S.; Katz, L.J. Iatrogenic Glaucoma Secondary to Medications. *Am. J. Med.* **2011**, *124*, 20–25. [CrossRef]
71. Schlingemann, R.O.; Smit, A.A.; Lunel, H.F.; Hijdra, A. Amaurosis Fugax on Standing and Angle-Closure Glaucoma with Clomipramine. *Lancet* **1996**, *347*, 465. [CrossRef]
72. Lowe, R.F. Amitriptyline and Glaucoma. *Med. J. Aust.* **1966**, *2*, 509–510. [CrossRef]

73. Ritch, R.; Krupin, T.; Henry, C.; Kurata, F. Oral Imipramine and Acute Angle Closure Glaucoma. *Arch. Ophthalmol.* **1994**, *112*, 67–68. [CrossRef]
74. Epstein, N.E.; Goldbloom, D.S. Oral Imipramine and Acute Angle-Closure Glaucoma. *Arch. Ophthalmol.* **1995**, *113*, 698. [CrossRef]
75. Kim, W.J.; Li, J.; Oh, I.-S.; Song, I.; Lee, E.; Namkoong, K.; Shin, J.-Y. Benzodiazepine Use and Risk of Acute Angle-Closure Glaucoma: A Population-Based Case-Crossover Study. *Drug Saf.* **2020**, *43*, 539–547. [CrossRef]
76. Park, M.Y.; Kim, W.J.; Lee, E.; Kim, C.; Son, S.J.; Yoon, J.S.; Kim, W.; Namkoong, K. Association between Use of Benzodiazepines and Occurrence of Acute Angle-Closure Glaucoma in the Elderly: A Population-Based Study. *J. Psychosom. Res.* **2019**, *122*, 1–5. [CrossRef] [PubMed]
77. Fragen, R.J.; Hauch, T. The Effect of Midazolam Maleate and Diazepam on Intraocular Pressure in Adults. *Arzneimittelforschung* **1981**, *31*, 2273–2275.
78. Nasrallah, H.A. Atypical Antipsychotic-Induced Metabolic Side Effects: Insights from Receptor-Binding Profiles. *Mol. Psychiatry* **2008**, *13*, 27–35. [CrossRef]
79. Souza, V.B.N.E.; Moura Filho, F.J.R.; de Souza, F.G.d.M.E.; Pereira Filho, S.A.C.; Coelho, S.S.; Furtado, F.A.M.L.; Gonçalves, T.B.A.; Vasconcelos, K.F.X. Intraocular Pressure in Schizophrenic Patients Treated with Psychiatric Medications. *Arq. Bras. Oftalmol.* **2008**, *71*, 660–664. [CrossRef]
80. Reid, W.H.; Blouin, P. Outpatient Psychiatric Medications and Glaucoma. *Psychosomatics* **1976**, *17*, 83–85. [CrossRef]
81. Khosla, P.; Kothari, S.; Gupta, M.C.; Srivastava, R.K. Evaluation of Haloperidol, a Dopamine Antagonist, on Intraocular Pressure in Experimental Glaucoma. *Indian J. Exp. Biol.* **1996**, *34*, 580–581. [PubMed]
82. Chiou, G.C. Ocular Hypotensive Actions of Haloperidol, a Dopaminergic Antagonist. *Arch. Ophthalmol.* **1984**, *102*, 143–145. [CrossRef] [PubMed]
83. Sheppard, J.D.; Schaid, D.J. Oral Haloperidol Lowers Human Intraocular Pressure. *J. Ocul. Pharmacol.* **1986**, *2*, 215–224. [CrossRef]
84. Joshi, S.V.; Patel, E.P.; Vyas, B.A.; Lodha, S.R.; Kalyankar, G.G. Repurposing of Iloperidone: Antihypertensive and Ocular Hypotensive Activity in Animals. *Eur. J. Pharm. Sci.* **2020**, *143*, 105173. [CrossRef]
85. Al-Amin, M.M.; Nasir-Uddin, M.M.; Mahmud Reza, H. Effects of Antipsychotics on the Inflammatory Response System of Patients with Schizophrenia in Peripheral Blood Mononuclear Cell Cultures. *Clin. Psychopharmacol. Neurosci.* **2013**, *11*, 144–151. [CrossRef]
86. Caruso, G.; Grasso, M.; Fidilio, A.; Tascedda, F.; Drago, F.; Caraci, F. Antioxidant Properties of Second-Generation Antipsychotics: Focus on Microglia. *Pharmaceuticals* **2020**, *13*, 457. [CrossRef] [PubMed]
87. Aringhieri, S.; Carli, M.; Kolachalam, S.; Verdesca, V.; Cini, E.; Rossi, M.; McCormick, P.J.; Corsini, G.U.; Maggio, R.; Scarselli, M. Molecular Targets of Atypical Antipsychotics: From Mechanism of Action to Clinical Differences. *Pharmacol. Ther.* **2018**, *192*, 20–41. [CrossRef] [PubMed]
88. Carli, M.; Aringhieri, S.; Kolachalam, S.; Longoni, B.; Grenno, G.; Rossi, M.; Gemignani, A.; Fornai, F.; Maggio, R.; Scarselli, M. Is Adult Hippocampal Neurogenesis Really Relevant for the Treatment of Psychiatric Disorders? *Curr. Neuropharmacol.* **2020**, *18*. [CrossRef]
89. Quigley, H.A.; McKinnon, S.J.; Zack, D.J.; Pease, M.E.; Kerrigan-Baumrind, L.A.; Kerrigan, D.F.; Mitchell, R.S. Retrograde Axonal Transport of BDNF in Retinal Ganglion Cells Is Blocked by Acute IOP Elevation in Rats. *Investig. Ophthalmol. Vis. Sci.* **2000**, *41*, 3460–3466.
90. Chew, M.L.; Mulsant, B.H.; Pollock, B.G.; Lehman, M.E.; Greenspan, A.; Kirshner, M.A.; Bies, R.R.; Kapur, S.; Gharabawi, G. A Model of Anticholinergic Activity of Atypical Antipsychotic Medications. *Schizophr. Res.* **2006**, *88*, 63–72. [CrossRef]
91. Narula, P.K.; Rehan, H.S.; Unni, K.E.S.; Gupta, N. Topiramate for Prevention of Olanzapine Associated Weight Gain and Metabolic Dysfunction in Schizophrenia: A Double-Blind, Placebo-Controlled Trial. *Schizophr. Res.* **2010**, *118*, 218–223. [CrossRef]
92. Rapoport, Y.; Benegas, N.; Kuchtey, R.W.; Joos, K.M. Acute Myopia and Angle Closure Glaucoma from Topiramate in a Seven-Year-Old: A Case Report and Review of the Literature. *BMC Pediatr.* **2014**, *14*, 96. [CrossRef]
93. Ho, J.-D.; Keller, J.J.; Tsai, C.-Y.; Liou, S.-W.; Chang, C.-J.; Lin, H.-C. Topiramate Use and the Risk of Glaucoma Development: A Population-Based Follow-up Study. *Am. J. Ophthalmol.* **2013**, *155*, 336–341. [CrossRef]
94. Fraunfelder, F.W.; Fraunfelder, F.T.; Keates, E.U. Topiramate-Associated Acute, Bilateral, Secondary Angle-Closure Glaucoma. *Ophthalmology* **2004**, *111*, 109–111. [CrossRef]
95. Etminan, M.; Maberley, D.; Mikelberg, F.S. Use of Topiramate and Risk of Glaucoma: A Case-Control Study. *Am. J. Ophthalmol.* **2012**, *153*, 827–830. [CrossRef] [PubMed]
96. Alzendi, N.; Badawi, A.; Alhazzaa, B.; Alshahrani, A.; Owaidhah, O. Topiramate-Induced Angle Closure Glaucoma: Two Unique Case Reports. *Saudi J. Ophthalmol.* **2020**, *34*, 202. [CrossRef] [PubMed]
97. Agarwal, A. Ciliochoroidal Effusion in Topiramate-Induced Bilateral Acute Angle Closure Glaucoma. *Indian J. Ophthalmol.* **2019**, *67*, 1466–1467. [CrossRef]
98. Mahendradas, P.; Parab, S.; Sasikumar, R.; Kawali, A.; Shetty, B.K. Topiramate-Induced Acute Angle Closure with Severe Panuveitis: A Challenging Case Report. *Indian J. Ophthalmol.* **2018**, *66*, 1342–1344. [CrossRef] [PubMed]
99. Sierra-Rodríguez, M.A.; Rodríguez-Vicente, L.; Chavarri-García, J.J.; Del Río-Mayor, J.L. Acute narrow-angle glaucoma induced by topiramate with acute myopia and macular striae: A case report. *Arch. Soc. Esp. Oftalmol. Engl. Ed.* **2019**, *94*, 130–133. [CrossRef]

100. Lan, Y.-W.; Hsieh, J.-W. Bilateral Acute Angle Closure Glaucoma and Myopic Shift by Topiramate-Induced Ciliochoroidal Effusion: Case Report and Literature Review. *Int. Ophthalmol.* **2018**, *38*, 2639–2648. [CrossRef]
101. Czyz, C.N.; Clark, C.M.; Justice, J.D.; Pokabla, M.J.; Weber, P.A. Delayed Topiramate-Induced Bilateral Angle-Closure Glaucoma. *J. Glaucoma* **2014**, *23*, 577–578. [CrossRef] [PubMed]
102. Pikkel, Y.Y. Acute Bilateral Glaucoma and Panuveitis as a Side Effect of Topiramate for Weight Loss Treatment. *BMJ Case Rep.* **2014**, *2014*, bcr2014203787. [CrossRef] [PubMed]
103. Katsimpris, J.M.; Katsimpris, A.; Theoulakis, P.E.; Lepidas, J.; Petropoulos, I.K. Bilateral Severe Anterior Uveitis and Acute Angle-Closure Glaucoma Following Topiramate Use for Migraine Crisis. *Klin. Monbl. Augenheilkd.* **2014**, *231*, 439–441. [CrossRef] [PubMed]
104. Quagliato, L.B.; Barella, K.; Abreu Neto, J.M.; Quagliato, E.M.A.B. Topiramate-Associated Acute, Bilateral, Angle-Closure Glaucoma: Case Report. *Arq. Bras. Oftalmol.* **2013**, *76*, 48–49. [CrossRef]
105. Caglar, C.; Yasar, T.; Ceyhan, D. Topiramate Induced Bilateral Angle-Closure Glaucoma: Low Dosage in a Short Time. *J. Ocul. Pharmacol. Ther.* **2012**, *28*, 205–207. [CrossRef]
106. Cole, K.L.; Wang, E.E.; Aronwald, R.M. Bilateral Acute Angle-Closure Glaucoma in a Migraine Patient Receiving Topiramate: A Case Report. *J. Emerg. Med.* **2012**, *43*, e89–e91. [CrossRef]
107. Van Issum, C.; Mavrakanas, N.; Schutz, J.S.; Shaarawy, T. Topiramate-Induced Acute Bilateral Angle Closure and Myopia: Pathophysiology and Treatment Controversies. *Eur. J. Ophthalmol.* **2011**, *21*, 404–409. [CrossRef] [PubMed]
108. Willett, M.C.; Edward, D.P. Refractory Topiramate-Induced Angle-Closure Glaucoma in a Man: A Case Report. *J. Med. Case Rep.* **2011**, *5*, 33. [CrossRef] [PubMed]
109. Natesh, S.; Rajashekhara, S.K.; Rao, A.S.D.; Shetty, B. Topiramate-Induced Angle Closure with Acute Myopia, Macular Striae. *Oman J. Ophthalmol.* **2010**, *3*, 26–28. [CrossRef]
110. Acharya, N.; Nithyanandam, S.; Kamat, S. Topiramate-Associated Bilateral Anterior Uveitis and Angle Closure Glaucoma. *Indian J. Ophthalmol.* **2010**, *58*, 557–559. [CrossRef]
111. Spaccapelo, L.; Leschiutta, S.; Aurea, C.; Ferrari, A. Topiramate-Associated Acute Angle Closure Glaucoma in a Migraine Patient Receiving Concomitant Citalopram Therapy: A Case-Report. *Cases J.* **2009**, *2*, 87. [CrossRef]
112. Sbeity, Z.; Gvozdyuk, N.; Amde, W.; Liebmann, J.M.; Ritch, R. Argon Laser Peripheral Iridoplasty for Topiramate-Induced Bilateral Acute Angle Closure. *J. Glaucoma* **2009**, *18*, 269–271. [CrossRef]
113. Chalam, K.V.; Tillis, T.; Syed, F.; Agarwal, S.; Brar, V.S. Acute Bilateral Simultaneous Angle Closure Glaucoma after Topiramate Administration: A Case Report. *J. Med. Case Rep.* **2008**, *2*, 1. [CrossRef]
114. Boonyaleephan, S. Bilateral Acute Onset Myopia and Angle Closure Glaucoma after Oral Topiramate: A Case Report. *J. Med. Assoc. Thai.* **2008**, *91*, 1904–1907. [PubMed]
115. Aminlari, A.; East, M.; Wei, W.; Quillen, D. Topiramate Induced Acute Angle Closure Glaucoma. *Open Ophthalmol. J.* **2008**, *2*, 46–47. [CrossRef]
116. Singh, S.K.; Thapa, S.S.; Badhu, B.P. Topiramate Induced Bilateral Angle-Closure Glaucoma. *Kathmandu Univ. Med. J. KUMJ* **2007**, *5*, 234–236. [PubMed]
117. Parikh, R.; Parikh, S.; Das, S.; Thomas, R. Choroidal Drainage in the Management of Acute Angle Closure after Topiramate Toxicity. *J. Glaucoma* **2007**, *16*, 691–693. [CrossRef] [PubMed]
118. Viet Tran, H.; Ravinet, E.; Schnyder, C.; Reichhart, M.; Guex-Crosier, Y. Blood-Brain Barrier Disruption Associated with Topiramate-Induced Angle-Closure Glaucoma of Acute Onset. *Klin. Monbl. Augenheilkd.* **2006**, *223*, 425–427. [CrossRef]
119. Sachi, D.; Vijaya, L. Topiramate Induced Secondary Angle Closure Glaucoma. *J. Postgrad. Med.* **2006**, *52*, 72–73.
120. Rhee, D.J.; Ramos-Esteban, J.C.; Nipper, K.S. Rapid Resolution of Topiramate-Induced Angle-Closure Glaucoma with Methylprednisolone and Mannitol. *Am. J. Ophthalmol.* **2006**, *141*, 1133–1134. [CrossRef]
121. Levy, J.; Yagev, R.; Petrova, A.; Lifshitz, T. Topiramate-Induced Bilateral Angle-Closure Glaucoma. *Can. J. Ophthalmol.* **2006**, *41*, 221–225. [CrossRef]
122. Desai, C.M.; Ramchandani, S.J.; Bhopale, S.G.; Ramchandani, S.S. Acute Myopia and Angle Closure Caused by Topiramate, a Drug Used for Prophylaxis of Migraine. *Indian J. Ophthalmol.* **2006**, *54*, 195–197.
123. Mansoor, Q.; Jain, S. Bilateral Angle-Closure Glaucoma Following Oral Topiramate Therapy. *Acta Ophthalmol. Scand.* **2005**, *83*, 627–628. [CrossRef]
124. Craig, J.E.; Ong, T.J.; Louis, D.L.; Wells, J.M. Mechanism of Topiramate-Induced Acute-Onset Myopia and Angle Closure Glaucoma. *Am. J. Ophthalmol.* **2004**, *137*, 193–195. [CrossRef]
125. Boentert, M.; Aretz, H.; Ludemann, P. Acute Myopia and Angle-Closure Glaucoma Induced by Topiramate. *Neurology* **2003**, *61*, 1306. [CrossRef] [PubMed]
126. Medeiros, F.A.; Zhang, X.Y.; Bernd, A.S.; Weinreb, R.N. Angle-Closure Glaucoma Associated with Ciliary Body Detachment in Patients Using Topiramate. *Arch. Ophthalmol.* **2003**, *12*, 282–285. [CrossRef]
127. Chen, T.C.; Chao, C.W.; Sorkin, J.A. Topiramate Induced Myopic Shift and Angle Closure Glaucoma. *Br. J. Ophthalmol.* **2003**, *87*, 648–649. [CrossRef] [PubMed]
128. Banta, J.T.; Hoffman, K.; Budenz, D.L.; Ceballos, E.; Greenfield, D.S. Presumed Topiramate-Induced Bilateral Acute Angle-Closure Glaucoma. *Am. J. Ophthalmol.* **2001**, *132*, 112–114. [CrossRef]

129. Sankar, P.S.; Pasquale, L.R.; Grosskreutz, C.L. Uveal Effusion and Secondary Angle-Closure Glaucoma Associated with Topiramate Use. *Arch. Ophthalmol.* **2001**, *119*, 1210–1211.
130. Rhee, D.J.; Goldberg, M.J.; Parrish, R.K. Bilateral Angle-Closure Glaucoma and Ciliary Body Swelling from Topiramate. *Arch. Ophthalmol.* **2001**, *119*, 1721–1723.

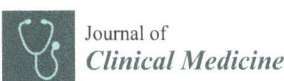

Review

Devices and Treatments to Address Low Adherence in Glaucoma Patients: A Narrative Review

Barbara Cvenkel [1,2,*] and Miriam Kolko [3,4]

1. Department of Ophthalmology, University Medical Centre Ljubljana, 1000 Ljubljana, Slovenia
2. Medical Faculty, University of Ljubljana, 1000 Ljubljana, Slovenia
3. Department of Drug Design and Pharmacology, University of Copenhagen, 2100 Copenhagen, Denmark
4. Department of Ophthalmology, Copenhagen University Hospital, Rigshospitalet, 2600 Glostrup, Denmark
* Correspondence: barbara.cvenkel@gmail.com

Abstract: Poor adherence to topical glaucoma medications has been linked to worse visual field outcomes in glaucoma patients. Therefore, identifying and overcoming the adherence barriers are expected to slow down the progression of disease. The most common barriers to adherence, in addition to the lack of knowledge, include forgetfulness, side effects of medications, difficulties with drop instillation and low self-efficacy. Symptoms and signs of ocular surface disease, which importantly reduce patients' quality of life, are decreased by using preservative-free topical medications. Sustained drug delivery systems using different vehicles seem promising for relieving the burden of drop administration. Currently, only the bimatoprost sustained-release intracameral implant is available for clinical use and single administration. In the era of digitalization, smart drug delivery-connected devices may aid adherence and, by sharing data with care providers, improve monitoring and adjusting treatment. Selective laser trabeculoplasty as first-line treatment delays the need for drops, whereas minimally invasive glaucoma procedures with and without devices combined with cataract surgery increase the likelihood of patients with early-to-moderate glaucoma to remain drop free or reduce the number of drops needed to control intraocular pressure. The aim of this narrative review is to present and discuss devices and treatments that may improve adherence by reducing the need for drops and side effects of medications and aiding in glaucoma monitoring. For the future, there is a need for studies focusing on clinically important outcomes, quality of life and the cost of intervention with longer post-interventional follow up.

Keywords: adherence; drug delivery system; glaucoma; laser trabeculoplasty; medical treatment; minimally invasive glaucoma surgery

1. Introduction

Lowering of intraocular pressure (IOP) is the only proven treatment to slow or delay the progression of glaucoma [1–4]. Medical treatment is the most common approach to achieving an individual eye "safe" IOP, followed by monitoring to determine the rate of progression [5]. As glaucoma is chronic optic neuropathy, and patients usually need to take lifelong medications. Therefore, adherence to a treatment regimen is crucial to maintain visual function. The reported rates of nonadherence to topical glaucoma medication vary widely from 16% to 67%, reflecting different methods to identify nonadherence as well as absence of a quantitative standard for measuring adherence to glaucoma medication [6]. Adherence over a longer period has been found to be even lower. Thus, only one-quarter of patients with newly diagnosed glaucoma continued their glaucoma medication after 2 years of follow up in Taiwan [7], whereas only 15% with newly diagnosed glaucoma in another study showed persistently good adherence over 4 years of follow up [8]. For most patients of newly prescribed glaucoma medications, adherence patterns observed in the first year of treatment mirror adherence patterns over the subsequent 3 years [8]. It is recognized that poorer adherence to glaucoma treatment leads to higher IOP, greater fluctuations in

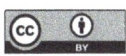

Citation: Cvenkel, B.; Kolko, M. Devices and Treatments to Address Low Adherence in Glaucoma Patients: A Narrative Review. *J. Clin. Med.* **2023**, *12*, 151. https://doi.org/10.3390/jcm12010151

Academic Editors: Michele Lanza and Luigi Fontana

Received: 7 November 2022
Revised: 5 December 2022
Accepted: 21 December 2022
Published: 24 December 2022

Copyright: © 2022 by the authors. Licensee MDPI, Basel, Switzerland. This article is an open access article distributed under the terms and conditions of the Creative Commons Attribution (CC BY) license (https://creativecommons.org/licenses/by/4.0/).

IOP and consequently progression of glaucoma [9–11]. Glaucoma patients who reported less than 80% adherence to their prescribed medications were significantly more likely to have worse visual field defects [11]. Few studies longitudinally assessed the relationship between medication adherence and visual field progression. A longitudinal study assessing adherence in 35 glaucoma patients reported that patients with a stable visual field had a significantly higher median adherence rate of 85% compared to progressing patients with a median medication adherence of 21% [12]. In another study, patients randomized to the treatment arm of the Collaborative Initial Glaucoma Treatment Study were assessed for medication adherence using telephone interviews scheduled at the same 6-month intervals as clinical visits but on different days and followed up for an average of 7.3 years [13]. Scheduling timing of telephone interviews independently of clinical visit represents a strength of the study as nonadherence is often not admitted in front of the treating physician. Patients who reported never missing a dose of medication over the follow up had an average mean deviation (MD) loss of 0.62 dB over time, consistent with age-related loss, whereas patients missing medication doses at one-third and two-thirds of visits had an average loss of 1.42 and 2.23 dB of MD, respectively [13]. These findings indicate a dose–response relationship between medication adherence and visual field progression. A range of factors affect adherence and persistence, with one study identifying 71 barriers to adherence over four categories: situation factors, medication regimen, individual patient factors and medical provider issues [14]. Patients with poor adherence cited several barriers to medication adherence, which varied between individuals. The most important barriers associated with nonadherence included forgetfulness, low self-efficacy, difficulties with drop instillation and treatment schedule, side effects of medication, lack of motivation, poor education and other specific individual and age differences [15–17]. In addition, certain types of disabilities such as having a limb disability, being in a vegetative state, and having dementia reduce glaucoma medication adherence by up to 17.6% [18]. Therefore, approaches addressing adherence to glaucoma medications need to be multifaceted and individually tailored [19].

The purpose of this narrative review is to discuss strategies that may improve adherence by reducing the side effects of drops, the number of instillations and the number of medications required to control intraocular pressure. These approaches include medical treatments using preservative-free drops, intracameral sustained drug delivery and various drug delivery systems still undergoing clinical trials, smart drug delivery-connected devices as well as selective laser trabeculoplasty and minimally invasive glaucoma surgery.

2. Materials and Methods

We conducted a literature search using the PubMed database. The following search terms were included "adherence" AND "glaucoma medication", "topical treatment" AND "glaucoma", drug delivery systems and glaucoma treatment, "selective laser trabeculoplasty", and "minimally invasive glaucoma surgery". The articles retrieved were reviewed for their title, abstract, and language. Articles included were in in English language published before August 2022 including clinical trials in humans, editorials, reviews, systematic reviews, and meta-analyses. We focused on randomized clinical trials (when available). After retrieving relevant articles using keywords, a search was performed through the reference lists of the chosen studies and additional papers were selected.

3. Medical Treatments

3.1. Preservative-Free Drops

Adverse drug reactions are a major barrier to adherence and persistence. Local side effects can vary from minor dry eye symptoms to allergic and toxic-inflammatory responses [20]. The use of preservatives, especially benzalkonium chloride (BAK), is a known cause of ocular surface disease (OSD) in patients taking topical IOP-lowering eye drops [21]. In a survey study in French glaucoma patients, 62% of the patients cited at least one OSD side effect and 19% of patients at least four such side effects [22]. The reported prevalence of OSD among glaucoma patients in other studies is similar, between 60% and 70%, which is much higher than in age-matched subjects without glaucoma (between 15% and 33%) [23–25]. Self-reported nonadherence over 9.4 years, defined as missing ≥5% of the prescribed eye drops, was reported by 30% of participants [26]. Individuals who experienced side effects reported significantly higher levels of nonadherence than those who did not (37.6% vs. 18.4%) [26]. The side effects of OSD were associated with a reduced quality of life and worsening of quality-of-life scores correlated with reduced adherence captured by a questionnaire [22]. Several studies reported that the severity and prevalence of OSD in glaucoma patients correlated with the number of preserved drops per day and duration of treatment [24,27,28].

The improvement of symptoms and signs of OSD after switching from preserved to preservative-free eye drops has been shown in many studies [29–33]. In a large prospective survey including 4107 participants, Pisella et al. reported that patients taking preserved eye drops had significantly more symptoms and signs of OSD than those taking preservative-free eye drops [29]. For patients experiencing more pronounced signs and symptoms of ocular irritation, a treatment change from preserved to preservative-free eye drops significantly decreased the prevalence of all symptoms and signs. Jaenen et al. in a cross-sectional study including 9658 patients assessed subjective symptoms and signs of ocular irritation [30]. Each symptom and all the signs (blepharitis, eczema, hyperemia, and fluorescein staining) were significantly more frequent in patients taking preserved than in patients on preservative-free eye drops [30]. At the time of these two studies, most patients used preserved hypotensive drops, and the choice of preservative-free formulations on the market was limited. Following the launch of preservative-free tafluprost and a preservative-free fixed combination of timolol with dorzolamide, preservative-free latanoprost and bimatoprost and later their fixed combinations with timolol became available. Several studies have compared the efficacy and tolerability of preservative-free prostaglandin analogues and their fixed combinations to their preserved counterpart and found that preservative-free formulations are noninferior in their IOP-lowering effect and associated with less signs and symptoms of OSD. Patients with ocular symptoms or signs of OSD on preserved latanoprost (Xalatan®; Pfizer, New York, NY, USA) were switched to preservative-free tafluprost (Taflotan®; Santen Oy, Finland) which had similar IOP-lowering effect as preserved latanoprost but was better tolerated and resulted in a decrease in symptoms and signs, and improved quality of life and patients' satisfaction [31,34]. The same efficacy and better tolerability have been shown for a preservative-free latanoprost (Monopost®, Thea Pharmaceuticals, France) compared with preserved latanoprost (Xalatan®; Pfizer, New York, NY, USA) [35]. Pillunat et al. [33] evaluated in an open-label study efficacy and tolerability of preservative-free fixed combination of tafluprost/timolol (Taptiqom®; Santen Oy, Tampere, Finland) in 1157 patients. Preservative-free fixed combination lowered IOP in all subgroups of patients: treatment naïve, prior monotherapy and prior fixed combinations. At the final visit at 16 weeks, symptoms, and signs of OSD improved in patients with prior medical therapy and, using a simple questionnaire, 90% of patients rated treatment comfort as very good or good [33].

3.2. Sustained Drug Delivery Systems

Development of sustained drug delivery vehicles has been an ongoing search to improve adherence among patients. These drug delivery systems may be applied onto the ocular surface (contact lenses, nanoparticles, microspheres, extraocular inserts), in the puncta (punctal plugs) or injected into the eye. Different novel drug delivery techniques are in different stages of development and only one, the intracameral bimatoprost SR ocular implant (Durysta®; Allergan, Irvine, CA, USA) has been recently approved by the FDA for sustained IOP reduction [36].

3.2.1. Nanoparticles

To overcome the limitations of topical antiglaucoma medications, nanoparticulate (NP) delivery systems may improve solubility of the drug and corneal penetration, increase concentration at the target tissue, reduce irritation and systemic side effects and provide dose accuracy and sustained release of the drug [37]. Nanoparticles, tiny structures ranging from 1 to 100 nm in size, can bypass biological barriers and deliver drug to the target tissue. Nanoparticles are used in different shapes such as nanoemulsions, dendrimers, liposomes, nanospheres, hydrogels, nanocrystals, nanodiamonds, microspheres, niosomes, nanofibers, and nanocapsules [37]. Lipid and polymer nanoparticles are usually used to carry the drugs, isolate their contents from degradation and regulate their release. Several drugs using a NP delivery system are under investigation, but currently none has been approved for clinical use [38].

3.2.2. Contact Lenses

The contact lens drug delivery system is also very attractive. As the bioavailability of drugs with drop instillations is very low, the incorporation of drugs into the contact lens matrix increases the drug residence time on the cornea and improves drug bioavailability by more than 50% compared to eye drops [39]. Achieving sustained or prolonged release of the drug from the contact lens allows for reduced frequency of drop instillation and potentially improved adherence. Different drug loading methods are used to incorporate drugs into polymeric support [39,40]. At present, most of the glaucoma drug-loaded therapeutic contact lenses are in the preclinical or clinical stages and data regarding safety, efficacy and pharmacokinetics are required [41].

3.2.3. Extraocular Inserts

Ocular inserts of different forms and sizes are shaped to fit into the conjunctival fornices. These inserts increase the ocular surface contact time of the drug, improve its bioavailability and reduce the need for frequent drop instillation. Among the first approved ocular inserts, Ocusert™ was placed under the eyelid and released pilocarpine over one week [42]. Although it was effective in reducing IOP, its use was limited by device dislodgement and high cost. Ocusert™ is not available on the market since 1993.

Another insert, bimatoprost sustained-release fornix ring-type insert, is in the late stage of development for clinical use. The insert achieved IOP reduction over 6 months similar to timolol 0.5% BID drops, was safe and well tolerated [43]. In a 13 months open-label extension study the bimatoprost ring showed good retention rate with a median IOP reduction of 4 mmHg (interquartile range 2–6) [44]. The most frequently reported adverse events from both studies were mucous eye discharge (16%), conjunctival hyperemia (14%) and punctate keratitis (12%).

3.2.4. Punctal Delivery Systems

Different solutions, suspensions, emulsions, nanoparticle or microparticle or liposome suspensions can be loaded into the core of the plug [45]. The latanoprost punctal plug delivery system (Mati Therapeutics) was loaded with 70.5 µg of latanoprost per device. When two such plugs were inserted in the upper and lower puncta, the mean IOP was reduced by 5.7 mmHg (22.3%) from baseline after 4 weeks [46]. The latanoprost-loaded punctal plug was well tolerated, with tearing reported as the most frequent adverse event.

The travoprost punctal plug (OTX-TP, Ocular Therapeutics, Bedford, MA, USA) is a rod-shaped hydrogel rod that swells in the canalliculus, thus preventing extrusion. Travoprost is encapsulated in polylactic acid microparticles for sustained release to the tear film over 90 days [47]. In the double-masked phase 2b study (NCT02312544) comparing the safety and efficacy of sustained-release travoprost plug delivery to timolol eyedrops in patients with open-angle glaucoma or ocular hypertension, OTX-TP plugs reduced IOP by 4.5–5.7 mmHg, whereas timolol reduced IOP by 6.4 mmHg–7.6 mmHg. The superb efficacy of timolol eye drops is likely the effect of decreased wash-out through the nasolacrimal ducts by inert punctal plugs. In an Asian population, sustained-release travoprost reduced IOP by 24% at 10 days, and by 15.6% at day 30 [48].

Among the major limitations of the punctal drug delivery system is that only low drug doses, typically required for potent drugs (e.g., prostaglandins and corticosteroids), can be embedded into the plug core matrix. At present the only punctal delivery system available on the market is dexamethasone 0.4 mg insert (Dextenza™, Ocular Therapeutix) approved by the FDA in 2018 for the treatment of ocular inflammation and pain following ophthalmic surgery.

3.2.5. The Periocular Drug Delivery System

For the subconjunctival route, several delivery systems can be used such as implants, microspheres, nanospheres, liposomes, and gels [45]. Most of the studies were performed in rabbits by injecting a subconjunctival formulation of timolol, brimonidine, latanoprost and carbonic anhydrase inhibitors and achieved good IOP reduction without signs of inflammation for up to 90 days, depending on the delivery system used [49–54]. In a pilot study (NCT01987323) including six patients, a nanoliposome-based latanoprost delivery system was well tolerated, and in five out of six patients IOP reduction achieved at 3 months was as effective as previous reports of latanoprost ophthalmic solution [55]. A recently completed randomized trial including 80 participants (NCT02466399) comparing the efficacy of subconjunctival liposomal latanoprost injection to latanoprost ophthalmic solution reported a mean change in IOP at month 3 of −2.3 mmHg (SD 4.6) and of −6.4 mmHg (SD 2.9), respectively. Adverse events were reported in the liposomal latanoprost group only, with the most frequent being conjunctival hemorrhage (26.4%), foreign body sensation (17.0%), and conjunctival hyperemia (13.2%). To date, no subconjunctival delivery system has been approved, suggesting inherent delivery and efficiency limitations associated with these delivery systems.

3.2.6. Intraocular/Intracameral Drug Delivery

Bimatoprost intracameral implant 10 µg (Durysta®; Allergan, Irvine, CA, USA) is the only sustained-release glaucoma therapy approved by the FDA in March 2020 for the lowering of IOP in patients with open-angle glaucoma or ocular hypertension [56]. It is a rod-shaped biodegradable implant based on a poly (lactic-co-glycol) acid matrix Novadur® platform, used in dexamethasone intravitreal implant (Ozurdex®, Allergan, Irvine, CA, USA) and provides steady bimatoprost release for up to 6 months [57]. A single-use, 28-gauge sterile applicator is used for intracameral administration. Several doses were studied in clinical trials with the 10 µg of bimatoprost having the best balance between safety and efficacy [58–60]. The 10 µg of drug released is equivalent to a single drop of bimatoprost 0.03% ophthalmic solution [61]. The FDA approval for a new drug application was based on the results of two phase 3 clinical studies comparing administration of 10 and 15 µg bimatoprost implant with twice daily timolol maleate 0.5% eye drops. Both implants showed noninferiority to topical timolol eye drops in lowering IOP through 12 weeks but with more adverse events such as corneal edema and endothelial cell loss than in the topical timolol group, especially with the 15-µg implant after repeated administration [60,62]. Long-term retention of the implant beyond the optimal drug effect period is another disadvantage when considering readministration. For this reason, the 10 µg bimatoprost implant with a better benefit–risk ratio was approved by the FDA and limited to a single intracameral administration. Pooled analysis of the two phase 3 studies reported that the percentage of bimatoprost 10 µg-treated patients with at least 20% IOP lowering from baseline in the study eye was 72% at week 12 and 57% at week 15 [63]. The IOP-lowering efficacy of the bimatoprost 10 µg implant declined from week 12 to week 15. In the 24-month phase 1/2 study, 21 patients received the 10 µg bimatoprost implant in the study eye and topical bimatoprost 0.03% in the fellow eye [59]. The percentage of eyes receiving the bimatoprost implant with at least 20% reduction from baseline was 76.2% (16/21) at week 12 and 52.4% (11/21) at week 16. Interestingly, in 5 patients who reached month 24 without re-treatment or additional hypotensive medication, the IOP-lowering effect at the final visit was similar to the effect of once-daily topical bimatoprost [59].

Ongoing clinical trials (NCT03891446, NCT03850782) are evaluating the efficacy of IOP lowering and the safety of readministration of the bimatoprost implant (Durysta®) over 24 to 48 months. Of interest are clinical trials comparing the efficacy and safety of bimatoprost SR to selective laser trabeculoplasty (SLT), of which one (NCT023636946) was completed last year. This study included 144 participants with open-angle glaucoma or ocular hypertension who were not adequately managed with topical IOP-lowering medications for reasons other than medication efficacy (e.g., due to intolerance or nonadherence) and were randomized to the bimatoprost SR 15 µg or SLT treatment groups. The primary outcome measure was change from baseline IOP at week 4, 12 and 24. The bimatoprost SR 15 µg was noninferior in IOP reduction to SLT at all scheduled visits. The second ongoing trial (NCT02507687) is comparing the IOP-lowering effect and the safety of bimatoprost SR (Durysta®) compared with SLT in patients with open-angle glaucoma or ocular hypertension who are not adequately managed with topical IOP-lowering medication. The findings of both aforementioned ongoing studies can support clinical decision, but also the long-term safety, repeatability and cost-effectiveness need to be considered. As a result of the prolonged IOP-lowering effect of bimatoprost SR, an ongoing trial is also investigating the efficacy and safety of treat and extend (NCT03850782) of Durysta®. No current results are available.

Another intracameral implant in a phase 2 clinical trial (NCT02371746) is the ENV515 travoprost extended release (XR) (Envisia therapeutics, Research Triangle Park, NC, USA), using a biodegradable polymer as the drug delivery system. Single intracameral administration of a low dose of the ENV515 reduced the mean IOP by 6.7 mmHg (SD 3.7) at 11 months. Lowering of IOP was comparable to latanoprost, bimatoprost (reports) and the in-study 0.5 timolol maleate topical daily drops. Ocular hyperemia, punctate keratitis and foreign body sensation were the most common adverse events (NCT02371746).

The iDose travoprost implant (Glaukos Inc., San Clemente, CA, USA) is a titanium intracameral delivery system that elutes travoprost. It is placed through a small corneal incision and anchored to trabecular meshwork. The membrane within the implant controls the release of travoprost into the anterior chamber. Once depleted, the implant can be removed and exchanged for continued treatment [47]. Ongoing clinical trials (NCT02754596, NCT03868124, and NCT03519386) are comparing different elution rates of the travoprost implant to topical timolol 0.5% dosed twice daily. In a phase 2b study (NCT02754596), mean IOP lowering at the 36 months was 8.3 and 8.5 mmHg in the fast and- slow-release travoprost implant, respectively, versus 8.2 mmHg in the timolol control arm. The 36-month phase 2 data did not show clinically significant corneal endothelial cell loss, no serious corneal adverse events and periorbital fat atrophy and conjunctival hyperemia in either elution arm [64]. Repeated procedures and presence of the implant in the angle for continued treatment may be associated with adverse events related to surgical procedure and long-term effect on the corneal endothelial cells. A phase 2 study is evaluating the safety of the operative and surgical exchange procedure of the travoprost intraocular implant (NCT04615403).

Travoprost for a slow and extended release, OTX-TIC (Ocular Therapeutix, Bedford, MA, USA), has also been incorporated in a fully biodegradable implant that is administered into the anterior chamber with a 27 G or 26 G needle. In OTX-TIC, travoprost-loaded microparticles are embedded in hydrogel, which allows for an extended release of travoprost for a 4–6-month duration. A phase 2 study (NCT05335122) is evaluating the efficacy and safety of the OTX-TIC low- and high-dose intracameral implant in patients with open-angle glaucoma or ocular hypertension and comparing 2 travoprost dose strength to a single injection of bimatoprost SR (Durysta®).

4. Monitoring Devices and Smart Drug Delivery Systems

The challenge of how to monitor adherence has been differently addressed and some studies used more than one method. The most common objective way of measuring adherence is electronic monitoring using a medication event monitoring system (MEMS), followed by pharmacy records [65]. A MEMS is a cap that fits on bottles and records the time and date each time the bottle is opened and closed. The Travatan Dosing Aid was among the first electronic monitoring devices designed to hold a bottle of travoprost. The device had attached base that recorded time when the lever that administered the medication was fully depressed, and the data were downloaded from the device [66]. Electronic monitoring using a MEMS has been used to assess the rate of adherence, identify patients' characteristics associated with poor adherence and evaluate its change after different interventions to improve adherence [67–73]. Adherence data collected by a MEMS have shown that patients with glaucoma, especially those newly diagnosed were likely to overreport the percentage of doses taken [70,74,75]. Recently, Japanese researchers have developed and evaluated an eye dropper bottle sensor system comprising motion sensor with automatic motion waveform analysis using deep learning to accurately measure adherence of patients with antiglaucoma ophthalmic solution therapy [76]. An eye dropper bottle sensor was installed at patients' homes, and they were asked to instill the medication and manually record each instillation time for 3 days. Waveform data were automatically collected from the eye dropper bottle sensor and judged as a complete instillation by the deep learning instillation assessment model. The eye dropper bottle sensor system successfully auto extracted the instillation data of 20 patients with glaucoma for 3 days with 100% accuracy in a moment and may be an option to objectively measure adherence in clinical practice [76].

Innovative solutions have been developed in the area of smart drug delivery. The benefits include better monitoring, user support, uploading data from different devices that are integrated using different platforms and made accessible to health care providers. Smart drug delivery makes treatment management for patients easier and may improve their adherence, integrated data shared with the eyecare providers can provide better monitoring and communications, all of which may increase treatment efficacy. In addition, smart drug delivery enhances treatment efficiency as the prescriptions are timely fulfilled without stopping therapy, which may lead to improved control of disease and less hospitalization. These innovations were introduced to improve adherence and monitoring of other chronic diseases, such as diabetes and asthma. Various smart insulin pens have been developed, including smart pen caps that automatically capture injection data and enable immediate transmission of data from the pen via Bluetooth or near-field communication to a smartphone application and into digital storage, so the stored data can be viewed by health care providers or caregivers [77–79]. Studies showed that patients preferred smart insulin pens as they increased their confidence in diabetes management, but there was a lack of published data regarding smart insulin pens with connectivity [77].

Kali Drop (Kali Care, Santa Clara, CA, USA) represents a potential improvement in the eye care by directly measuring regimen adherence in patients using topical medications [80]. This device is a compact, 3G wireless monitor that electronically transmits medication use (e.g., number of drops dispensed, time, and date taken) in real time through wireless networks to a user-friendly interface that may be used by patients, caregivers, and providers to view and track adherence to topical therapy. The device was used in a pilot study comparing use of topical medications for 2 months between a wireless monitoring device and validated self-reported measures of glaucoma medication adherence [81]. Median adherence as measured by the device and self-report differed and dropped slightly after 1 month for both. This suggests that despite participating in a study and knowing they will be monitored, adherence wanes over short time. The majority of subjects found the device easy to use and reported that it did not interfere with their daily activities, and they were not bothered by the physician tracking their eye administration. However, this study included a small sample (23 subjects) with a short follow up. Studies including more patients in a real-world setting with longer monitoring would add additional information about usability of this device.

E-Novelia® (Nemera, La Verpillière, France) is a smart drug delivery-connected device. It is designed as an add-on to existing preservative-free formulations for glaucoma or dry eye treatment and is applicable across different medications. It has the potential to improve an already existing way of drop instillation and adherence [82]. This approach requires the use of the company's own custom eye drop medication bottles to latch to a system that contains the embedded sensors. The device has several electronic features that could be transferred across multiple device platforms: tilt sensor and LED indication for device positioning, location tracking, remaining drug indicator, treatment history and compliance, shelf-life management, drop detection, electronic instructions for use, smartphone application and notification, shaking formulation indication, and RFID tag on eyedropper bottle to collect data.

In the United States, an intelligent sleeve, a monitoring system capable of detecting and quantifying eye drop medication use without altering the original medication packaging has been developed [83]. The prescription bottle is placed in the sleeve with the embedded sensors and electronics that measure fluid level, dropper orientation, the state of the dropper top (on/off), and rates of angular motion during an application. The sleeve was tested with ten patients (age $\geq$ 65) and successfully identified and timestamped 94% of use events [83]. Data from the sensors are transmitted from the system to a smart phone or another Bluetooth-connected device. Health care providers can use this information to support clinical decisions.

This technology has the potential to be useful for patients, and health care providers that will benefit from following and adjusting treatment. The limitation of these devices is that they measure drop dispensing and not really drop instillation into the eye itself. A pilot study using imaging system to record video of the drop technique has shown that few patients were able to properly apply the drops. Most had issues either getting the drops in their eyes, applying the correct number of drops, touching the bottle to the eye or adnexa or some combination of the above [84]. We did not find any studies evaluating adherence in the real world using smart drug delivery-connected devices in glaucoma patients.

5. Selective Laser Trabeculoplasty

Selective laser trabeculoplasty (SLT) has fewer adverse events, improved repeatability and ease of use compared to its predecessor argon laser trabeculoplasty. It is an outpatient laser procedure which lowers IOP by increasing aqueous outflow through the trabecular meshwork. The procedure is indicated to lower IOP in open-angle glaucoma and ocular hypertension as first-line treatment or as an add-on or replacement treatment (e.g., nonadherence or intolerance) [5]. The LiGHT trial showed that there was no difference between SLT and eye drops used for first-line therapy over the 36 months period in achieving target IOP (20% or 30% IOP reduction), health-related quality of life, adverse events and treatment adherence in newly diagnosed patients with open-angle glaucoma and ocular hypertension [85]. This trial also reported that people who were given eye drops as first-line treatment, used more eye drops and required the use of more than 1 eye drop medication at 12 months, compared with people who were given SLT as first-line treatment. Furthermore, three-quarters of the patients initially treated with laser did not need any eye drops for the first 3 years of treatment and had a reduced need for surgery [86]. To achieve target IOP over 36 months, SLT needed to be repeated in approximately 15% of people in the SLT arm within the first year [86]. Visual field outcomes (median 9 visual fields over 48 months) showed that a slightly greater number of eyes (56 eyes (9.5%)) treated with medical therapy first had fast visual field progression defined as total deviation progression < -1 dB/year compared with those treated first with SLT (32 eyes (5.4%)) [87]. Cost-effectiveness analysis, pertinent to the United Kingdom, where the trial was conducted, showed that first-line treatment with 360° SLT was more effective and less costly compared with eye drops and should be offered as initial treatment in patients with open-angle glaucoma and ocular hypertension meeting the inclusion criteria of this trial [85]. No difference in adherence between the medical and SLT first-treated arm in the LiGHT trial may be due to patient selection, including highly motivated people with extensive support, which is not the case in practice [7,75,88]. Another prospective multicenter clinical trial comparing the effectiveness of SLT with topical medication as initial treatment did not find that SLT was superior over medication in improving glaucoma-specific health-related quality of life in newly diagnosed primary open-angle and exfoliative glaucoma patients over 2-year follow up [89]. More individuals in the medication arm had conjunctival hyperemia and eyelid erythema compared with the SLT at 24 months. Successful IOP reduction, defined as IOP-lowering of 25% or more from baseline, was superior in the medication arm compared with the SLT arm. The differences in findings between the two studies are probably caused by the differences in trial design, population and sample size. For participants with early to moderate primary open-angle and exfoliation glaucoma, no separate analysis by the subtype of glaucoma was performed [89,90].

Based on the evidence of the LiGHT trial regarding cost effectiveness, the National Institute for Health and Care Excellence (NICE) guidelines recommends that 360° SLT should be offered as first-line treatment to people with newly diagnosed ocular hypertension with IOP of 24 mmHg or more (and if they are at risk of visual impairment during their lifetime) or chronic open-angle glaucoma [91]. In the published literature, the most common adverse events are transient elevation of IOP, especially in eyes with heavily pigmented trabecular meshwork within the first 2 h after SLT (greater than 6 mmHg in 3.4% of eyes) and mild iritis which resolves in a few days [92,93]. Rare adverse events described in case reports include transient changes in the corneal endothelium on specular microscopy in eyes with pigment on endothelium [94], recurrence or worsening of macular edema [95–97] and hyphema [98,99].

In practice, adherence to topical eye drops is often overestimated and SLT relieves the burden of topical instillation, which is of concern especially in older people with co-morbidities and low-self efficacy [100,101]. There is a reduction in SLT effect over time, with approximately 50% of failure after 2 years [102]. Most commonly, the success of SLT has been defined as IOP reduction from a baseline of at least 20% or of 3 mmHg or greater and not by achieving target IOP [103–105]. The recommendation for repeating SLT are required, because repeat SLT treatment is usually performed in clinical setting. Most of the studies evaluating retreatments with SLT after prior SLT or ALT were retrospective and performed in a small number of patients with medically uncontrolled glaucoma [106–111]. They reported that repeat SLT effectively lowered IOP in eyes with initial successful SLT [106–108,111] and controlled IOP up to 24 months in approximately 30% of eyes [108], whereas in one study [109] the effect of repeat SLT was half of the effect of the initial treatment.

The post hoc analysis of the LiGHT trial also investigated whether IOP-lowering efficacy and duration of effect of repeat SLT were comparable to initial SLT in medication-naïve open-angle glaucoma and ocular hypertensive eyes [112]. A total of 115 eyes of 90 patients received repeat SLT during the first 18 months of the trial. Absolute IOP reduction at 2 months was greater after initial SLT compared to repeat SLT, but when adjusting for pretreatment IOP (greater IOP in the initial SLT than in the repeat SLT), the absolute IOP reduction was greater in repeat SLT [112]. However, the comparison between retrospective studies and the LiGHT trial regarding the efficacy of repeat SLT is difficult due to different populations and criteria of success. At this moment, there are no randomized clinical trials to recommend how many times SLT can be repeated and is still effective. However, based on clinical experience, effect from SLT might be reduced after repeating it more than 2 or 3 times. As glaucoma is a lifelong disease, for the future, we need knowledge about long-term SLT outcomes such as visual field progression at 5- or 10-year follow up.

6. Minimally Invasive Glaucoma Surgery

Minimally or microinvasive glaucoma surgery (MIGS) is a term collectively used to define a number of surgical procedures that involve a microincisional approach with minimal tissue trauma, have a higher safety profile than conventional drainage surgery and allow for rapid recovery with less impact on patients' quality of life [113]. In recent years many of these surgical procedures have been implemented in clinical practice. MIGS procedures and devices lower IOP by draining aqueous into Schlemm canal, the subconjunctival space, or the suprachoroidal space [114]. By reducing the number of or the need for drops these procedures have the potential to reduce side effects of topical treatment and improve adherence [6].

MIGS procedures are bleb forming or non-bleb. In order to differentiate, the term microinvasive bleb surgery (MIBS) has been introduced. The distinction is important as bleb-forming procedures need meticulous post-operative management and experience in filtering surgery. To prevent scarring and establish flow, adherence to a topical anti-inflammatory treatment regimen is important. MIBS can be placed ab externo or ab interno (within the eye). Only those procedures with an ab interno approach with clear corneal incision and sparing of conjunctiva are considered MIGS [115,116].

The only MIBS with ab interno approach is XEN gel stent microshunt (Allergan, Dublin, Ireland). Meta-analysis of 78 studies found that XEN gel stent effectively reduced IOP and number of glaucoma drops till 48 months after surgery, but had a higher needling rate compared to trabeculectomy [117]. Three-year outcomes of ab interno XEN gel standalone procedure or combined phaco-XEN showed similar IOP-lowering from baseline and decrease in the number of eye drops (approximately halved) in both groups [118]. Needling over 3 years was required in 93 out of total 212 eyes (44%), with the mean number of needling of 1.3 per eye [118]. This suggests that careful post-operative follow up and interventions are important to maintain functioning bleb, all of which require patients' adherence. Meta-analysis on the standalone XEN45 gel stent implantation in the treatment of open-angle glaucoma reported that the overall quality of current evidence is low, and there is the need for more randomized controlled trials and outcomes measured with a clinically meaningful definition of success [119].

MIGS implanted ab interno are required by the FDA to be performed at the time of cataract surgery. Therefore, the trial protocols compared a reduction in IOP and number of drops in eyes with MIGS combined with cataract surgery to cataract surgery alone [115]. MIGS implants that increase Schlemm canal outflow by either removing or bypassing juxtacanalicular trabecular meshwork tissue and inner wall of Schlemm canal include Trabectome® (NeoMedix Corporation, Tustin, CA, USA), iStent inject (Glaukos Inc., San Clemente, CA, USA) and Hydrus microstent (Ivantis, Inc., Irvine, CA, USA). Although Trabectome was approved by the FDA in 2004 there has been only one randomized trial comparing ab interno removal of angle tissue with trabectome combined with cataract surgery to trabeculectomy combined with cataract surgery [120]. Phaco-trabectome achieved similar IOP lowering at 6 and 12 months compared to phaco-trabeculectomy with similar medications required at 1 year and no serious complications in the phaco-trabectome group. The trial has low quality evidence for the outcomes of ab interno trabectome surgery for open-angle glaucoma, with only 19 patients included and termination before the intended sample was reached [121]. Another procedure, also termed ab interno goniotomy or trabeculectomy, uses Kahook dual blade device (KDB, New World Medical Inc., Rancho Cucamonga, CA, USA) to excise and remove trabecular meshwork tissue, thus increasing aqueous outflow via Schlemm canal. In patients with mild to moderate glaucoma, adding ab interno trabeculectomy with Kahook dual blade to phacoemuslification was not more effective than phacoemulsification alone, with a similar safety profile [122]. Some studies found greater IOP reduction for goniotomy with Kahook dual blade [123,124]. However, the findings cannot be compared, as studies have different designs, study populations and criteria of success. It seems that this procedure modestly reduces IOP and the number of eye drops at 12 months, comparable to iStent [125,126].

Data from two RCTs suggested that iStent in combination with phacoemulsification was more effective in lowering IOP than phacoemulsification alone and reduced required daily topical medications by 0.4 drops more than cataract surgery alone at 1 year [127,128]. A greater reduction in IOP without medication for iStent inject (a second generation of iStent delivering 2 implants) combined with cataract surgery than for cataract surgery alone was sustained and present at 2 year-follow up [129]. The iStent inject trial captured patient reported outcomes using Visual Function Questionnaire 25 and Ocular Surface Disease Questionnaire [130]. The responses from both questionnaires suggest that reducing medication burden with iStent inject may improve quality of life by improving ocular surface symptoms and thus facilitating vision-related activities.

Hydrus microstent (Ivantis Inc., Irvine, CA, USA), an 8 mm intracanalicular scaffold device inserted through a corneal incision in the trabecular meshwork, lowers IOP by increasing aqueous outflow via Schlemm canal. It was approved by the FDA in 2018 with cataract surgery to treat mild to moderate glaucoma. A study comparing real-world 24-month outcomes for Hydrus (120 eyes) or iStent inject (224 eyes) combined with cataract surgery in patients with mild to moderate open-angle glaucoma or ocular hypertension showed sustained IOP reduction with a good safety profile and no significant difference in IOP reduction between the groups [131]. There may be a small additional reduction in glaucoma medication usage following cataract surgery with iStent inject compared to Hydrus [131]. Recent meta-analysis found moderate certainty evidence that adding a Hydrus safely improved the likelihood of drop-free glaucoma control at medium-term (6–18 months) and long-term (>18 months) follow up and conferred 2.0 mmHg greater IOP reduction at long-term follow-up, compared with cataract surgery alone [132,133]. The latest systematic review and network meta-analysis including 6 prospective RCTs reported that the Hydrus implantation may have a slight advantage to achieve drop-free status versus the 1-iStent or 2-iStent implantation in combination with phacoemulsification [134]. Both device-augmented MIGS can reduce or delay the need for more invasive filtration surgery.

MIGS devices inserted ab interno that target the suprachoroidal route include the Cypass® microstent (Alcon, Laboratories, Texas, Inc., Texas, USA), iStent SUPRA® model G3 (Glaukos Inc., San Clemente, CA, USA) and the MINIject™ (iStar Medical, Wavre, Belgium). Cypass microstent combined with cataract surgery reduced IOP and the number of eye drops more than cataract surgery alone, but was associated with corneal endothelial cells loss and was withdrawn from the market by Alcon [135,136]. A study evaluating the efficacy and safety of suprachoroidal iStent SUPRA in conjunction with cataract surgery compared to cataract surgery alone has not published the results (NCT01461278). The MINIject, undergoing clinical trials, as a standalone procedure achieved 20% IOP reduction in all patients at 2 years [137], but a longer follow up to evaluate safety is required. MIGS devices using the suprachoridal pathway have not been a long-term success due to fibrosis and/or complications, hence improvement of material biocompatibility to limit foreign body reaction may overcome these barriers.

7. Discussion

Similarly to other chronic diseases, nonadherence to medication is a challenge to effective treatment of glaucoma. There are many barriers to adherence that need to be detected and the approach individually tailored [19]. The purpose of this review is to highlight different approaches to address adherence and relieve the burden of long-term frequent drop administration (Table 1). However, many of these approaches are still undergoing clinical trials.

Table 1. Summary of treatment options to address low adherence.

Treatment Option	Type	Advantages	Disadvantages/Limitations	Clinical Setting
1. Medical treatment				
Topical PF drugs		Reduce signs and symptoms of OSD, thus may improve adherence	Drop instillation is not reduced	PF drugs available for most of the drug classes
Sustained DDS		No or reduced need of drop instillation depending on the DDS; reduction in systemic and local side effects	Depends on the DDS; Lack of data on the dosage and administration regimen of these formulations, metabolic ways and ocular toxicity of all formulation components, their pharmacokinetics and pharmacodynamics, the release of the drug in different eye tissues, formulation stability, the influence of the method of the synthesis not only on physio-chemical properties of formulation but also on its physiological effect, the suitability of nanocarriers with respect to biodegradability and patient comfort, safety issues	Only 1 sustained DDS approved for clinical use, single drug loading
	Nanoparticles	Different forms: liposomes, dendrimers	Improved corneal penetration, higher concentration at target tissue, longer retention, sustained release; different NP systems investigated carrying different glaucoma drugs	See above limitations	Not approved for clinical use; in preclinical and clinical trials
	Contact lenses	Various types of drugs or delivery systems can be placed into the periphery of lens	Increased drug residence time > 30 min improves bioavailability, prolonged drug release	Changes in contact lens swelling and water content, transmittance, protein adherence, surface roughness, tensile strength, ion, and oxygen permeability and leaching of the drug during contact lens manufacture and storage	Preclinical studies: contact lens eluting latanoprost starting human trial
	Extraocular inserts	Bimatoprost ring insert	As above, IOP-lowering effect over 6 months similar to timolol eye drops	Foreign body reaction to insert? Long-term acceptance-dislodgement. Cost	Not approved for clinical use
	Punctal DDS	Different pharmaceutical forms loaded into the core of the plug	Reduced need of drop instillation	Only low drug doses of potent drugs (e.g., prostaglandins) can be loaded into the plug matrix. Long-term acceptance. Side effects	Not approved for clinical use; in clinical trials
	Periocular DDS	Different DDS, subconjunctival injections	Reduced need of drop instillation	Efficacy and safety issues depending on the DDS	Most studies in animals. Not approved for clinical use
	Intraocular/intracameral drug delivery	Biodegradable implants using different DDS (bimatoprost, travoprost); titanium implant eluting travoprost (needs to be exchanged)	No or reduced need of drop instillation, effective IOP lowering ≥ 6 months	Retention of implant beyond the optimal drug effect, long-term safety, and repeatability	Bimatoprost SR intracameral biodegradable implant approved for single administration. Ongoing trials

Table 1. *Cont.*

Treatment Option	Type	Advantages	Disadvantages/Limitations	Clinical Setting
2. Monitoring systems and smart DDS	MEMS caps for electronic monitoring. Smart drug delivery-connected devices	Supporting adherence by providing information to patients (alerts, remaining drug volume, positioning), health care providers	Studies showing improved adherence over short-term, measure drop dispensing and not drops landing into the eye. No real-world data, cost Data protection issues	Smart drug delivery-connected devices
3. SLT		Postpones the need for medical treatment, safe, can be repeated	Greater effect in eyes with higher pre-SLT IOP; reduction in effect over time. Lack of data about long-term SLT outcomes (visual field), how many times can be repeated and is still efficacious	As first treatment in open-angle glaucoma or high-risk ocular hypertension
4. MIGS	Microinvasive bleb surgery. Non-bleb forming	No drops or reduce the number of drops needed over 2 years; delay the need for more invasive surgery	Lack of large RCTs with long-term outcomes and real-world data on clinical and economic effectiveness	Available, combined with cataract surgery to treat mild to moderate glaucoma

DDS, drug delivery system; MIGS, minimally invasive glaucoma surgery; NP, nanoparticle; OSD, ocular surface disease; PF, preservative free; RCT, randomized controlled trial; SLT, selective laser trabeculoplasty.

Side effects of treatment are often reduced when switching from preserved to preservative-free eye drops and decreasing the number of daily drop instillations in patients with signs and symptoms of OSD. The toxic-inflammatory effects of BAK are well known and preservative-free drops should be a reference standard for all [138]. However, there is less information about the long-term influence of excipients on ocular surface. Freiberg et al. [139] observed that among preservative-free latanoprost products there were significant differences in pH value, osmolality, and surface tension which may lead to unstable tear film and ocular surface adverse effects. For the future, long-term clinical studies are required to evaluate the safety and efficacy of formulations with different physicochemical properties using a consensus-based series of outcomes and assessment methods [140].

In sustained drug delivery, nanotechnology-based treatments may have the potential to overcome the limitations of currently available glaucoma therapy as they enable targeted delivery, accurate dosing, less side effects, sustained release and increased bioavailability. Several glaucoma drugs have been investigated in nanomedicine formulation, but none of them is available for clinical use.

Of the sustained delivery systems, only the bimatoprost SR (Durysta®) intracameral implant has been approved for single administration due to safety issues until the results of the ongoing clinical trials on the long-term safety and efficacy of the implant are available. With the effect lasting up to 6 months, patients would need multiple administrations in aseptic conditions, which increases the risk of infections.

An important limitation of different drug delivery systems is that only one drug can be loaded, whereas the majority of glaucoma patients need more than one drug to achieve target IOP. Moreover, no studies on cost-effectiveness have been published, possibly because many of these new drug delivery systems are in the preclinical or clinical trials.

In the era of eHealth, smart drug delivery-connected devices in treatment of glaucoma have the potential to improve adherence and for the care provider to detect nonadherence and highlight the risk of progression. Smart drug delivery systems have been used only in research setting including small number of motivated subjects with a short follow up [141]. The size of these devices is still large, which may be inconvenient to adopt. Protection of data and sharing are important issues in digital health care and also fiduciary physician-patient relationship.

The SLT as first-line treatment was shown to be more cost effective compared to medication in the UK setting. It delays the need for eye drops in patients with OHT, early and moderate open-angle glaucoma. A retrospective study in a real-world setting found that 70% of patients initially responded to SLT, but approximately three-quarters of eyes failed treatment within 2 years post-SLT [142]. In this study, definition of failure included IOP > 21 mmHg, IOP reduction < 20% from baseline and further glaucoma procedures (including repeat SLT) or medication increase from baseline.

Although there is increasing use of MIGS and MIBS devices and procedures, there is a lack of large randomized controlled trials and real-world observational studies to determine clinical and economic effectiveness. It is not clear whether the costs of using MIGS and MIBS are outweighed by the reduced number of medication and further intervention [143]. Cost-utility analysis using Markov model over lifetime horizon showed that iStent inject combined with cataract surgery is a cost-effective option for the treatment of patients with early to moderate glaucoma from the Italian NHS perspective [144]. MIGS may offer the advantage of a less rigorous follow up and post-op treatment regimen compared to bleb-forming procedures and some (Hydrus microstent, iStent inject) confer better IOP lowering and no or reduced medication need in early to moderate glaucoma compared to cataract surgery alone.

Finally, identifying issues for poor adherence and addressing them in individual patient care using clear communication is critical [145]. A multifaceted approach including education, reminders, a regimen, and instillation techniques seems to work better in aiding adherence [65,72]. Future studies should focus on clinically important outcomes (e.g., VF progression), quality of life as well as the costs of intervention with longer post-interventional follow up.

Author Contributions: Conceptualization, B.C. and M.K.; methodology, B.C. and M.K.; software, B.C. and M.K.; validation, B.C. and M.K.; formal analysis, B.C.; investigation, B.C. and M.K.; resources, B.C. and M.K.; data curation, B.C. and M.K.; writing—original draft preparation, B.C. and M.K.; writing—B.C. and M.K.; review and editing, B.C. and M.K.; visualization, B.C. and M.K.; supervision, B.C. and M.K.; project administration, B.C. and M.K.; funding acquisition, B.C. All authors have read and agreed to the published version of the manuscript.

Funding: This research received no external funding. The APC was funded by the Slovenian Research Agency (ARRS) (grant no. P3-0333).

Institutional Review Board Statement: Not applicable.

Informed Consent Statement: Not applicable.

Data Availability Statement: Not applicable.

Conflicts of Interest: B.C. is a consultant and speaker for Thea. M.K. is a consultant and speaker for Abbvie, Santen and Thea. M.K. receives research support from Thea.

References

1. Kass, M.A.; Heuer, D.K.; Higginbotham, E.J.; Johnson, C.A.; Keltner, J.L.; Miller, J.P.; Parrish, R.K., II; Wilson, M.R.; Gordon, M.O. The Ocular Hypertension Treatment Study: A randomized trial determines that topical ocular hypotensive medication delays or prevents the onset of primary open-angle glaucoma. *Arch. Ophthalmol.* **2002**, *120*, 701–713. [CrossRef] [PubMed]
2. Agis Investigators. The Advanced Glaucoma Intervention Study (AGIS): 7. The relationship between control of intraocular pressure and visual field deterioration. *Am. J. Ophthalmol.* **2000**, *130*, 429–440. [CrossRef] [PubMed]
3. The effectiveness of intraocular pressure reduction in the treatment of normal-tension glaucoma. *Am. J. Ophthalmol.* **1998**, *126*, 498–505. [CrossRef] [PubMed]
4. Heijl, A.; Leske, M.C.; Bengtsson, B.; Hyman, L.; Bengtsson, B.; Hussein, M. Reduction of intraocular pressure and glaucoma progression: Results from the Early Manifest Glaucoma Trial. *Arch. Ophthalmol.* **2002**, *120*, 1268–1279. [CrossRef]
5. European Glaucoma Society Terminology and Guidelines for Glaucoma, 4th Edition—Chapter 3: Treatment principles and optionsSupported by the EGS Foundation: Part 1: Foreword; Introduction; Glossary; Chapter 3 Treatment principles and options. *Br. J. Ophthalmol.* **2017**, *101*, 130–195. [CrossRef]
6. Robin, A.L.; Muir, K.W. Medication adherence in patients with ocular hypertension or glaucoma. *Expert Rev. Ophthalmol.* **2019**, *14*, 199–210. [CrossRef]
7. Hwang, D.-K.; Liu, C.J.-L.; Pu, C.-Y.; Chou, Y.-J.; Chou, P. Persistence of Topical Glaucoma Medication: A nationwide population-based cohort study in Taiwan. *JAMA Ophthalmol.* **2014**, *132*, 1446–1452. [CrossRef]

8. Newman-Casey, P.A.; Blachley, T.; Lee, P.P.; Heisler, M.; Farris, K.B.; Stein, J.D. Patterns of Glaucoma Medication Adherence over Four Years of Follow-Up. *Ophthalmology* **2015**, *122*, 2010–2021. [CrossRef]
9. Caprioli, J.; Coleman, A.L. Intraocular Pressure Fluctuation: A Risk Factor for Visual Field Progression at Low Intraocular Pressures in the Advanced Glaucoma Intervention Study. *Ophthalmology* **2008**, *115*, 1123–1129.e3. [CrossRef]
10. De Moraes, C.G.V.; Juthani, V.J.; Liebmann, J.M.; Teng, C.C.; Tello, C.; Susanna, R., Jr.; Ritch, R. Risk Factors for Visual Field Progression in Treated Glaucoma. *Arch. Ophthalmol.* **2010**, *129*, 562–568. [CrossRef]
11. Sleath, B.; Blalock, S.; Covert, D.; Stone, J.L.; Skinner, A.C.; Muir, K.; Robin, A.L. The Relationship between Glaucoma Medication Adherence, Eye Drop Technique, and Visual Field Defect Severity. *Ophthalmology* **2011**, *118*, 2398–2402. [CrossRef] [PubMed]
12. Rossi, G.C.; Pasinetti, G.M.; Scudeller, L.; Radaelli, R.; Bianchi, P.E. Do Adherence Rates and Glaucomatous Visual Field Progression Correlate? *Eur. J. Ophthalmol.* **2011**, *21*, 410–414. [CrossRef] [PubMed]
13. Newman-Casey, P.A.; Niziol, L.M.; Gillespie, B.W.; Janz, N.K.; Lichter, P.R.; Musch, D.C. The Association between Medication Adherence and Visual Field Progression in the Collaborative Initial Glaucoma Treatment Study. *Ophthalmology* **2020**, *127*, 477–483. [CrossRef] [PubMed]
14. Tsai, J.C.; McClure, C.A.; Ramos, S.E.; Schlundt, D.G.; Pichert, J.W. Compliance Barriers in Glaucoma: A Systematic Classification. *Eur. J. Gastroenterol. Hepatol.* **2003**, *12*, 393–398. [CrossRef] [PubMed]
15. Lacey, J.; Cate, H.T.; Broadway, D.C. Barriers to adherence with glaucoma medications: A qualitative research study. *Eye* **2009**, *23*, 924–932. [CrossRef] [PubMed]
16. Newman-Casey, P.A.; Robin, A.L.; Blachley, T.; Farris, K.; Heisler, M.; Resnicow, K.; Lee, P.P. The Most Common Barriers to Glaucoma Medication Adherence: A Cross-Sectional Survey. *Ophthalmology* **2015**, *122*, 1308–1316. [CrossRef] [PubMed]
17. Robin, A.L.; Novack, G.D.; Covert, D.W.; Crockett, R.S.; Marcic, T.S. Adherence in Glaucoma: Objective Measurements of Once-Daily and Adjunctive Medication Use. *Am. J. Ophthalmol.* **2007**, *144*, 533–540.e2. [CrossRef]
18. Hou, C.-H.; Pu, C. Medication Adherence in Patients with Glaucoma and Disability. *JAMA Ophthalmol.* **2021**, *139*, 1292–1298. [CrossRef]
19. Tapply, I.; Broadway, D.C. Improving Adherence to Topical Medication in Patients with Glaucoma. *Patient Prefer. Adherence* **2021**, *15*, 1477–1489. [CrossRef]
20. Anwar, Z.; Wellik, S.R.; Galor, A. Glaucoma therapy and ocular surface disease: Current literature and recommendations. *Curr. Opin. Ophthalmol.* **2013**, *24*, 136–143. [CrossRef]
21. Baudouin, C.; Labbé, A.; Liang, H.; Pauly, A.; Brignole-Baudouin, F. Preservatives in eyedrops: The good, the bad and the ugly. *Prog. Retin. Eye Res.* **2010**, *29*, 312–334. [CrossRef] [PubMed]
22. Nordmann, J.-P.; Auzanneau, N.; Ricard, S.; Berdeaux, G. Vision related quality of life and topical glaucoma treatment side effects. *Health Qual. Life Outcomes* **2003**, *1*, 75. [CrossRef] [PubMed]
23. Leung, E.W.; Medeiros, F.A.; Weinreb, R.N. Prevalence of Ocular Surface Disease in Glaucoma Patients. *J. Glaucoma* **2008**, *17*, 350–355. [CrossRef] [PubMed]
24. Ghosh, S.; O'Hare, F.; Lamoureux, E.; Vajpayee, R.B.; Crowston, J.G. Prevalence of signs and symptoms of ocular surface disease in individuals treated and not treated with glaucoma medication. *Clin. Exp. Ophthalmol.* **2012**, *40*, 675–681. [CrossRef]
25. Moss, S.E.; Klein, R.; Klein, B.E. Prevalence of and Risk Factors for Dry Eye Syndrome. *Arch. Ophthalmol.* **2000**, *118*, 1264–1268. [CrossRef]
26. Wolfram, C.; Stahlberg, E.; Pfeiffer, N. Patient-Reported Nonadherence with Glaucoma Therapy. *J. Ocul. Pharmacol. Ther.* **2019**, *35*, 223–228. [CrossRef]
27. Rossi, G.C.M.; Pasinetti, G.M.; Scudeller, L.; Raimondi, M.; Lanteri, S.; Bianchi, P.E. Risk Factors to Develop Ocular Surface Disease in Treated Glaucoma or Ocular Hypertension Patients. *Eur. J. Ophthalmol.* **2013**, *23*, 296–302. [CrossRef]
28. Valente, C.; Iester, M.; Corsi, E.; Rolando, M. Symptoms and Signs of Tear Film Dysfunction in Glaucomatous Patients. *J. Ocul. Pharmacol. Ther.* **2011**, *27*, 281–285. [CrossRef]
29. Pisella, P.J.; Pouliquen, P.; Baudouin, C. Prevalence of ocular symptoms and signs with preserved and preservative free glaucoma medication. *Br. J. Ophthalmol.* **2002**, *86*, 418–423. [CrossRef]
30. Jaenen, N.; Baudouin, C.; Pouliquen, P.; Manni, G.; Figueiredo, A.; Zeyen, T. Ocular Symptoms and Signs with Preserved and Preservative-Free Glaucoma Medications. *Eur. J. Ophthalmol.* **2007**, *17*, 341–349. [CrossRef]
31. Uusitalo, H.; Chen, E.; Pfeiffer, N.; Brignole-Baudouin, F.; Kaarniranta, K.; Leino, M.; Puska, P.; Palmgren, E.; Hamacher, T.; Hofmann, G.; et al. Switching from a preserved to a preservative-free prostaglandin preparation in topical glaucoma medication. *Acta Ophthalmol.* **2010**, *88*, 329–336. [CrossRef] [PubMed]
32. Munoz-Negrete, F.J.; Lemij, H.G.; Erb, C. Switching to preservative-free latanoprost: Impact on tolerability and patient satisfaction. *Clin. Ophthalmol.* **2017**, *11*, 557–566. [CrossRef] [PubMed]
33. Pillunat, L.E.; Erb, C.; Ropo, A.; Kimmich, F.; Pfeiffer, N. Preservative-free fixed combination of tafluprost 0.0015% and timolol 0.5% in patients with open-angle glaucoma and ocular hypertension: Results of an open-label observational study. *Clin. Ophthalmol.* **2017**, *11*, 1051–1064. [CrossRef] [PubMed]
34. Uusitalo, H.; Egorov, E.; Kaarniranta, K.; Astakhov, Y.; Ropo, A. Benefits of switching from latanoprost to preservative-free tafluprost eye drops: A meta-analysis of two Phase IIIb clinical trials. *Clin. Ophthalmol.* **2016**, *10*, 445–454. [CrossRef]

35. Rouland, J.-F.; Traverso, C.E.; Stalmans, I.; El Fekih, L.; Delval, L.; Renault, D.; Baudouin, C. Efficacy and safety of preservative-free latanoprost eyedrops, compared with BAK-preserved latanoprost in patients with ocular hypertension or glaucoma. *Br. J. Ophthalmol.* **2012**, *97*, 196–200. [CrossRef]
36. Shirley, M. Bimatoprost Implant: First Approval. *Drugs Aging* **2020**, *37*, 457–462. [CrossRef]
37. Occhiutto, M.L.; Maranhão, R.C.; Costa, V.P.; Konstas, A.G. Nanotechnology for Medical and Surgical Glaucoma Therapy—A Review. *Adv. Ther.* **2020**, *37*, 155–199. [CrossRef]
38. González-Fernández, F.M.; Bianchera, A.; Gasco, P.; Nicoli, S.; Pescina, S. Lipid-Based Nanocarriers for Ophthalmic Administration: Towards Experimental Design Implementation. *Pharmaceutics* **2021**, *13*, 447. [CrossRef]
39. Franco, P.; De Marco, I. Contact Lenses as Ophthalmic Drug Delivery Systems: A Review. *Polymers* **2021**, *13*, 1102. [CrossRef]
40. Toffoletto, N.; Saramago, B.; Serro, A.P. Therapeutic Ophthalmic Lenses: A Review. *Pharmaceutics* **2020**, *13*, 36. [CrossRef]
41. Xu, J.; Ge, Y.; Bu, R.; Zhang, A.; Feng, S.; Wang, J.; Gou, J.; Yin, T.; He, H.; Zhang, Y.; et al. Co-delivery of latanoprost and timolol from micelles-laden contact lenses for the treatment of glaucoma. *J. Control. Release* **2019**, *305*, 18–28. [CrossRef]
42. Macoul, K.L.; Pavan-Langston, D. Pilocarpine Ocusert System for Sustained Control of Ocular Hypertension. *Arch. Ophthalmol.* **1975**, *93*, 587–590. [CrossRef] [PubMed]
43. Brandt, J.D.; Sall, K.; DuBiner, H.; Benza, R.; Alster, Y.; Walker, G.; Semba, C.P.; Budenz, D.; Day, D.; Flowers, B.; et al. Six-Month Intraocular Pressure Reduction with a Topical Bimatoprost Ocular Insert: Results of a Phase II Randomized Controlled Study. *Ophthalmology* **2016**, *123*, 1685–1694. [CrossRef]
44. Brandt, J.D.; DuBiner, H.B.; Benza, R.; Sall, K.N.; Walker, G.A.; Semba, C.P.; Budenz, D.; Day, D.; Flowers, B.; Lee, S.; et al. Long-term Safety and Efficacy of a Sustained-Release Bimatoprost Ocular Ring. *Ophthalmology* **2017**, *124*, 1565–1566. [CrossRef] [PubMed]
45. Kompella, U.B.; Hartman, R.R.; Patil, M.A. Extraocular, periocular, and intraocular routes for sustained drug delivery for glaucoma. *Prog. Retin. Eye Res.* **2021**, *82*, 100901. [CrossRef] [PubMed]
46. Goldberg, D.F.; Williams, R. A Phase 2 Study Evaluating Safety and Efficacy of the Latanoprost Punctal Plug Delivery System (L-PPDS) in Subjects with Ocular Hypertension (OH) or Open-Angle Glaucoma (OAG). *Investig. Ophthalmol. Vis. Sci.* **2012**, *53*, 5095.
47. Kesav, N.P.; Young, C.E.C.; Ertel, M.K.; Seibold, L.K.; Kahook, M.Y. Sustained-release drug delivery systems for the treatment of glaucoma. *Int. J. Ophthalmol.* **2021**, *14*, 148–159. [CrossRef] [PubMed]
48. Perera, S.A.; Ting, D.S.; Nongpiur, M.E.; Chew, P.T.; Aquino, M.C.D.; Sng, C.C.; Ho, S.-W.; Aung, T. Feasibility study of sustained-release travoprost punctum plug for intraocular pressure reduction in an Asian population. *Clin. Ophthalmol.* **2016**, *10*, 757–764. [CrossRef]
49. Fahmy, H.M.; Saad, E.A.E.-M.S.; Sabra, N.M.; El-Gohary, A.A.; Mohamed, F.F.; Gaber, M.H. Treatment merits of Latanoprost/Thymoquinone—Encapsulated liposome for glaucomatus rabbits. *Int. J. Pharm.* **2018**, *548*, 597–608. [CrossRef]
50. Lavik, E.; Kuehn, M.H.; Shoffstall, A.J.; Atkins, K.; Dumitrescu, A.; Kwon, Y. Sustained Delivery of Timolol Maleate for Over 90 Days by Subconjunctival Injection. *J. Ocul. Pharmacol. Ther.* **2016**, *32*, 642–649. [CrossRef]
51. Pek, Y.S.; Wu, H.; Mohamed, S.T.; Ying, J.Y. Long-Term Subconjunctival Delivery of Brimonidine Tartrate for Glaucoma Treatment Using a Microspheres/Carrier System. *Adv. Healthc. Mater.* **2016**, *5*, 2823–2831. [CrossRef] [PubMed]
52. Fu, J.; Sun, F.; Liu, W.; Liu, Y.; Gedam, M.; Hu, Q.; Fridley, C.; Quigley, H.A.; Hanes, J.; Pitha, I. Subconjunctival Delivery of Dorzolamide-Loaded Poly(ether-anhydride) Microparticles Produces Sustained Lowering of Intraocular Pressure in Rabbits. *Mol. Pharm.* **2016**, *13*, 2987–2995. [CrossRef] [PubMed]
53. Voss, K.; Falke, K.; Bernsdorf, A.; Grabow, N.; Kastner, C.; Sternberg, K.; Minrath, I.; Eickner, T.; Wree, A.; Schmitz, K.-P.; et al. Development of a novel injectable drug delivery system for subconjunctival glaucoma treatment. *J. Control. Release* **2015**, *214*, 1–11. [CrossRef] [PubMed]
54. Natarajan, J.V.; Chattopadhyay, S.; Ang, M.; Darwitan, A.; Foo, S.; Zhen, M.; Koo, M.; Wong, T.T.; Venkatraman, S.S. Sustained Release of an Anti-Glaucoma Drug: Demonstration of Efficacy of a Liposomal Formulation in the Rabbit Eye. *PLoS ONE* **2011**, *6*, e24371. [CrossRef] [PubMed]
55. Wong, T.T.; Novack, G.D.; Natarajan, J.V.; Ho, C.L.; Htoon, H.M.; Venkatraman, S.S. Nanomedicine for glaucoma: Sustained release latanoprost offers a new therapeutic option with substantial benefits over eyedrops. *Drug Deliv. Transl. Res.* **2014**, *4*, 303–309. [CrossRef] [PubMed]
56. Sirinek, P.E.; Lin, M.M. Intracameral sustained release bimatoprost implants (Durysta). *Semin. Ophthalmol.* **2022**, *37*, 385–390. [CrossRef]
57. Lee, S.S.; Hughes, P.; Ross, A.D.; Robinson, M.R. Biodegradable Implants for Sustained Drug Release in the Eye. *Pharm. Res.* **2010**, *27*, 2043–2053. [CrossRef] [PubMed]
58. Lewis, R.A.; Christie, W.C.; Day, D.G.; Craven, E.R.; Walters, T.; Bejanian, M.; Lee, S.S.; Goodkin, M.L.; Zhang, J.; Whitcup, S.M.; et al. Bimatoprost Sustained-Release Implants for Glaucoma Therapy: 6-Month Results From a Phase I/II Clinical Trial. *Am. J. Ophthalmol.* **2017**, *175*, 137–147. [CrossRef]
59. Craven, E.R.; Walters, T.; Christie, W.C.; Day, D.G.; Lewis, R.A.; Goodkin, M.L.; Chen, M.; Wangsadipura, V.; Robinson, M.R.; Bejanian, M.; et al. 24-Month Phase I/II Clinical Trial of Bimatoprost Sustained-Release Implant (Bimatoprost SR) in Glaucoma Patients. *Drugs* **2020**, *80*, 167–179. [CrossRef]

60. Medeiros, F.A.; Walters, T.R.; Kolko, M.; Coote, M.; Bejanian, M.; Goodkin, M.L.; Guo, Q.; Zhang, J.; Robinson, M.R.; Weinreb, R.N.; et al. Phase 3, Randomized, 20-Month Study of Bimatoprost Implant in Open-Angle Glaucoma and Ocular Hypertension (ARTEMIS 1). *Ophthalmology* **2020**, *127*, 1627–1641. [CrossRef]
61. Seal, J.R.; Robinson, M.R.; Burke, J.; Bejanian, M.; Coote, M.; Attar, M. Intracameral Sustained-Release Bimatoprost Implant Delivers Bimatoprost to Target Tissues with Reduced Drug Exposure to Off-Target Tissues. *J. Ocul. Pharmacol. Ther.* **2019**, *35*, 50–57. [CrossRef]
62. Bacharach, J.; Tatham, A.; Ferguson, G.; Belalcázar, S.; Thieme, H.; Goodkin, M.L.; Chen, M.Y.; Guo, Q.; Liu, J.; Robinson, M.R.; et al. Phase 3, Randomized, 20-Month Study of the Efficacy and Safety of Bimatoprost Implant in Patients with Open-Angle Glaucoma and Ocular Hypertension (ARTEMIS 2). *Drugs* **2021**, *81*, 2017–2033. [CrossRef] [PubMed]
63. Medeiros, F.A.; Sheybani, A.; Shah, M.M.; Rivas, M.; Bai, Z.; Werts, E.; Ahmed, I.I.K.; Craven, E.R. Single Administration of Intracameral Bimatoprost Implant 10 µg in Patients with Open-Angle Glaucoma or Ocular Hypertension. *Ophthalmol. Ther.* **2022**, *11*, 1517–1537. [CrossRef] [PubMed]
64. Glaukos' iDose TR Demonstrates Sustained IOP Reduction and Favorable Safety Profile Over 36 Months in Phase 2b Study. Available online: https://eyewire.news/news/glaukos-idose-tr-demonstrates-sustained-iop-reduction-and-favorable-safety-profile-over-36-months-in-phase-2b-study?c4src=article:infinite-scroll (accessed on 18 July 2022).
65. Buehne, K.L.; Rosdahl, J.A.; Muir, K.W. Aiding Adherence to Glaucoma Medications: A Systematic Review. *Semin. Ophthalmol.* **2022**, *37*, 313–323. [CrossRef] [PubMed]
66. Friedman, D.S.; Jampel, H.D.; Congdon, N.G.; Miller, R.; Quigley, H.A. The TRAVATAN Dosing Aid Accurately Records When Drops Are Taken. *Am. J. Ophthalmol.* **2007**, *143*, 699–701. [CrossRef]
67. Chang, D.S.; Friedman, D.S.; Frazier, T.; Plyler, R.; Boland, M.V. Development and Validation of a Predictive Model for Nonadherence with Once-Daily Glaucoma Medications. *Ophthalmology* **2013**, *120*, 1396–1402. [CrossRef]
68. Boland, M.V.; Chang, D.S.; Frazier, T.; Plyler, R.; Jefferys, J.L.; Friedman, D.S. Automated Telecommunication-Based Reminders and Adherence with Once-Daily Glaucoma Medication Dosing: The automated dosing reminder study. *JAMA Ophthalmol.* **2014**, *132*, 845–850. [CrossRef]
69. Boland, M.V.; Chang, D.S.; Frazier, T.; Plyler, R.; Friedman, D.S. Electronic Monitoring to Assess Adherence with Once-Daily Glaucoma Medications and Risk Factors for Nonadherence: The automated dosing reminder study. *JAMA Ophthalmol.* **2014**, *132*, 838–844. [CrossRef]
70. Cook, P.F.; Schmiege, S.J.; Mansberger, S.L.; Kammer, J.; Fitzgerald, T.; Kahook, M.Y. Predictors of Adherence to Glaucoma Treatment in a Multisite Study. *Ann. Behav. Med.* **2015**, *49*, 29–39. [CrossRef]
71. Cook, P.F.; Schmiege, S.J.; Mansberger, S.L.; Sheppler, C.; Kammer, J.; Fitzgerald, T.; Kahook, M.Y. Motivational interviewing or reminders for glaucoma medication adherence: Results of a multi-site randomised controlled trial. *Psychol. Health* **2017**, *32*, 145–165. [CrossRef]
72. Muir, K.W.; Rosdahl, J.A.; Hein, A.M.; Woolson, S.; Olsen, M.K.; Kirshner, M.; Sexton, M.; Bosworth, H.B. Improved Glaucoma Medication Adherence in a Randomized Controlled Trial. *Ophthalmol. Glaucoma* **2022**, *5*, 40–46. [CrossRef] [PubMed]
73. Miller, D.J.; Niziol, L.M.; Elam, A.R.; Heisler, M.; Lee, P.P.; Resnicow, K.; Musch, D.C.; Darnley-Fisch, D.; Mitchell, J.; Newman-Casey, P.A. Demographic, Clinical, and Psychosocial Predictors of Change in Medication Adherence in the Support, Educate, Empower Program. *Ophthalmol. Glaucoma* **2021**, *5*, 47–57. [CrossRef] [PubMed]
74. Richardson, C.; Brunton, L.; Olleveant, N.; Henson, D.B.; Pilling, M.; Mottershead, J.; Fenerty, C.H.; Spencer, A.F.; Waterman, H. A study to assess the feasibility of undertaking a randomized controlled trial of adherence with eye drops in glaucoma patients. *Patient Prefer. Adherence* **2013**, *7*, 1025–1039. [CrossRef] [PubMed]
75. Sayner, R.; Carpenter, D.M.; Blalock, S.J.; Robin, A.L.; Muir, K.W.; Hartnett, M.E.; Giangiacomo, A.L.; Tudor, G.; Sleath, B. Accuracy of Patient-reported Adherence to Glaucoma Medications on a Visual Analog Scale Compared with Electronic Monitors. *Clin. Ther.* **2015**, *37*, 1975–1985. [CrossRef] [PubMed]
76. Nishimura, K.; Tabuchi, H.; Nakakura, S.; Nakatani, Y.; Yorihiro, A.; Hasegawa, S.; Tanabe, H.; Noguchi, A.; Aoki, R.; Kiuchi, Y. Evaluation of Automatic Monitoring of Instillation Adherence Using Eye Dropper Bottle Sensor and Deep Learning in Patients with Glaucoma. *Transl. Vis. Sci. Technol.* **2019**, *8*, 55. [CrossRef]
77. Heinemann, L.; Schnell, O.; Gehr, B.; Schloot, N.C.; Görgens, S.W.; Görgen, C. Digital Diabetes Management: A Literature Review of Smart Insulin Pens. *J. Diabetes Sci. Technol.* **2022**, *16*, 587–595. [CrossRef]
78. Gomez-Peralta, F.; Abreu, C.; Gomez-Rodriguez, S.; Ruiz, L. Insulclock: A Novel Insulin Delivery Optimization and Tracking System. *Diabetes Technol. Ther.* **2019**, *21*, 209–214. [CrossRef]
79. BIOCORP. Mallya. Available online: https://biocorpsys.com/en/our-products/connected-devices/mallya/ (accessed on 2 August 2022).
80. Kali Homepage. Available online: https://www.kali.care/ (accessed on 2 August 2022).
81. Gatwood, J.D.; Johnson, J.; Jerkins, B. Comparisons of Self-reported Glaucoma Medication Adherence with a New Wireless Device: A Pilot Study. *J. Glaucoma* **2017**, *26*, 1056–1061. [CrossRef]
82. Nemera. e-Novelia. Available online: https://www.nemera.net/products/ophthalmic/e-novelia/ (accessed on 3 August 2022).
83. Payne, N.; Gangwani, R.; Barton, K.; Sample, A.P.; Cain, S.M.; Burke, D.T.; Newman-Casey, P.A.; Shorter, K.A. Medication Adherence and Liquid Level Tracking System for Healthcare Provider Feedback. *Sensors* **2020**, *20*, 2435. [CrossRef]

84. Eaton, A.M.; Gordon, G.M.; Konowal, A.; Allen, A.; Allen, M.; Sgarlata, A.; Gao, G.; Wafapoor, H.; Avery, R.L. A novel eye drop application monitor to assess patient compliance with a prescribed regimen: A pilot study. *Eye* **2015**, *29*, 1383–1391. [CrossRef]
85. Gazzard, G.; Konstantakopoulou, E.; Garway-Heath, D.; Garg, A.; Vickerstaff, V.; Hunter, R.; Ambler, G.; Bunce, C.; Wormald, R.; Nathwani, N.; et al. Selective laser trabeculoplasty versus eye drops for first-line traetment of ocular hypertension and glaucoma (LiGHT): A multicentre randomised controlled trial. *Lancet* **2019**, *393*, 1505–1516. [CrossRef] [PubMed]
86. Gazzard, G.; Konstantakopoulou, E.; Garway-Heath, D.; Garg, A.; Vickerstaff, V.; Hunter, R.; Ambler, G.; Bunce, C.; Wormald, R.; Nathwani, N.; et al. Selective laser trabeculoplasty versus drops for newly diagnosed ocular hypertension and glaucoma: The LiGHT RCT. *Health Technol. Assess.* **2019**, *23*, 1–102. [CrossRef] [PubMed]
87. Wright, D.M.; Konstantakopoulou, E.; Montesano, G.; Nathwani, N.; Garg, A.; Garway-Heath, D.; Crabb, D.P.; Gazzard, G. Laser in Glaucoma and Ocular Hypertension Trial (LiGHT) Study Group. Visual Field Outcomes from the Multicenter, Randomized Controlled Laser in Glaucoma and Ocular Hypertension Trial (LiGHT). *Ophthalmology* **2020**, *127*, 1313–1321. [CrossRef] [PubMed]
88. Kim, C.Y.; Park, K.H.; Ahn, J.; Ahn, M.-D.; Cha, S.C.; Kim, H.S.; Kim, J.M.; Kim, M.J.; Kim, T.-W.; Kim, Y.Y.; et al. Treatment patterns and medication adherence of patients with glaucoma in South Korea. *Br. J. Ophthalmol.* **2017**, *101*, 801–807. [CrossRef]
89. Ang, G.S.; Fenwick, E.K.; Constantinou, M.; Gan, A.T.L.; Man, R.E.K.; Casson, R.J.; Finkelstein, E.A.; Goldberg, I.; Healey, P.R.; Pesudovs, K.; et al. Selective laser trabeculoplasty versus topical medication as initial glaucoma treatment: The glaucoma initial treatment study randomised clinical trial. *Br. J. Ophthalmol.* **2020**, *104*, 813–821. [CrossRef]
90. Lamoureux, E.L.; Mcintosh, R.; Constantinou, M.; Fenwick, E.K.; Xie, J.; Casson, R.; Finkelstein, E.; Goldberg, I.; Healey, P.; Thomas, R.; et al. Comparing the effectiveness of selective laser trabeculoplasty with topical medication as initial treatment (the Glaucoma Initial Treatment Study): Study protocol for a randomised controlled trial. *Trials* **2015**, *16*, 406. [CrossRef]
91. Shalaby, W.S.; Ahmed, O.M.; Waisbourd, M.; Katz, L.J. A review of potential novel glaucoma therapeutic options independent of intraocular pressure. *Surv. Ophthalmol.* **2022**, *67*, 1062–1080. [CrossRef]
92. Damji, K.F.; Shah, K.C.; Rock, W.J.; Bains, H.S.; Hodge, W.G. Selective laser trabeculoplasty v argon laser trabeculoplasty: A prospective randomised clinical trial. *Br. J. Ophthalmol.* **1999**, *83*, 718–722. [CrossRef]
93. Song, J. Complications of selective laser trabeculoplasty: A review. *Clin. Ophthalmol.* **2016**, *10*, 137–143. [CrossRef]
94. Ong, K.; Ong, L. Selective laser trabeculoplasty may compromise corneas with pigment on endothelium. *Clin. Exp. Ophthalmol.* **2013**, *41*, 109–110. [CrossRef]
95. Ha, J.H.I.; Bowling, B.; Chen, S.D. Cystoid macular oedema following selective laser trabeculoplasty in a diabetic patient. *Clin. Exp. Ophthalmol.* **2013**, *42*, 200–201. [CrossRef] [PubMed]
96. Wechsler, D.Z.; Wechsler, I.B. Cystoid macular oedema after selective laser trabeculoplasty. *Eye* **2010**, *24*, 1113. [CrossRef] [PubMed]
97. Wu, Z.Q.; Huang, J.; Sadda, S. Selective laser trabeculoplasty complicated by cystoid macular edema: Report of two cases. *Eye Sci.* **2012**, *27*, 193–197. [CrossRef] [PubMed]
98. Shihadeh, W.A.; Ritch, R.; Liebmann, J.M. Hyphema Occurring During Selective Laser Trabeculoplasty. *Ophthalmic Surg. Lasers Imaging Retin.* **2006**, *37*, 432–433. [CrossRef] [PubMed]
99. Rhee, D.J.; Krad, O.; Pasquale, L.R. Hyphema Following Selective Laser Trabeculoplasty. *Ophthalmic Surg. Lasers Imaging Retin.* **2009**, *40*, 493–494. [CrossRef] [PubMed]
100. Okeke, C.O.; Quigley, H.A.; Jampel, H.D.; Ying, G.-S.; Plyler, R.J.; Jiang, Y.; Friedman, D.S. Adherence with Topical Glaucoma Medication Monitored Electronically: The Travatan Dosing Aid Study. *Ophthalmology* **2009**, *116*, 191–199. [CrossRef] [PubMed]
101. Gatwood, J.P.; Brooks, C.; Meacham, R.; Abou-Rahma, J.; Cernasev, A.; Brown, E.; Kuchtey, R.W.M. Facilitators and Barriers to Glaucoma Medication Adherence. *J. Glaucoma* **2022**, *31*, 31–36. [CrossRef]
102. Bovell, A.M.; Damji, K.F.; Hodge, W.G.; Rock, W.J.; Buhrmann, R.R.; Pan, Y.I. Long term effects on the lowering of intraocular pressure: Selective laser or argon laser trabeculoplasty? *Can. J. Ophthalmol.* **2011**, *46*, 408–413. [CrossRef]
103. Damji, K.F.; Bovell, A.M.; Hodge, W.G.; Rock, W.; Shah, K.; Buhrmann, R.; Pan, Y.I. Selective laser trabeculoplasty versus argon laser trabeculoplasty: Results from a 1-year randomised clinical trial. *Br. J. Ophthalmol.* **2006**, *90*, 1490–1494. [CrossRef]
104. Koucheki, B.; Hashemi, H. Selective Laser Trabeculoplasty in the Treatment of Open-angle Glaucoma. *J. Glaucoma* **2012**, *21*, 65–70. [CrossRef]
105. Liu, Y.; Birt, C.M. Argon Versus Selective Laser Trabeculoplasty in Younger Patients: 2-year results. *J. Glaucoma* **2012**, *21*, 112–115. [CrossRef] [PubMed]
106. Hong, B.K.; Winer, J.C.; Martone, J.F.; Wand, M.; Altman, B.; Shields, B. Repeat Selective Laser Trabeculoplasty. *J. Glaucoma* **2009**, *18*, 180–183. [CrossRef] [PubMed]
107. Avery, N.; Ang, G.S.; Nicholas, S.; Wells, A. Repeatability of primary selective laser trabeculoplasty in patients with primary open-angle glaucoma. *Int. Ophthalmol.* **2013**, *33*, 501–506. [CrossRef] [PubMed]
108. Khouri, A.S.; Lari, H.B.; Berezina, T.L.; Maltzman, B.; Fechtner, R.D. Long term efficacy of repeat selective laser trabeculoplasty. *J. Ophthalmic Vis. Res.* **2014**, *9*, 444–448. [CrossRef] [PubMed]
109. Hutnik, C.; Crichton, A.; Ford, B.; Nicolela, M.; Shuba, L.; Birt, C.; Sogbesan, E.; Damji, K.F.; Dorey, M.; Saheb, H.; et al. Selective Laser Trabeculoplasty versus Argon Laser Trabeculoplasty in Glaucoma Patients Treated Previously with 360° Selective Laser Trabeculoplasty: A Randomized, Single-Blind, Equivalence Clinical Trial. *Ophthalmology* **2019**, *126*, 223–232. [CrossRef] [PubMed]
110. Ilveskoski, L.; Taipale, C.; Tuuminen, R. Selective laser trabeculoplasty in exfoliative glaucoma eyes with prior argon laser trabeculoplasty. *Acta Ophthalmol.* **2019**, *98*, 58–64. [CrossRef] [PubMed]

111. Polat, J.; Grantham, L.; Mitchell, K.; Realini, T. Repeatability of selective laser trabeculoplasty. *Br. J. Ophthalmol.* **2016**, *100*, 1437–1441. [CrossRef]
112. Garg, A.; Vickerstaff, V.; Nathwani, N.; Garway-Heath, D.; Konstantakopoulou, E.; Ambler, G.; Bunce, C.; Wormald, R.; Barton, K.; Gazzard, G.; et al. Efficacy of Repeat Selective Laser Trabeculoplasty in Medication-Naive Open-Angle Glaucoma and Ocular Hypertension during the LiGHT Trial. *Ophthalmology* **2020**, *127*, 467–476. [CrossRef]
113. Richter, G.M.; Coleman, A.L. Minimally invasive glaucoma surgery: Current status and future prospects. *Clin. Ophthalmol.* **2016**, *10*, 189–206. [CrossRef]
114. Kerr, N.M.; Wang, J.; Barton, K. Minimally invasive glaucoma surgery as primary stand-alone surgery for glaucoma. *Clin. Exp. Ophthalmol.* **2017**, *45*, 393–400. [CrossRef]
115. Fellman, R.L.; Mattox, C.; Singh, K.; Flowers, B.; Francis, B.A.; Robin, A.L.; Butler, M.R.; Shah, M.M.; Giaconi, J.A.; Sheybani, A.; et al. American Glaucoma Society Position Paper: Microinvasive Glaucoma Surgery. *Ophthalmol. Glaucoma* **2020**, *3*, 1–6. [CrossRef] [PubMed]
116. European Glaucoma Society Terminology and Guidelines for Glaucoma, 5th Edition. *Br. J. Ophthalmol.* **2021**, *105*, 1–169. [CrossRef] [PubMed]
117. Yang, X.; Zhao, Y.; Zhong, Y.; Duan, X. The efficacy of XEN gel stent implantation in glaucoma: A systematic review and meta-analysis. *BMC Ophthalmol.* **2022**, *22*, 305. [CrossRef] [PubMed]
118. Reitsamer, H.; Vera, V.; Ruben, S.; Au, L.; Vila-Arteaga, J.; Teus, M.; Lenzhofer, M.; Shirlaw, A.; Bai, Z.; Balaram, M.; et al. Three-year effectiveness and safety of the XEN gel stent as a solo procedure or in combination with phacoemulsification in open-angle glaucoma: A multicentre study. *Acta Ophthalmol.* **2022**, *100*, e233–e245. [CrossRef] [PubMed]
119. Lim, S.Y.; Betzler, B.K.; Yip, L.W.L.; Dorairaj, S.; Ang, B.C.H. Standalone XEN45 Gel Stent implantation in the treatment of open-angle glaucoma: A systematic review and meta-analysis. *Surv. Ophthalmol.* **2022**, *67*, 1048–1061. [CrossRef] [PubMed]
120. Ting, J.L.M.; Rudnisky, C.J.; Damji, K.F. Prospective randomized controlled trial of phaco-trabectome versus phaco-trabeculectomy in patients with open angle glaucoma. *Can. J. Ophthalmol.* **2018**, *53*, 588–594. [CrossRef]
121. Hu, K.; Shah, A.; Virgili, G.; Bunce, C.; Gazzard, G. Ab interno trabecular bypass surgery with Trabectome for open-angle glaucoma. *Cochrane Database Syst. Rev.* **2021**, *2021*, CD011693. [CrossRef]
122. Ventura-Abreu, N.; García-Feijoo, J.; Pazos, M.; Biarnés, M.; Morales-Fernández, L.; Martínez-De-La-Casa, J.M. Twelve-month results of ab interno trabeculectomy with Kahook Dual Blade: An interventional, randomized, controlled clinical study. *Graefe's Arch. Clin. Exp. Ophthalmol.* **2021**, *259*, 2771–2781. [CrossRef]
123. ElMallah, M.K.; Berdahl, J.P.; Williamson, B.K.; Dorairaj, S.K.; Kahook, M.Y.; Gallardo, M.J.; Mahootchi, A.; Smith, S.N.; Rappaport, L.A.; Diaz-Robles, D.; et al. Twelve-Month Outcomes of Stand-Alone Excisional Goniotomy in Mild to Severe Glaucoma. *Clin. Ophthalmol.* **2020**, *14*, 1891–1897. [CrossRef]
124. Iwasaki, K.; Kakimoto, H.; Orii, Y.; Arimura, S.; Takamura, Y.; Inatani, M. Long-Term Outcomes of a Kahook Dual Blade Procedure Combined with Phacoemulsification in Japanese Patients with Open-Angle Glaucoma. *J. Clin. Med.* **2022**, *11*, 1354. [CrossRef]
125. Le, C.; Kazaryan, S.; Hubbell, M.; Zurakowski, D.; Ayyala, R.S. Surgical Outcomes of Phacoemulsification Followed by iStent Implantation Versus Goniotomy with the Kahook Dual Blade in Patients with Mild Primary Open-angle Glaucoma with a Minimum of 12-Month Follow-up. *J. Glaucoma* **2019**, *28*, 411–414. [CrossRef] [PubMed]
126. Arnljots, T.S.; Economou, M.A. Kahook Dual Blade Goniotomy vs iStent inject: Long-Term Results in Patients with Open-Angle Glaucoma. *Clin. Ophthalmol.* **2021**, *15*, 541–550. [CrossRef] [PubMed]
127. Fea, A.M. Phacoemulsification versus phacoemulsification with micro-bypass stent implantation in primary open-angle glaucoma: Randomized double-masked clinical trial. *J. Cataract. Refract. Surg.* **2010**, *36*, 407–412. [CrossRef] [PubMed]
128. Samuelson, T.W.; Katz, L.J.; Wells, J.M.; Duh, Y.-J.; Giamporcaro, J.E.; US iStent Study Group. Randomized Evaluation of the Trabecular Micro-Bypass Stent with Phacoemulsification in Patients with Glaucoma and Cataract. *Ophthalmology* **2011**, *118*, 459–467. [CrossRef]
129. Samuelson, T.W.; Sarkisian, S.R., Jr.; Lubeck, D.M.; Stiles, M.C.; Duh, Y.-J.; Romo, E.A.; Giamporcaro, J.E.; Hornbeak, D.M.; Katz, L.J.; Bartlett, W.; et al. Prospective, Randomized, Controlled Pivotal Trial of an Ab Interno Implanted Trabecular Micro-Bypass in Primary Open-Angle Glaucoma and Cataract: Two-Year Results. *Ophthalmology* **2019**, *126*, 811–821. [CrossRef]
130. Samuelson, T.W.; Singh, I.P.; Williamson, B.K.; Falvey, H.; Lee, W.C.; Odom, D.; McSorley, D.; Katz, L.J. Quality of Life in Primary Open-Angle Glaucoma and Cataract: An Analysis of VFQ-25 and OSDI from the iStent inject® Pivotal Trial. *Am. J. Ophthalmol.* **2021**, *229*, 220–229. [CrossRef]
131. Holmes, D.P.; Clement, C.I.; Nguyen, V.; Healey, P.R.; Lim, R.; White, A.; Yuen, J.; Lawlor, M.; Franzco, R.L.; Franzco, J.Y. Comparative study of 2-year outcomes for Hydrus or iStent inject microinvasive glaucoma surgery implants with cataract surgery. *Clin. Exp. Ophthalmol.* **2022**, *50*, 303–311. [CrossRef]
132. Bicket, A.K.; Le, J.T.; Azuara-Blanco, A.; Gazzard, G.; Wormald, R.; Bunce, C.; Hu, K.; Jayaram, H.; King, A.; Otárola, F.; et al. Minimally Invasive Glaucoma Surgical Techniques for Open-Angle Glaucoma: An Overview of Cochrane Systematic Reviews and Network Meta-analysis. *JAMA Ophthalmol.* **2021**, *139*, 983–989. [CrossRef]
133. Otarola, F.; Virgili, G.; Shah, A.; Hu, K.; Bunce, C.; Gazzard, G. Ab interno trabecular bypass surgery with Schlemm´s canal microstent (Hydrus) for open angle glaucoma. *Cochrane Database Syst. Rev.* **2020**, *2020*, CD012740. [CrossRef]

134. Hu, R.; Guo, D.; Hong, N.; Xuan, X.; Wang, X. Comparison of Hydrus and iStent microinvasive glaucoma surgery implants in combination with phacoemulsification for treatment of open-angle glaucoma: Systematic review and network meta-analysis. *BMJ Open* **2022**, *12*, e051496. [CrossRef]
135. Reiss, G.; Clifford, B.; Vold, S.; He, J.; Hamilton, C.; Dickerson, J.; Lane, S. Safety and Effectiveness of CyPass Supraciliary Micro-Stent in Primary Open-Angle Glaucoma: 5-Year Results from the COMPASS XT Study. *Am. J. Ophthalmol.* **2019**, *208*, 219–225. [CrossRef] [PubMed]
136. Sandhu, A.; Jayaram, H.; Hu, K.; Bunce, C.; Gazzard, G. Ab interno supraciliary microstent surgery for open-angle glaucoma. *Cochrane Database Syst. Rev.* **2021**, *2021*, CD012802. [CrossRef]
137. Denis, P.; Hirneiß, C.; Durr, G.M.; Reddy, K.P.; Kamarthy, A.; Calvo, E.; Hussain, Z.; Ahmed, I.K. Two-year outcomes of the MINIject drainage system for uncontrolled glaucoma from the STAR-I first-in-human trial. *Br. J. Ophthalmol.* **2022**, *106*, 65–70. [CrossRef] [PubMed]
138. Baudouin, C.; Kolko, M.; Melik-Parsadaniantz, S.; Messmer, E.M. Inflammation in Glaucoma: From the back to the front of the eye, and beyond. *Prog. Retin. Eye Res.* **2021**, *83*, 100916. [CrossRef] [PubMed]
139. Freiberg, J.C.; Hedengran, A.; Heegaard, S.; Petrovski, G.; Jacobsen, J.; Cvenkel, B.; Kolko, M. An Evaluation of the Physicochemical Properties of Preservative-Free 0.005% (w/v) Latanoprost Ophthalmic Solutions, and the Impact on In Vitro Human Conjunctival Goblet Cell Survival. *J. Clin. Med.* **2022**, *11*, 3137. [CrossRef]
140. Thein, A.-S.; Hedengran, A.; Azuara-Blanco, A.; Arita, R.; Cvenkel, B.; Gazzard, G.; Heegaard, S.; de Paiva, C.S.; Petrovski, G.; Prokosch-Willing, V.; et al. Adverse Effects and Safety in Glaucoma Patients: Agreement on Clinical Trial Outcomes for Reports on Eye Drops (ASGARD)—A Delphi Consensus Statement. *Am. J. Ophthalmol.* **2022**, *241*, 190–197. [CrossRef] [PubMed]
141. Erras, A.; Shahrvini, B.; Weinreb, R.N.; Baxter, S.L. Review of glaucoma medication adherence monitoring in the digital health era. *Br. J. Ophthalmol.* **2021**. [CrossRef] [PubMed]
142. Khawaja, A.P.; Campbell, J.H.; Kirby, N.; Chandwani, H.S.; Keyzor, I.; Parekh, M.; McNaught, A.I.; Vincent, D.; Angela, K.; Nitin, A.; et al. Real-World Outcomes of Selective Laser Trabeculoplasty in the United Kingdom. *Ophthalmology* **2020**, *127*, 748–757. [CrossRef]
143. Agrawal, P.; Bradshaw, S.E. Systematic Literature Review of Clinical and Economic Outcomes of Micro-Invasive Glaucoma Surgery (MIGS) in Primary Open-Angle Glaucoma. *Ophthalmol. Ther.* **2018**, *7*, 49–73. [CrossRef]
144. Fea, A.M.; Cattel, F.; Gandolfi, S.; Buseghin, G.; Furneri, G.; Costagliola, C. Cost-utility analysis of trabecular micro-bypass stents (TBS) in patients with mild-to-moderate open-angle Glaucoma in Italy. *BMC Health Serv. Res.* **2021**, *21*, 1–12. [CrossRef]
145. Buller, A.J.; Connell, B.; Spencer, A.F. Compliance: Clear communication's critical. *Br. J. Ophthalmol.* **2005**, *89*, 1370. [CrossRef] [PubMed]

Disclaimer/Publisher's Note: The statements, opinions and data contained in all publications are solely those of the individual author(s) and contributor(s) and not of MDPI and/or the editor(s). MDPI and/or the editor(s) disclaim responsibility for any injury to people or property resulting from any ideas, methods, instructions or products referred to in the content.

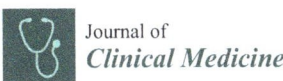

Article

An Evaluation of the Physicochemical Properties of Preservative-Free 0.005% (*w*/*v*) Latanoprost Ophthalmic Solutions, and the Impact on In Vitro Human Conjunctival Goblet Cell Survival

Josefine C. Freiberg [1], Anne Hedengran [1,2], Steffen Heegaard [2,3], Goran Petrovski [4,5], Jette Jacobsen [6], Barbara Cvenkel [7,8] and Miriam Kolko [1,2,*]

[1] Department of Drug Design and Pharmacology, University of Copenhagen, 2100 Copenhagen, Denmark; josefine.freiberg@sund.ku.dk (J.C.F.); anne.hedengran.nagstrup@regionh.dk (A.H.)
[2] Department of Ophthalmology, Copenhagen University Hospital, Rigshospitalet-Glostrup, 2600 Glostrup, Denmark; steffen.heegaard@regionh.dk
[3] Department of Pathology, Copenhagen University Hospital, Rigshospitalet, 2100 Copenhagen, Denmark
[4] Center for Eye Research, Department of Ophthalmology, Oslo University Hospital, 0450 Oslo, Norway; gokipepo@gmail.com
[5] Institute for Clinical Medicine, Faculty of Medicine, University of Oslo, 0372 Oslo, Norway
[6] Department of Pharmacy, University of Copenhagen, 2100 Copenhagen, Denmark; jette.jacobsen@sund.ku.dk
[7] Glaucoma Unit, Department of Ophthalmology, University Medical Centre Ljubljana, 1000 Ljubljana, Slovenia; barbara.cvenkel@gmail.com
[8] Medical Faculty, University of Ljubljana, 1000 Ljubljana, Slovenia
* Correspondence: miriamk@sund.ku.dk

Abstract: Purpose: To examine the physicochemical properties of five preservative-free (PF) 0.005% latanoprost ophthalmic products; Monoprost®, Latanest®, Gaap Ofteno®, Xalmono®, and Xaloptic® Free. Furthermore, the study investigated the mucin production and cell survival of primary cultured human conjunctival goblet cells when treated with PF eye drops. Method: The pH value, osmolality, and surface tension were examined. Cell survival was analyzed using lactate dehydrogenase and tetrazolium dye colorimetric assays. Mucin production was analyzed with immunohistochemical staining. Results: Monoprost® (pH value 6.84 ± 0.032) had a pH value closest to the pH value of tear fluid (pH value 7.4–7.6), whereas Gaap Ofteno® (pH value 6.34 ± 0.004) and Latanest® (pH value 6.33 ± 0.003) had the lowest pH values. Gaap Ofteno® (325.9 ± 2.9 mosmol/kg) showed iso-osmolar probabilities, whereas the other products were hypo-osmolar. Gaap Ofteno® (60.31 ± 0.35 mN/m) had a higher surface tension compared to the tear fluid (40 to 46 mN/m), as described in the literature. No significant differences in goblet cell survival or mucin release were observed between the treatments and control. Conclusion: Significant differences in pH value, osmolality, and surface tension were observed. However, this did not affect the viability of the goblet cells or the release of mucin. Clinical studies are required to evaluate the long-term effects of use on efficacy and safety.

Keywords: latanoprost; preservative-free (PF); pH value; osmolality; surface tension; goblet cells; cell viability; tear film

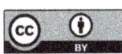

1. Introduction

Glaucoma is one of the leading causes of blindness worldwide, with an overall global prevalence of 3.54% (95%CI 2.09–5.82) in patients aged 40–80 years [1]. Elevated intraocular pressure (IOP) is a recognized risk factor in the development of glaucoma, and lifelong treatment is essential to prevent the progression of the disease [2–4]. Prostaglandin analog (PGA) eye drops are often the first choice when prescribing anti-glaucomatous eye drops because of their well-documented IOP-lowering effect and high tolerability [4].

Several studies have shown that long-term treatment with preservative-containing eye drops induces ocular surface inflammation, instability of the tear film, and damage to the corneal surface [5–7].

The tear film consists of a mucin/aqueous layer and an external lipid layer [8]. Mucin is produced by the conjunctival goblet cells. Goblet cells are essential for obtaining a stable tear film, as well as protecting and lubricating the ocular surface [8–10].

Various clinical, animal, and cellular studies document the finding that preservative agents, such as benzalkonium chloride (BAK), harm the ocular tissue and induce an inflammatory response [11–14].

Prostaglandins are lipophilic molecules and, thus, demand a solubilizing agent that is compatible with the tear film [15]. Besides the solution's antibacterial properties, preservative agents such as BAK solubilize the ophthalmic solution. If preservative agents are removed from an ophthalmic solution, they should be replaced with other solubilizing or stabilizing agents. In 2012, a preservative-free (PF) 0.005% latanoprost ophthalmic solution with Macrogol glycerol hydroxy stearate 40 (MGH40) as a solubilizing agent was developed, patented, and marketed by Laboratoires Théa (Clermont-Ferrand, France) (Monoprost®) [16]. PF formulations can be dispensed as single-dose units or multidose bottles. To prevent contamination of the formulations with a water content above 20% (w/w), multidose containers have incorporated systems, such as filters or two-layer bottles, to protect against contamination. Pharmaceutical companies have patented multi-dose bottles, e.g., ABAK® and EASYGRIP®, developed by Laboratoires Théa, Novelia®, developed by Nemerand (La Verpillière, France), and the 3K® pump/COMOD® device developed by Ursapharm (Saarbrücken, Germany) [17–19].

The European Medicines Agency (EMA, Amsterdam, The Netherlands) requires the active drug used in generics to be identical to the original preparation, with the same concentration, indication, route of administration, and bioavailability. However, the excipients may differ from the original preparation, and generics are not tested with the same efficacy and safety studies as the original products [20,21]. Differences in the physicochemical properties of preserved PGA eye drops have been identified [22,23], but little is known about the differences among PF PGA eye drops and their effect on the ocular surface, cells, and tissue.

In this pre-clinical study, five PF 0.005% latanoprost eye drops were investigated in terms of their chemical and physical properties: the pH value, osmolality, and surface tension. As a proxy for the eye drops' effect on the viability of human conjunctival goblet cells, lactate dehydrogenase (LDH) and tetrazolium dye (MTT) colorimetric assays were conducted on cultured human conjunctival goblet cells. The presence of mucin in the goblet cells was evaluated with immunohistochemical staining.

2. Materials and Methods

2.1. Materials and Reagents

We used the same methods as previously described by Müllerts et al. and Hendegran et al. [24,25]. The following 0.005% (w/v) PF latanoprost products were included: Monoprost® (Laboratoires Théa—France), Latanest® (Esteve—Spain), Gaap Ofteno® (Laboratorios SOPHIA—Mexico), Xalmono® (Rockmed—Belgium) and Xaloptic® Free (Polpharma, Poland)

In brief, human goblet cells from donors were cultured in Roswell Park Memorial Institute (RPMI) media 1640 1x (32404-014; Gibco, Life Technologies, Waltham, MA, USA) with 10% fetal bovine serum (FBS) (10270-106; Gibco, Life Technologies, Waltham, MA, USA) and 1% of the following mentioned solutions: penicillin/streptomycin (15140-122; Gibco, Life Technologies, Waltham, MA, USA), non-essential amino acid (NEAA) solution (M7145; Sigma-Aldrich, St. Louis, MO, USA), 1 M HEPES (15630-080; Gibco, Life Technologies, Waltham, MA, USA), L-glutamine (25030-024; Gibco, Life Technologies, Waltham, MA, USA) and sodium pyruvate (11360-039; Gibco, Life Technologies, Waltham, MA, USA).

When performing LDH and MTT assays, phosphate-buffered saline (PBS) was prepared with 137 mM NaCl, 2.7 mM KCl, 10 mM Na_2HPO_4, and 1.8 mM KH_2PO_4 with a pH value of 7.4, adjusted with either 1 M HCl or 1 M NaOH. Then, 1 M EDTA (E5134; Sigma-Aldrich, St. Louis, MO, USA) in PBS, 0.48 mM versene (15040-033; Gibco, Life Technologies, Waltham, MA, USA), and trypsin (T4799; Sigma-Aldrich, St. Louis, MO, USA) were used when trypsinizing the goblet cells. An LDH cytotoxicity detection kit from Takara BIO, Kusatsu Shiga, Japan (MK401) was utilized, and the MTT assay was performed using 12.5 mM thiazolyl blue tetrazolium bromide (M5655; Sigma-Aldrich, St. Louis, MO, USA) in PBS.

For immunohistochemical staining, 4% (w/v) of paraformaldehyde in PBS (provided by the RegionH pharmacy) was used to fixate the cells. PBS, Triton-X (1001325622; Sigma-Aldrich, St. Louis, MO, USA), bovine serum albumin (ab181831; Sigma-Aldrich, St. Louis, MO, USA), and saponin from Quillaja Bark (1001658552; Sigma-Aldrich, St. Louis, MO, USA) were used for immunohistochemical staining with the primary antibodies, Cytokeratin7 (ab181831; Abcam, Cambridge, UK) and monoclonal anti-human gastric mucin (M5293; Sigma-Aldrich, St. Louis, MO, USA). The secondary antibodies used were Alexa488 (A11034; Gibco, Life Technologies, Waltham, MA, USA), Texas red (T862; Gibco, Life Technologies, Waltham, MA, USA), and DAPI (D3571; Invitrogen, Waltham, MA, USA).

2.2. Physicochemical Characterization

The osmolality and pH values were measured in triplicate for both diluted and undiluted eye drops. The eye drops were diluted at 1:7 (v/v) in RPMI media. The pH value was measured at room temperature using a calibrated 744 pH meter (Metrohm; Nordic ApS, Herisau, Switzerland), and the freezing point depression (Osmomat 3000; Gonotec, Berlin, Germany) measured the osmolality. The Wilhelmy method was used to detect the surface tension with a force tensiometer, K-100c (Krüss GmbH, Hamburg, Germany), and the Laboratory Desktop software, version 3.2.2.3068 (Laboratory Desktop, Krüss GmbH). The measurements were performed in triplicate with the undiluted products at room temperature and with a standard deviation of less than 0.1 mN/m.

2.3. Human Conjunctival Goblet Cell Cultivation

With approval from the Danish National Committee on Health Research (H-17007902) and the Norwegian Regional Committees for Medical and Health Research Ethics (REK: 2013/803), the conjunctiva from post-mortem human donors was cultivated to generate primary goblet cell cultures. Conjunctiva pieces were incubated for 14 days at 37 °C and 5% CO_2. Media was added to the cultures every day for the first three days and, thereafter, was changed every other day. To keep the purified cell cultures, microscopy of the cells was performed before every media change using light microscopy. If any fibroblasts appeared in the cultures, they were removed manually.

2.4. Cell Survival Analysis

The goblet cells were trypsinized after 14 days of cultivation, counted, and replated in a 96-well plate with a cell density of 25,000 cells/cm^2 for LDH and 50,000 cells/cm^2 for the MTT assay. Cells were incubated for an additional four to five days at 37 °C and 5% CO_2, to ensure adhesion before they were treated for 30 min with eye drops that were diluted at 1:7 (v/v) in media. After 30 min of treatment, the eye drops were removed, fresh media was added, and the cells were incubated for various time periods, depending on the assay performed thereafter. The LDH assay was performed 20 h after treatment with eye drops. LDH solution was prepared immediately before the experiment, added to the cells, and incubated at room temperature in the dark for 15–20 min before the stop solution (10% HCL, v/v) was added. Concerning the MTT assay, 12 mM MTT (w/v) in PBS was added to the cells, immediately after treatment with the diluted eye drops. The cells were incubated at 37 °C and 5% CO_2 for one hour, followed by adding 0.01% (v/v) HCL in 10% (w/v) SDS, in PBS solution. The cells were then incubated in the dark for 18 h at room temperature. A SpectraMax i3X multi-mode microplate reader (Molecular Devices, San Jose, CA, USA) with an absorbance of 490 nm for LDH and 560 nm for MTT was applied. To secure the reproducibility of the results, a minimum of three batches from a minimum of four different donors was required for analysis. For every experiment, a control treated with only RPMI media was included. The cell survival data was calculated as the mean percentage change in absorbance, compared to the control ± standard deviation (SD).

2.5. Immunohistochemical Staining

The goblets cells were cultivated on slides and treated with RPMI media or diluted eye drops 1:7 (v/v) for 30 min at 37 °C 5% CO. With the use of paraformaldehyde 4% (v/v), the slides were fixated and stored at 4 °C. The cell membranes of the goblet cells were permeated using 0.1% v/v Triton X-100 in PBS, and by using 3% (w/v) bovine serum albumin in PBS, unspecific binding was blocked. The cells were treated with the primary antibodies Cytokeratin-7 (anti-cytokeratin7, 1:500 v/v) and monoclonal anti-human gastric mucin (anti-mucin, 1:200 v/v), diluted in 0.25% bovine serum albumin/0.1% saponin in PBS and washed with PBS thereafter. The fluorescent secondary antibodies, Alexa488 (anti-rabbit, 1:500 v/v) and Texas red (anti-mouse, 1:200 v/v), both diluted in 0.25% bovine serum albumin/0.1% saponin in PBS, were added. Then, 0.3 µM of DAPI in PBS stained the nuclei of the goblet cells. Imaging was performed using an Axioskop 2 (Zeiss; Göttingen, Germany) with an Axio Cam MRm camera (Zeiss; Göttingen, Germany) and an HXP 120 lighting unit (Zeiss; Göttingen, Germany). Image scaling and the merging of pictures were conducted using ImageJ 1.52q (Wayne Rasband, National Institute of Health, Bethesda, MD, USA).

2.6. Statistics

The software program, GraphPad Prism 9 (GraphPad Software, San Diego, California USA), was used for the statistical analyses and graphs. Descriptive statistics and a comparative one-way analysis of variance (ANOVA) were chosen as the statistical analyses for all data sets. To estimate the differences in cell survival, osmolality, pH value, and surface tension among the treatments, Tukey's multiple comparison test was applied. All results were expressed as mean ± SD, and a p-value of ≤ 0.05 was considered statistically significant.

3. Results

3.1. pH Value

The pH value was examined in both undiluted and diluted products, while the goblet cell cultures were treated with diluted products (Figure 1). Of the undiluted eye drops (Figure 1a), Monoprost® had the highest pH value of 6.84 ± 0.032, while Latanest® had the lowest pH value of 6.33 ± 0.003. The pH value of the remaining eye drops was 6.34 ± 0.004 (Gaap Ofteno®), 6.70 ± 0.003 (Xalmono®), and 6.71 ± 0.000 (Xaloptic® Free). Significant differences ($p \leq 0.0001$) were observed between all eye drops, except between Latanest® and Gaap Ofteno®, and between Xalmono® and Xaloptic® Free. As presented in Figure 1b, the pH value of the diluted formulations was 7.62 ± 0.002 (Monoprost®), 6.89 ± 0.007 (Latanest®), 7.34 ± 0.004 (Gaap Ofteno®), 7.34 ± 0.009 (Xalmono®) and 7.37 ± 0.002 (Xaloptic® Free). Significant differences were observed between the eye drops with $p \leq 0.001$ or $p \leq 0.0001$. Gaap Ofteno® and Xalmono® were not significantly different.

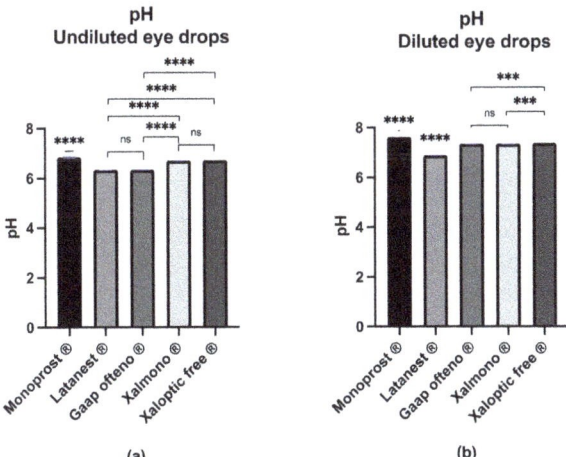

Figure 1. The pH value characterization of preservative-free 0.005% latanoprost products Monoprost®, Latanest®, Gaap Ofteno®, Xalmono®, and Xaloptic® Free: (**a**) pH value of the undiluted eye drops; (**b**) pH value of the diluted eye drops (1:7, v/v). Values are listed as mean ± SD, and $n = 3$. A one-way ANOVA with a Tukey multiple-comparison test ($p = 0.05$) was performed. ns = not significant, with $p \geq 0.05$, *** $p \leq 0.001$, **** $p \leq 0.0001$.

3.2. Osmolality

The osmolality was examined in both undiluted and diluted products, while the goblet cell cultures were treated with diluted products (Figure 2). The osmolality of the undiluted Gaap Ofteno® was 325.9 ± 2.9 mosmol/kg and was significantly higher, compared to the four other products ($p \leq 0.0001$) (Figure 2a). The osmolality of the other eye drops was 275.8 ± 0.7 mosmol/kg (Monoprost®), 278.9 ± 1.3 mosmol/kg (Latanest®), 261.0 ± 1.2 mosmol/kg (Xalmono®) and 261.2 ± 0.3 mosmol/kg (Xaloptic® Free), as visualized in Figure 2a. There were no significant differences between Monoprost® and Latanest® or between Xalmono® and Xaloptic Free®.

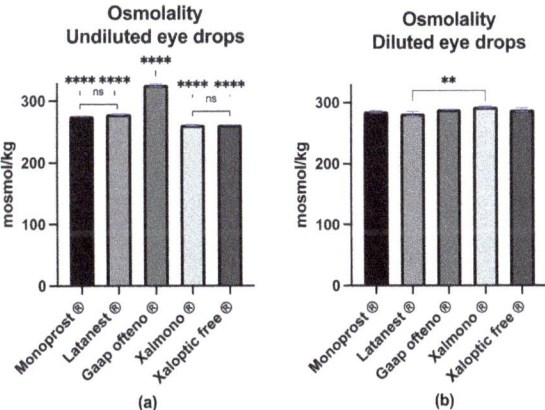

Figure 2. Osmolality characterization of preservative-free 0.005% latanoprost eye drops Monoprost®, Latanest®, Gaap Ofteno®, Xalmono® and Xaloptic® Free: (**a**) osmolality of the undiluted eye drops; (**b**) osmolality of the diluted eye drops (1:7, v/v). Values are listed as mean ± SD, and $n = 3$. A one-way ANOVA with a Tukey multiple-comparison test ($p = 0.05$) was performed. ns = not significant with $p \geq 0.05$, ** $p \leq 0.01$, **** $p \leq 0.0001$.

Of the diluted eye drops (Figure 2b), Latanest® had the lowest osmolality of 281.9 ± 4.2 mosmol/kg, and Xalmono® had the highest osmolality of 292.7 ± 2.1 mosmol/kg. Monoprost® had an osmolality of 285.3 ± 2.2 mosmol/kg, Xaloptic® Free, osmolality of 288.1 ± 3.5 mosmol/kg, and Gaap Ofteno®, osmolality of 288.9 ± 0.5 mosmol/kg (Figure 2b). Significant differences ($p \leq 0.01$) were observed between Latanest® and Xalmono®.

No significant differences were observed among the other eye drops.

3.3. Surface Tension

Gaap Ofteno® demonstrated a surface tension of 60.31 ± 0.35 mN/m, which was significantly higher compared to the other products ($p \leq 0.0001$) (Figure 3). Xalmono® had the lowest surface tension of 39.00 ± 0.38 mN/m, and was significantly lower compared to the other products ($p \leq 0.0001$). No significant differences were observed between Monoprost® (42.44 ± 0.75 mN/m) and Xaloptic® Free (42.76 ± 0.36 mN/m), or between Latanest® (43.15 ± 1.13 mN/m) and Xaloptic® Free.

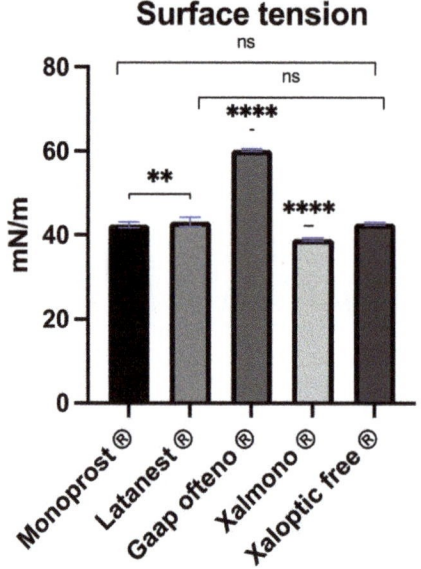

Figure 3. Surface tension characterization of preservative-free 0.005% latanoprost products; Monoprost®, Latanest®, Gaap Ofteno®, Xalmono® and Xaloptic® Free. Values are listed as mean ± SD, n = 3. A one-way ANOVA with a Tukey multiple-comparison test (p = 0.05) were performed. ns = not significant with $p \geq 0.05$, ** $p \leq 0.01$, **** $p \leq 0.0001$.

3.4. Cell Survival

LDH and MTT analyses were performed on primary cultured human conjunctival goblet cells treated with diluted PF 0.005% latanoprost products. Cell survival was reported relative to the control, these being goblet cells treated with RPMI media. According to the results of the LDH assays, the mean cell survival after treatment with eye drops was 100.70 ± 12.8% (Monoprost®), 98.17 ± 9.4% (Latanest®), 101.40 ± 5.9% (Gaap Ofteno®), 99.36 ± 5.7% (Xalmono®) and 93.66 ± 6.0% (Xaloptic® Free). As seen in Figure 4a, the LDH assay showed no significant differences in cell survival between treatments. Similar results were obtained from the MTT analysis, showing no significant differences in cell survival between the treatments (Figure 4b). The mean cell survival compared to the control was 86.40 ± 9.1% (Monoprost®), 83.53 ± 9.9% (Latanest®), 89.84 ± 18.2% (Gaap Ofteno®), 89.30 ± 12.7% (Xalmono®), and 89.51 ± 11.0% (Xaloptic® Free).

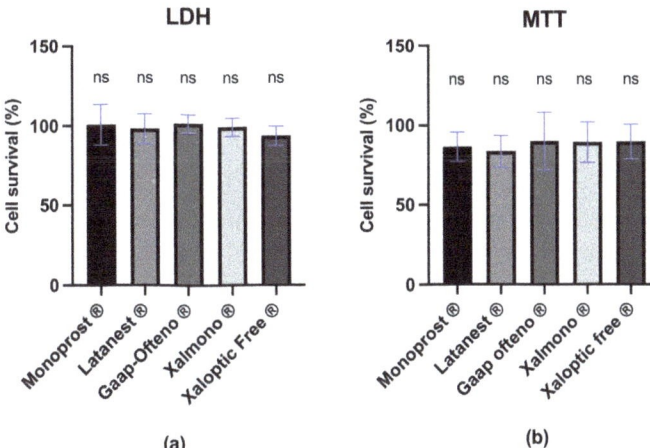

Figure 4. Mean cell survival analysis of human conjunctival goblet cells in % ± SD, relative to control, after 30 min of treatment with preservative-free 0.005% latanoprost eye drops. (**a**) Cell survival, examined with the LDH assay; (**b**) cell survival, examined with the MTT assay. Goblet cells were treated with diluted (1:7, v/v) preservative-free 0.005% latanoprost products: Monoprost®, Latanest®, Gaap Ofteno®, Xalmono®, and Xaloptic® Free. A one-way ANOVA with a Tukey multiple-comparison test was performed (p = 0.05), $n \geq 4$; ns = not significant; $p \geq 0.05$.

3.5. Immunohistochemical Staining

Immunohistochemical staining was used to visualize the cytoskeleton of the goblet cells, the nuclei, and mucin, as seen in Figure 5. Goblet cells treated with RPMI media showed mucin allocated around the nuclei (Figure 5A). Figure 5B–F demonstrated a similar pattern, showing mucin allocated near the nuclei when the cell cultures were treated with diluted PF 0.005% latanoprost eye drops: Monoprost®, Latanest®, Gaap Ofteno®, Xalmono®, and Xaloptic® Free.

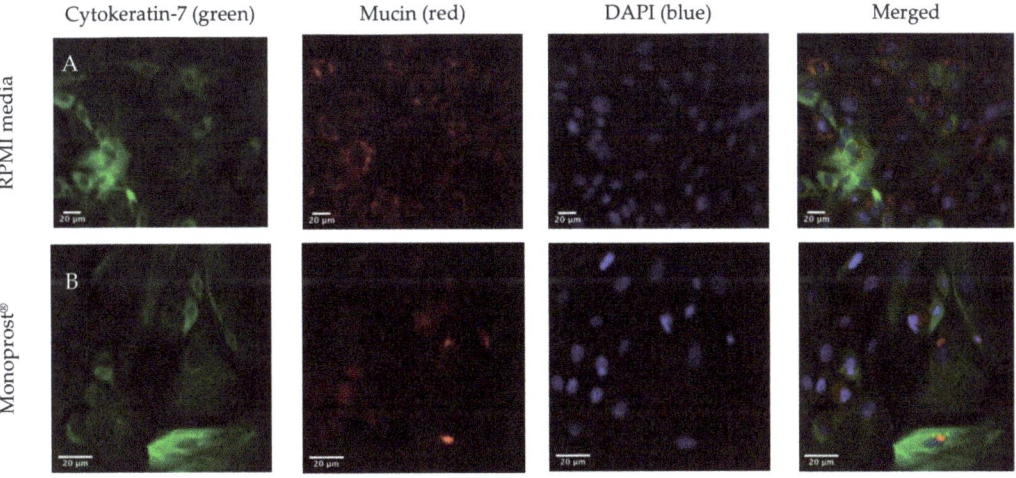

Figure 5. *Cont.*

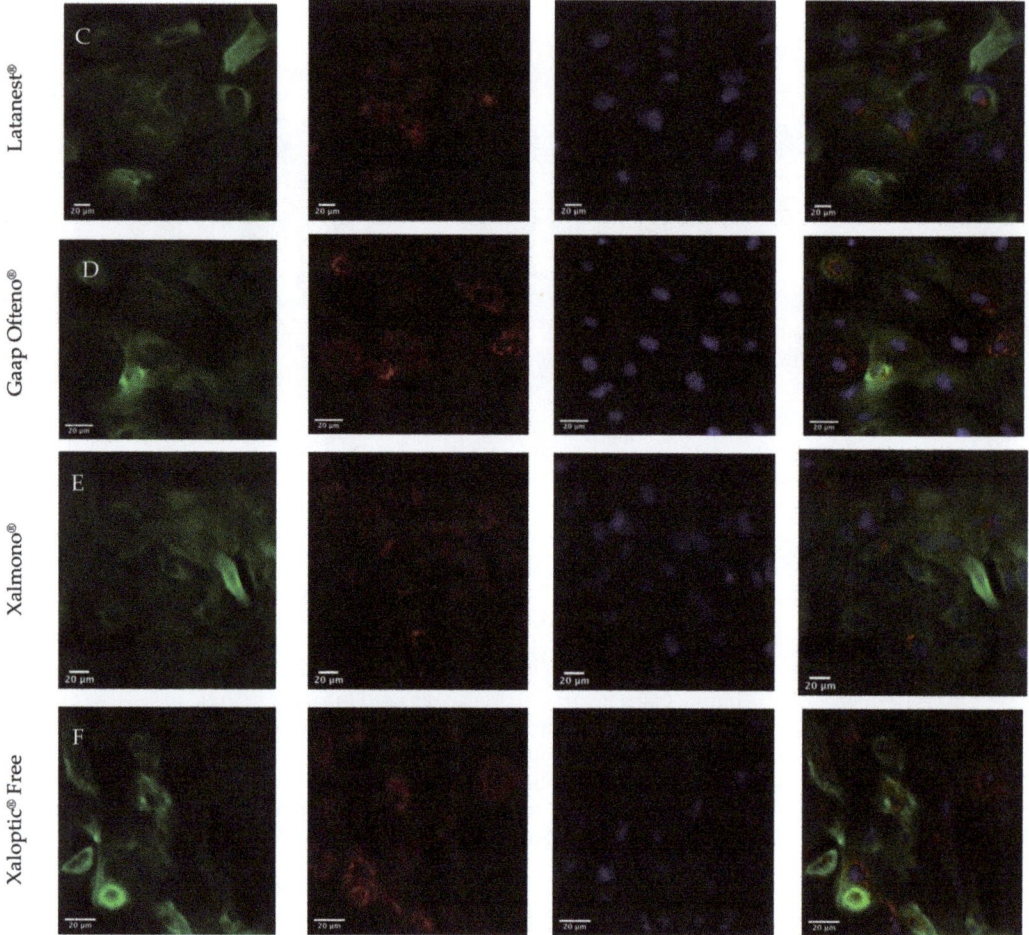

Figure 5. Immunohistochemical staining of human goblet cells, visualizing the cytoskeleton (column 1: Cytokeratin-7, green), mucin (column 2: mucin, red), the nucleus (column 3: DAPI, blue), and merged stainings (column 4: cytokeratin-7 (green), mucin (red) and DAPI (blue)). Cells were treated with diluted (1:7, v/v) 0.005% latanoprost preservative-free products. (**A**): RPMI media, (**B**): Monoprost®, (**C**): Latanest®, (**D**): Gaap Ofteno®, (**E**): Xalmono®, and (**F**): Xaloptic® Free. $n = 3$.

4. Discussion

Anti-glaucomatous treatment is lifelong, and the importance of minimizing adverse effects is crucial to increasing patients' adherence to the treatment regimen and for health-related quality of life [26]. Glaucoma patients experience side effects from the treatment, such as dry eye disease (DED), a foreign-body sensation, and a stinging or burning sensation in the eye [27]. The cause of DED is either reduced lacrimation or increased evaporation from the ocular surface. Changes in the ocular surface may lead to a hyperosmolar condition, which is a recognized risk factor for inducing proinflammatory stress [8,28,29]. The instability of the tear film can cause ocular discomfort or irritation, while pH value, osmolality, and surface tension all play a role in achieving a healthy ocular surface. The current study revealed significant differences in the physicochemical properties of pH value, osmolality, and surface tension. Some of the variations may be due to the product formulation, as Monoprost®, Xaloptic® Free, and Xalmono® were dispensed from single-dose units, whereas Gaap Ofteno® and Latanest® were dispensed from multi-dose bottles. Osmolality, pH value, and surface tension may vary due to variations in the solvents or stabilizers caused by the removal of preservatives. The physicochemical properties of the undiluted eye drops illustrated the properties of the eye drops immediately after application to the ocular surface in patients.

The pH value of tear fluid is 7.4–7.6 [30–32]. To optimize ocular comfort, the pH value of the ophthalmic formulations should match the tear film or at least be in the ocular range of 6.6–7.8, as an acidic or alkaline pH value induces lacrimation, ocular pain, and discomfort [23,32]. In this study, we found that Latanest® (pH value 6.33 ± 0.003) and Gaap Ofteno® (pH value 6.34 ± 0.004) were acidic, with pH values below the ocular range. The remaining three products, Monoprost® (pH value 6.84 ± 0.032), Xalmono® (6.70 ± 0.003), and Xaloptic® Free (6.71 ± 0.000), had pH values within the ocular range, with Monoprost® closest to the pH value of the tear film. An acidic pH value may cause side effects, such as ocular discomfort and increased lacrimation upon instillation, whereas a pH within the recommended range should not provide any discomfort related to the pH value. When the products were diluted with RPMI media, the pH values of all products were within the recommended pH range. Our findings imply that it would be of great interest to investigate the pH value of PF PGA products upon dilution with tear fluid in patients, to elucidate if differences in pH value may cause prolonged ocular discomfort.

The osmolality of the tear fluid varies from 310 to 350 mosmol/kg [31]. All products except Gaap Ofteno® (325.9 ± 2.9 mosmol/kg) were hypo-osmolar, compared to the tear fluid. As previously mentioned, a hyperosmolar tear film is related to ocular irritation and DED. Based on our findings, the osmolality of the tested products should not be of particular concern, as they demonstrated iso- or hypo-osmolar properties.

The surface tension of the tear fluid varies from 40 to 46 mN/m and ensures a stable tear film and tear film break-up time [33,34]. Furthermore, the surface tension influences the eye drops' ability to spread and adhere to the cornea, once applied [34]. We found that Monoprost® (42.44 ± 0.75 mN/m), Xaloptic® Free (42.76 ± 0.36 mN/m), and Latanest® (43.15 ± 1.13 mN/m) had a surface tension in the physiological range of the tear fluid. Gaap Ofteno® (60.31 ± 0.35 mN/m) had a surface tension well above the physiological range, while Xalmono® had a surface tension just below 40 (39.0 ± 0.38 mN/m). Surface tension exceeding the physiological range may cause instability of the tear film and is associated with dry eyes [34]. In addition, higher surface tension will increase the drop volume released from the bottle [35]. The drop volume will also affect the amount of latanoprost released [23]. A greater drop volume will increase the washout and may result in less uptake of latanoprost and reduced efficacy in terms of lowering IOP. Thus, increased surface tension in ophthalmic solutions may lead to both the ocular adverse effects caused by a destabilized tear film and potentially reduce the efficacy of the eye drops.

Keeping goblet cells unharmed and unstressed is essential for maintaining a stable tear film for a healthy ocular surface [9,10]. Diluted PF 0.005% latanoprost eye drops showed no negative effects on either cell survival or mucin release after treatment, according to the LDH assay, MTT assay, and immunohistochemical staining. Other studies have investigated the differences between preserved and preservative-free PGAs. Treatment with PF tafluprost showed reduced pro-apoptotic and pro-oxidative stress in a conjunctival epithelial cell line, compared to preserved PGAs [36]. In patients, the goblet cell density was significantly increased after six months of treatment with PF tafluprost, compared to the baseline. In comparison, patients treated with preserved tafluprost showed increased goblet cell density after one month of treatment, but no significant long-term effects were reported [37].

As previously mentioned, it is of great interest to minimize the adverse effects of treatment, since glaucoma is a chronic condition. A frequently reported side effect of PGAs is conjunctival hyperemia [38,39]. PF PGAs, e.g., Monoprost® and Gaap Ofteno®, have previously been examined and compared to preserved PGAs. A meta-analysis of 21 studies found that conjunctival hyperemia was significantly reduced in Monoprost® compared to preserved PGAs, with no significant differences in IOP between treatments [40].

In addition, Rouland et al. showed noninferiority in IOP efficacy and a significantly reduced conjunctival hyperemia after treatment with Monoprost®, compared to treatment with Xalatan® [41].

Gonzales et al. compared the stability, efficacy, and adverse effects of Gaap Ofteno® with the preserved brand product, Xalatan® [42]. As Gaap Ofteno® is dispensed from a multidose bottle, the stability of the drug was also examined. The study showed that the two products were comparable in terms of IOP reduction and safety, evaluated as conjunctival hyperemia, with a similar prevalence of 11.3% (Gaap Ofteno®) and 11.9% (Xalatan®). The above-mentioned studies support our findings that PF 0.005% latanoprost products are non-toxic to human conjunctival goblet cells under experimental conditions.

When patients instill ophthalmic solutions in the eye, the tear film dilutes the ophthalmic solutions and only 1–7% of the instilled drug reaches the aqueous humor [43]. We chose to treat goblet cell cultures with diluted eye drops at a constant concentration for 30 min. In patients, the tear film dilutes the eye drops gradually upon administration, with a reduced expected exposure time (less than 30 min) as the fluid turnover rate of the conjunctival cul-de-sac in the eye is 0.5–2.2 µL/min. With this turnover rate, the drug remains in the conjunctival cul-de-sac for approximately 3–5 min [43]. The RPMI media used in this study was not identical to the tear film and will have different capacities, for instance, in buffering. Therefore, the physicochemical properties of eye drops diluted with tear film may affect the goblet cells in other ways than those identified in this study.

The in vitro model used in this study has some limitations since it cannot be directly compared to the conditions in patients. We did not quantify the amount of mucin released from goblet cells; the immunohistochemical staining that was performed only detected the presence of mucin. In addition, we did not evaluate the long-term effects of treating human conjunctival goblet cells with PF products. Thus, clinical trials would be desirable to examine whether the physicochemical differences addressed in this study may influence the long-term efficacy and safety profile of PF eye drops.

5. Conclusions

In conclusion, this study identified significant differences in pH value, osmolality, and surface tension among five PF 0.005% latanoprost products. The variations in physicochemical properties, such as acidic pH values or high surface tension, may potentially destabilize the tear film and reduce the tolerability of eye drops on the ocular surface. However, the variations in the physicochemical properties of the PF eye drops had no negative effects on either cell survival or mucin release. Since the efficacy was not examined in this in vitro experiment, clinical studies would be of great interest in elucidating the potential differences among PF PGA treatments, in terms of efficacy, tolerability, and the side effects related to long-term treatment with PF 0.005% latanoprost products.

Author Contributions: Conceptualization, M.K., J.C.F., A.H., S.H., G.P. and J.J.; methodology, M.K. and J.J.; investigation and data curation, J.C.F.; formal analysis, J.C.F., A.H. and M.K.; writing—original draft preparation, J.C.F.; writing—review and editing, J.C.F., A.H., J.J., G.P., S.H., B.C. and M.K.; supervision, M.K., J.J., A.H.; funding acquisition, M.K. All authors have read and agreed to the published version of the manuscript.

Funding: This research was funded by Laboratoires Théa (France).

Institutional Review Board Statement: The study was conducted in accordance with the Declaration of Helsinki, and approved by the Danish National Committee on Health Research (H-17007902) and the Norwegian Regional Committees for Medical and Health Research Ethics (REK: 2013/803).

Informed Consent Statement: Patient consent for publication not applicable.

Data Availability Statement: Datasets are available on reasonable request.

Acknowledgments: Special thanks to laboratory technician Charlotte Taul for her laboratory assistance. We acknowledge the Hørslev-Fonden for their equipment grant for a tensiometer. We also acknowledge the Vissing-Fonden for their project support grant to meet the running costs. The study at the Center for Eye Research, Oslo, Norway, was partially supported by funding from the Norwegian Association of the Blind and Partially Sighted.

Conflicts of Interest: M.K. is speaker and in advisory boards for Abbvie, Santen and Thea. M.K. has a collaborative grant from Thea and serve as a consultant for Abbvie and Thea.

References

1. Tham, Y.C.; Li, X.; Wong, T.Y.; Quigley, H.A.; Aung, T.; Cheng, C.Y. Global prevalence of glaucoma and projections of glaucoma burden through 2040: A systematic review and meta-analysis. *Ophthalmology* **2014**, *121*, 2081–2090. [CrossRef] [PubMed]
2. Caprioli, J.; Varma, R. Intraocular Pressure: Modulation as Treatment for Glaucoma. *Am. J. Ophthalmol.* **2011**, *152*, 340–344.e2. [CrossRef] [PubMed]
3. Heijl, A.; Leske, M.C.; Bengtsson, B.; Hyman, L.; Bengtsson, B.; Hussein, M. Reduction of intraocular pressure and glaucoma progression: Results from the Early Manifest Glaucoma Trial. *Arch. Ophthalmol.* **2002**, *120*, 1268–1279. [CrossRef] [PubMed]
4. Li, T.; Lindsley, K.; Rouse, B.; Hong, H.; Shi, Q.; Friedman, D.S.; Friedman, D.S.; Wormald, R.; Dickersin, K. Comparative Effectiveness of First-Line Medications for Primary Open-Angle Glaucoma: A Systematic Review and Network Meta-analysis. *Ophthalmology* **2016**, *123*, 129–140. [CrossRef] [PubMed]
5. Baudouin, C. Allergic reaction to topical eyedrops. *Curr. Opin. Allergy Clin. Immunol.* **2005**, *5*, 459–463. [CrossRef]
6. Manni, G.; Centofanti, M.; Oddone, F.; Parravano, M.; Bucci, M.G. Interleukin-1β tear concentration in glaucomatous and ocular hypertensive patients treated with preservative-free nonselective beta-blockers. *Am. J. Ophthalmol.* **2005**, *139*, 72–77. [CrossRef]
7. Baudouin, C.; Hamard, P.; Liang, H.; Creuzot-Garcher, C.; Bensoussan, L.; Brignole, F. Conjunctival epithelial cell expression of interleukins and inflammatory markers in glaucoma patients treated over the long term. *Ophthalmology* **2004**, *111*, 2186–2192. [CrossRef]
8. Stahl, U.; Willcox, M.; Stapleton, F. Osmolality and tear film dynamics. *Clin. Exp. Optom.* **2012**, *95*, 3–11. [CrossRef]
9. Portal, C.; Gouyer, V.; Gottrand, F.; Desseyn, J.L. Ocular mucins in dry eye disease. *Exp. Eye Res.* **2019**, *186*, 107724. [CrossRef]
10. Gipson, I.K. Goblet cells of the conjunctiva: A review of recent findings. *Prog. Retin. Eye Res.* **2016**, *54*, 49–63. [CrossRef]
11. Lee, H.J.; Jun, R.M.; Cho, M.S.; Choi, K.R. Comparison of the ocular surface changes following the use of two different prostaglandin F2? analogues containing benzalkonium chloride or polyquad in rabbit eyes. *Cutan. Ocul. Toxicol.* **2015**, *34*, 195–202. [CrossRef]
12. Anwar, Z.; Wellik, S.R.; Galor, A. Glaucoma therapy and ocular surface disease: Current literature and recommendations. *Curr. Opin. Ophthalmol.* **2013**, *24*, 136–143. [CrossRef] [PubMed]
13. Baudouin, C. Detrimental effect of preservatives in eyedrops: Implications for the treatment of glaucoma. *Acta Ophthalmol.* **2008**, *86*, 716–726. [CrossRef] [PubMed]
14. Ayaki, M.; Iwasawa, A. Cytotoxicity of prostaglandin analog eye drops preserved with benzalkonium chloride in multiple corneoconjunctival cell lines. *Clin. Ophthalmol. (Auckl. NZ)* **2010**, *4*, 919–924. [CrossRef] [PubMed]
15. Rodriguez-Aller, M.; Guinchard, S.; Guillarme, D.; Pupier, M.; Jeannerat, D.; Rivara-Minten, E.; Veuthey, J.-L.; Gurny, R. New prostaglandin analog formulation for glaucoma treatment containing cyclodextrins for improved stability, solubility and ocular tolerance. *Eur. J. Pharm. Biopharm.* **2015**, *95*, 203–214. [CrossRef] [PubMed]
16. Fabrice Mercier, C.-F.F. inventor; Laboratoires Thea, Clermont Ferrand (FR), assignee. Polymeric Delivery System for A Nonviscous Prostaglandin-Based Solution without Preservatives. U.S. Patent 8637054-B2, 20 December 2012.
17. Baudouin, C.; Labbé, A.; Liang, H.; Pauly, A.; Brignole-Baudouin, F. Preservatives in eyedrops: The good, the bad and the ugly. *Prog. Retin. Eye Res.* **2010**, *29*, 312–334. [CrossRef]
18. Hsu, K.H.; Gupta, K.; Nayaka, H.; Donthi, A.; Kaul, S.; Chauhan, A. Multidose Preservative Free Eyedrops by Selective Removal of Benzalkonium Chloride from Ocular Formulations. *Pharm. Res.* **2017**, *34*, 2862–2872. [CrossRef]
19. SAIDANE, L.P.B. How to deliver preservative-free eye drops in a multidose system with a safer alternative to filters? *Investig. Ophthalmol. Vis. Sci.* **2017**, *58*, 4460.
20. EMA. Questions and Answers on Generic Medicines. Available online: https://www.ema.europa.eu/en/documents/medicine-qa/questions-answers-generic-medicines_en.pdf (accessed on 3 August 2021).
21. EMA. Generic and Hybrid Medicines. Available online: https://www.ema.europa.eu/en/human-regulatory/marketing-authorisation/generic-hybrid-medicines (accessed on 3 August 2021).
22. Kolko, M.; Koch Jensen, P. The physical properties of generic latanoprost ophthalmic solutions are not identical. *Acta Ophthalmol.* **2017**, *95*, 370–373. [CrossRef]
23. Angmo, D.; Wadhwani, M.; Velpandian, T.; Kotnala, A.; Sihota, R.; Dada, T. Evaluation of physical properties and dose equivalency of generic versus branded latanoprost formulations. *Int. Ophthalmol.* **2017**, *37*, 423–428. [CrossRef]
24. Müllertz, O.; Hedengran, A.; Mouhammad, Z.A.; Freiberg, J.; Nagymihály, R.; Jacobsen, J.; Larsen, S.W.; Bair, J.; Utheim, T.P.; Dartt, D.A.; et al. Impact of benzalkonium chloride-preserved and preservative-free latanoprost eye drops on cultured

human conjunctival goblet cells upon acute exposure and differences in physicochemical properties of the eye drops. *BMJ Open Ophthalmol.* **2021**, *6*, e000892. [CrossRef] [PubMed]
25. Hedengran, A.; Begun, X.; Müllertz, O.; Mouhammad, Z.; Vohra, R.; Bair, J.; Dartt, D.A.; Cvenkel, B.; Heegaard, S.; Petrovski, G.; et al. Benzalkonium Chloride-Preserved Anti-Glaucomatous Eye Drops and Their Effect on Human Conjunctival Goblet Cells in vitro. *Biomed. Hub* **2021**, *6*, 69–75. [CrossRef]
26. Skalicky, S.E.; Goldberg, I.; McCluskey, P. Ocular Surface Disease and Quality of Life in Patients With Glaucoma. *Am. J. Ophthalmol.* **2012**, *153*, 1–9.e2. [CrossRef] [PubMed]
27. Zhang, X.; Vadoothker, S.; Munir, W.M.; Saeedi, O. Ocular Surface Disease and Glaucoma Medications: A Clinical Approach. *Eye Contact Lens* **2019**, *45*, 11–18. [CrossRef]
28. Evangelista, M.; Koverech, A.; Messano, M.; Pescosolido, N. Comparison of Three Lubricant Eye Drop Solutions in Dry Eye Patients. *Optom. Vis. Sci.* **2011**, *88*, 1439–1444. [CrossRef] [PubMed]
29. Foulks, G.N. The Correlation Between the Tear Film Lipid Layer and Dry Eye Disease. *Surv. Ophthalmol.* **2007**, *52*, 369–374. [CrossRef]
30. Fischer, F.H.; Wiederholt, M. Human precorneal tear film pH measured by microelectrodes. *Graefes Arch. Clin. Exp. Ophthalmol.* **1982**, *218*, 168–170. [CrossRef] [PubMed]
31. Jitendra, S.P.; Banik, A.; Dixit, S. A new trend: Ocular drug delivery system. *Pharm. Sci.* **2011**, *2*, 720–744.
32. Garcia-Valldecabres, M.; López-Alemany, A.; Refojo, M.F. pH Stability of ophthalmic solutions. *Optom. J. Am. Optom. Assoc.* **2004**, *75*, 161–168. [CrossRef]
33. Nagyová, B.; Tiffany, J.M. Components responsible for the surface tension of human tears. *Curr. Eye Res.* **1999**, *19*, 4–11. [CrossRef]
34. Hotujac Grgurević, M.; Juretić, M.; Hafner, A.; Lovrić, J.; Pepić, I. Tear fluid-eye drops compatibility assessment using surface tension. *Drug Dev. Ind. Pharm.* **2017**, *43*, 275–282. [CrossRef]
35. Van Santvliet, L.; Ludwig, A. Determinants of eye drop size. *Surv. Ophthalmol.* **2004**, *49*, 197–213. [CrossRef] [PubMed]
36. Brasnu, E.; Brignole-Baudouin, F.; Riancho, L.; Guenoun, J.-M.; Warnet, J.-M.; Baudouin, C. In Vitro Effects of Preservative-Free Tafluprost and Preserved Latanoprost, Travoprost, and Bimatoprost in a Conjunctival Epithelial Cell Line. *Curr. Eye Res.* **2008**, *33*, 303–312. [CrossRef] [PubMed]
37. Mastropasqua, L.; Agnifili, L.; Fasanella, V.; Curcio, C.; Ciabattoni, C.; Mastropasqua, R.; Toto, L.; Ciancaglini, M. Conjunctival goblet cells density and preservative-free tafluprost therapy for glaucoma: An in vivo confocal microscopy and impression cytology study. *Acta Ophthalmol.* **2013**, *91*, e397–e405. [CrossRef] [PubMed]
38. Susanna, R., Jr.; Medeiros, F.A. The pros and cons of different prostanoids in the medical management of glaucoma. *Curr. Opin. Ophthalmol.* **2001**, *12*, 149–156. [CrossRef]
39. Honrubia, F.; Garcia-Sanchez, J.; Polo, V.; De La Casa, J.M.M.; Soto, J. Conjunctival hyperaemia with the use of latanoprost versus other prostaglandin analogues in patients with ocular hypertension or glaucoma: A meta-analysis of randomised clinical trials. *Br. J. Ophthalmol.* **2009**, *93*, 316–321. [CrossRef]
40. Cucherat, M.; Stalmans, I.; Rouland, J.F. Relative efficacy and safety of preservative-free latanoprost (T2345) for the treatment of open-angle glaucoma and ocular hypertension: An adjusted Indirect comparison meta-analysis of randomized clinical trials. *J. Glaucoma* **2014**, *23*, e69–e75. [CrossRef]
41. Rouland, J.-F.; Traverso, C.E.; Stalmans, I.; El Fekih, L.; Delval, L.; Renault, D.; Baudouin, C. Efficacy and safety of preservative-free latanoprost eyedrops, compared with BAK-preserved latanoprost in patients with ocular hypertension or glaucoma. *Br. J. Ophthalmol.* **2013**, *97*, 196–200. [CrossRef]
42. Gonzalez, J.R.; Baiza-Duran, L.; Quintana-Hau, J.; Tornero-Montano, R.; Castaneda-Hernandez, G.; Ortiz, M.; Oceguera, F.A.; Loustaunau, M.B.; Gastelum, M.C.; Mejia, J.G.; et al. Comparison of the stability, efficacy, and adverse effect profile of the innovator 0.005% latanoprost ophthalmic solution and a novel cyclodextrin-containing formulation. (Clinical report). *J. Clin. Pharmacol.* **2007**, *47*, 121–126. [CrossRef]
43. Ghate, D.; Edelhauser, H.F. Barriers to Glaucoma Drug Delivery. *J. Glaucoma* **2008**, *17*, 147–156. [CrossRef]

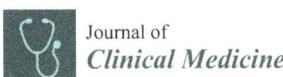

Article

Impact of Short-Term Topical Steroid Therapy on Selective Laser Trabeculoplasty Efficacy

Tomaž Gračner [1,2]

[1] Faculty of Medicine, University of Maribor, 2000 Maribor, Slovenia; tomaz.gracner@ukc-mb.si; Tel.: +386-40-522765; Fax: +386-23-312393
[2] Department of Ophthalmology, University Clinical Centre Maribor, 2000 Maribor, Slovenia

Abstract: Background: To evaluate whether short-term use of topical steroid therapy affected the efficacy of selective laser trabeculoplasty (SLT) for primary open-glaucoma (POAG). Methods: 25 eyes of 25 patients, who used a drop of dexamethasone 0.1% 4 times a day for 7 days as post-laser therapy, formed the Steroid SLT group and 24 eyes of 24 patients, where no topical steroids or nonsteroidal anti-inflammatory agents as post-laser therapy were used, formed the No-steroid SLT group. Success was defined as an intraocular pressure (IOP) lowering exceeding 20% of pretreatment IOP. Results: The mean follow-up time was 21.24 months for the Steroid SLT group and 20.25 months for the No-steroid SLT group ($p = 0.990$). No significant difference was found between the two groups for mean pretreatment IOP (22.20 mmHg vs. 22.33 mmHg), and for mean IOP reductions during whole follow-up period. At all follow-up visits, the mean IOP reductions were smaller in the Steroid SLT group than in the No-steroid SLT group. At all follow-up visits, the mean percent IOP reduction was smaller in the Steroid SLT group than in the No-steroid SLT group, and such a difference was significant at 12 months (25.4% vs. 29.6%, $p = 0.047$) and 24 months (25.3% vs. 29.7%, $p = 0.024$). According to the Kaplan–Meier survival analysis, the 24-month success rate was 84% in the Steroid SLT group and 79.2% in the No-steroid SLT group, with no differences between the groups ($p = 0.675$). Conclusion: Short-term use of topical steroid therapy had no impact on the efficacy of SLT for POAG.

Keywords: selective laser trabeculoplasty; topical steroid therapy; primary open-angle glaucoma; intraocular pressure

Citation: Gračner, T. Impact of Short-Term Topical Steroid Therapy on Selective Laser Trabeculoplasty Efficacy. *J. Clin. Med.* **2021**, *10*, 4249. https://doi.org/10.3390/jcm10184249

Academic Editors: Miriam Kolko and Barbara Cvenkel

Received: 24 August 2021
Accepted: 16 September 2021
Published: 19 September 2021

Publisher's Note: MDPI stays neutral with regard to jurisdictional claims in published maps and institutional affiliations.

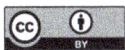

Copyright: © 2021 by the author. Licensee MDPI, Basel, Switzerland. This article is an open access article distributed under the terms and conditions of the Creative Commons Attribution (CC BY) license (https://creativecommons.org/licenses/by/4.0/).

1. Introduction

Selective laser trabeculoplasty (SLT), used since 1998 when the first successful protocol was described, has become an established method for lowering the intraocular pressure (IOP) in the treatment of open-angle glaucoma (OAG) and ocular hypertension (OH) [1–5]. Multiple prospective or retrospective studies clear demonstrated the safety and efficacy of SLT in reducing the IOP in eyes with OAG or OH [6–17]. Therefore, topical medical treatment and SLT are stated as initial, first line treatment options, and SLT is also an adjunctive treatment option in the treatment for OAG or OH in the latest 5th edition of *Terminology and Guidelines for Glaucoma* from the European Glaucoma Society [18].

Anti-inflammatory topical medication four times a day for 7 days after SLT treatment is described in many studies, although there is little evidence to support this [1,6–14]. Symptomatic or asymptomatic anterior chamber inflammation after SLT may occur, but usually resolves without treatment [1,5,19–23]. Treatment with topical steroids or non-steroidal anti-inflammatory agents after SLT in most reports has not shown to cause a significant reduction in inflammation or improved efficacy, but it still remains a controversy in clinical practice [20–25].

This retrospective chart review evaluates whether short-term use of topical steroid therapy affected the efficacy of SLT for primary open-glaucoma (POAG) patients.

2. Materials and Methods

The patients selected for this retrospective chart review were recruited from the glaucoma unit of the Department of Ophthalmology, University Clinical Centre Maribor, Slovenia. All the eyes of the patients had POAG with uncontrolled IOP (>18 mmHg) on uppermost tolerated topical antiglaucoma medication and were treated with 180 degrees SLT. In the study we included consecutive patients, between January and December 2004, who used a drop of dexamethasone 0.1% four times a day for 7 days as post-laser therapy and they formed the Steroid SLT group. In the study we also included consecutive patients, between January and December 2014, where no topical steroids or nonsteroidal anti-inflammatory agents as post-laser therapy were used and they formed the No-steroid SLT group. We included patients of both genders, older than 50 years. Data such as age, sex, past and present ocular medication and ocular history were recorded. Exclusion criterion included a history of previous ocular surgery within 6 months, any previous glaucoma surgery, eye trauma, glaucoma laser therapy or uveitis to the study eye and any other form of glaucoma aside from POAG, such as normal-pressure glaucoma (NTG), pseudoexfoliative glaucoma (PXFG), or ocular hypertension (OH). Hazards, advantages, and substitutes of SLT treatment for POAG were explained to every patient and informed consent was obtained. Thus 43 eyes of 25 patients (18 bilateral) formed the Steroid SLT group and 41 eyes of 24 patients (17 bilateral) formed the No-steroid SLT group. There was just one eye per patient incorporated in every bilateral case in the study. The selection of eyes was random using a random numbers table, where the right eye was combined with even numbers and the left eye with odd numbers. The data of best corrected visual acuity, results of slit lamp examination, ophthalmoscopy, automated static perimetry (Swedish Interactive Threshold Algorithm [SITA] standard 30-2 program of the Humphrey Field Analyzer), and gonioscopy were collected. Trabecular meshwork pigmentation was graded according to a standard scale (graded from 0 to 4+ where 0 = no pigment and 4+ = dense homogeneous pigment). The IOP was measured with a Goldmann applanation tonometer. The baseline IOP presented the mean of three times measured preoperative IOPs in the 3 weeks prior to SLT treatment. One hour prior to SLT treatment IOP was measured and one drop of 0.5% apraclonidine was applied in the treated eye. The trabecular meshwork of every eye was treated with 50 adjacent but not overlapping spots in the inferior 180 degrees with a 532 nm frequency doubled Q-switched Nd:YAG laser (Selecta 7000; Coherent, Palo Alto, CA, USA). The same laser was used for all the procedures done in the year 2004 and also in the year 2014. The pulse duration was 3 ns with a single pulse and the spot size was 400 microns. The SLT treatment started using energy of 0.8 mJ, which was increased or decreased until only intermittent cavitation bubbles formation appeared. After SLT treatment, a drop of 0.5% apraclonidine and 0.1% dexamethasone were applied in the treated eye. All SLTs were performed by the same glaucoma specialist (G.T.) All the eyes underwent a slit lamp examination and applanation tonometry 1 h post-laser to assess the anterior chamber reaction and IOP spikes. Patients were evaluated 1, 3, 6, 12, 18, and 24 months after treatment. A failure was defined as any eye with IOP lowering less than 20% from baseline IOP 1 month post-laser. Hypotensive antiglaucoma medical therapy was not modified during study period. When any eye required either an alteration of hypotensive medical therapy, and thus failed to respond to SLT, that eye was excluded from further analysis at that point. Independent sample t tests were used in statistical analyses of comparing the groups. Significant *p* values were considered to be less than 0.05. All tests were performed two-tailed. Because of the variability in length of follow-up among patients, Kaplan–Maier life-table (survival) analysis was used to estimate the success rates for the groups. The two survival curves (success rates) were compared using the log-rank test. Statistical analysis was carried out with IBM SPSS Statistics version 22.0 for Windows.

3. Results

In the Steroid SLT group were 25 eyes of 25 patients, and in the No-steroid SLT group were 24 eyes of 24 patients. The baseline characteristics including number of patients, number of eyes, age, sex, vertical Cup/Disc ratio, mean deviation, number of hypotensive medications, best corrected visual acuity, trabecular meshwork pigmentation, and mean baseline IOP of the Steroid SLT group and the No-steroid SLT group are listed in Table 1. The mean pretreatment IOP in the Steroid SLT group was 22.20 mmHg (SD 2.5) and 22.33 mmHg (SD 2.6) in the No-steroid SLT group ($p = 0.856$). The differences between those baseline characteristics were statistically not significant, except the difference between mean energy used for each spot ($p < 0.001$) and total energy used ($p < 0.001$), which were higher in the No-steroid SLT group.

Table 1. Baseline characteristics—all patients.

	Steroid SLT Group	No-Steroid SLT Group	p
Patients (No)	25	24	0.911
Eyes (No)	25	24	0.911
Mean age (years) (SD)	70.44 (8.6)	67.00 (12.0)	0.255
Sex: Male	12	12	
Female	13	12	0.855
Vertical Cup/Disc Ratio (mean) (SD)	0.75 (0.3)	0.85 (0.2)	0.173
Mean Deviation (mean) (dB) (SD)	−9.22 (1.3)	−10.33 (1.4)	0.754
Hypotensive medication (mean) (SD)	2.4 (0.7)	2.3 (0.5)	0.875
Best corrected visual acuity (SD)	0.78 (0.3)	0.71 (0.4)	0.413
Trabecular meshwork pigmentation (mean) (SD)	1.92 (0.8)	2.17 (0.8)	0.265
Mean energy/spot (mJ) (SD)	0.76 (0.2)	1.25 (0.1)	<0.001
Total energy (mJ) (SD)	37.63 (19.1)	70.96 (13.8)	<0.001
Mean baseline IOP (mmHg) (SD)	22.20 (2.5)	22.33 (2.6)	0.856

No—Number; (SD)—Standard deviation; p—Independent sample t test; SLT—selective laser trabeculoplasty.

Treatment with SLT was conducted in all eyes with adjacent 50 spots in the inferior 180 degrees of the trabecular meshwork. The mean energy used for each spot was in the Steroid SLT group 0.76 mJ (SD 0.2) and 1.25 mJ (SD 0.1) in the No-steroid SLT group; the difference was statistically significant ($p < 0.001$). The total energy used was in the Steroid SLT group 37.63 mJ (SD 10.1) and 70.96 mJ (SD 13.8) in the No-steroid SLT group; the difference was statistically significant ($p < 0.001$).

Ophthalmic Nd:YAG laser is a solid-state laser and is pumped by a pulsed flashlamp. The lifetime of the Nd:YAG laser can last for 10 or more years. The limiting component, the one that needs to be replaced occasionally, is the flashlamp. Over the working years of the Nd:YAG laser, the function of the pulsed flashlamp slowly diminishes, so to achieve the desired laser effect, the energy of the laser spot must be increased. In our study, the same laser was used for all the procedures done in the year 2004 and also in the year 2014. The treatment protocol of the trabecular meshwork of every eye in our study was the same, the energy of the laser spot was set at the level of the appearance of intermittent cavitation formation. This explains the significant difference between mean energy used for each spot and total energy used, which were higher in the No-steroid SLT group treated in the year 2014.

Hypotensive antiglaucoma medical therapy in both groups was not modified during whole study period.

The mean follow-up time was for the Steroid SLT group 21.24 (SD 7.0) months and for the No-steroid SLT group 20.25 (SD 7.6) months; the difference was statistically not significant ($p = 0.990$).

The mean IOPs, mean IOP reduction and mean percent IOP reduction from baseline IOP 1, 3, 6, 12, 18 and 24 months after treatment for the Steroid SLT group and the No-steroid SLT group are listed in Table 2. The differences in the mean IOPs and the mean IOP reductions at different time intervals following SLT between the two groups were statistically not significant ($p > 0.05$). At all follow-up visits, the mean IOP reduction was smaller in the Steroid SLT group than in the No-steroid SLT group.

At all follow-up visits, the mean percent IOP reduction was smaller in the Steroid SLT group than in the No-steroid SLT group, and such a difference was statistically significant at 12 months (25.4% (SD 4.8) vs. 29.6% (SD 8.2) ($p = 0.047$)), and 24 months (25.3% (SD 5.5) vs. 29.7% (SD 6.5) ($p = 0.024$)).

In the Steroid SLT group, 4 eyes failed to respond to SLT (3 eyes after 3 months and 1 eye after 18 months), and in the No-steroid SLT group 5 eyes failed to respond to SLT (2 eyes after 3 months, 2 eyes after 6 months and 1 eye after 12 months). The success rate after 24 months determined from Kaplan–Meier life-table (survival) analysis was 84% in the Steroid SLT group and 79.2% in the No-steroid SLT group. By the comparison of the two survival curves (success rates) with the log-rank test there was no statistically significant difference ($p = 0.675$) between the groups (Figure 1).

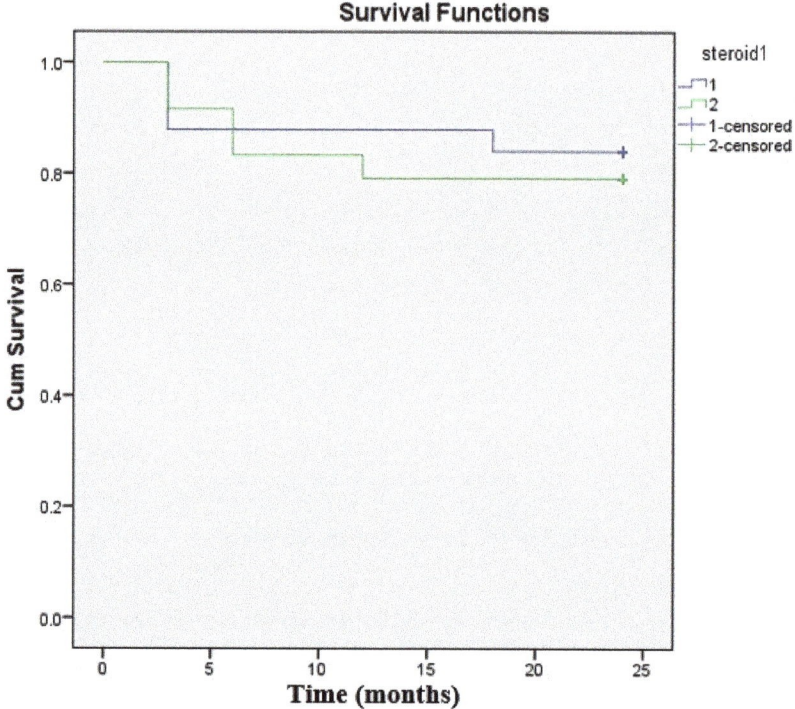

Figure 1. Kaplan–Meier survival analysis for the Steroid SLT group (group1) and the No-steroid SLT group (group 2).

After SLT there was no significant anterior segment inflammation or a transient increase in IOP in any of the treated eyes detected. No patient suffered any pain or inconvenience whilst they were treated.

Table 2. Mean IOP, mean IOP reduction, and mean percent IOP reduction from baseline IOP at different time intervals following SLT–all patients.

Follow-Up Time	Eyes (No) Steroid SLT Group	Eyes (No) No-Steroid SLT Group	Mean IOP (mm Hg) (SD) Steroid SLT Group	Mean IOP (mm Hg) (SD) No-Steroid SLT Group	p	Mean IOP Reduction (mm Hg) (SD) Steroid SLT Group	Mean IOP Reduction (mm Hg) (SD) No-Steroid SLT Group	p	Mean % IOP Reduction (mm Hg) (SD) Steroid SLT Group	Mean % IOP Reduction (mm Hg) (SD) No-Steroid SLT Group	p
BASELINE	25	24	22.20 (2.5)	22.33 (2.6)	0.856	-	-	-	-	-	-
1 month	25	24	16.72 (2.7)	17.10 (3.8)	0.699	5.48 (1.9)	5.49 (3.8)	0.976	25.1 (7.9)	26.6 (10.2)	0.547
3 months	22	22	16.14 (2.3)	15.90 (2.5)	0.705	6.09 (1.8)	6.45 (1.8)	0.520	27.4 (7.2)	28.9 (6.5)	0.459
6 months	22	20	16.00 (2.3)	15.60 (2.2)	0.570	6.23 (2.2)	6.55 (2.2)	0.633	27.8 (8.1)	29.5 (7.5)	0.505
12 months	22	19	16.64 (2.0)	15.26 (2.6)	0.053	5.59 (1.5)	6.68 (2.6)	0.102	25.4 (4.8)	29.6 (8.2)	0.047
18 months	21	19	16.05 (1.9)	15.05 (1.6)	0.080	6.19 (1.9)	6.95 (2.4)	0.274	27.7 (6.3)	30.8 (7.3)	0.154
24 months	21	19	16.62 (2.1)	15.32 (1.4)	0.051	5.62 (1.5)	6.58 (2.4)	0.137	25.3 (5.5)	29.7 (6.5)	0.024

No—Number; (SD)—Standard deviation; p—Independent sample t test; IOP—intraocular pressure.

4. Discussion

SLT is a laser procedure that selectively targets pigmented trabecular meshwork cells without causing thermal damage or collateral damage to nonpigmented cells or structures [26–30]. A 532 nm Q-switched frequency doubled Nd:YAG laser with a fixed spot size of 400 microns and pulse duration of 3 nanoseconds is used for SLT. The power range for treatment using currently available laser platforms is 0.3 to 2.0 mJ. The exact mechanism of action of reducing the IOP in this procedure is not completely understood and is likely multifactorial. The demonstrable clinical efficacy of SLT, despite the absence of coagulation of the trabecular meshwork suggests that laser trabeculoplasty works on the cellular level either through migration and phagocytosis of trabecular meshwork debris by the macrophages, or by stimulation of formation of healthy trabecular tissue, which may enhance the outflow properties of the trabecular meshwork [31]. Alvorado et al. has observed a five to eight fold increase in the number of monocytes and macrophages present in the trabecular meshwork of monkey eyes treated with SLT as compared with untreated controls [32]. They theorized that injury to the pigmented trabecular meshwork cells after SLT results in the release of factors and chemoatractants, which recruit monocytes which are activated and transformed into macrophages upon interacting with the injured tissues. These macrophages then engulf and clear the pigment granules from the trabecular meshwork tissues and exit the eye to return to the circulation via the Schlemm's canal [32]. The biological theory of SLT action implies a cascade of events (interleukins-1, tumor necrosis factor-a, matrix metalloproteinases, recruitment and increase in number of macrophages) triggered by the laser that causes the remodeling of the extracellular matrix in the non-treated areas of TM, so this remodeling presumably decreases the outflow resistance and hence decreases IOP [33–39]. All these events have been postulated to play a role in the IOP lowering effect of SLT. Short-term anti-inflammatory topical medication is commonly prescribed post SLT to ease early inflammation. Because of the proposed mechanism of action of SLT including production of pro-inflammatory cytokines, the potential counterproductive nature of prescribing topical anti-inflammatory medication has been considered.

Realini et al., in their prospective, randomized study, evaluated 25 POAG patients following bilateral 360° SLT, who in one randomly selected eye (25 eyes) used prednisolone acetate 1% 4 times daily for 1 week; the other eye (25 eyes) did not receive any anti-inflammatory treatment [20]. No significant difference in IOP-lowering effect was found between groups after a follow-up of 3 months [20].

Jinapriya et al., in their randomized, double-masked, placebo-controlled clinical trial, evaluated 125 patients with POAG or PXFG, 46 eyes treated with prednisolone acetate 1%, 41 eyes with ketorolac tromethamine 0.5%, or 38 eyes with placebo 4 times per day for 5 days after 180° SLT [21]. No significant difference in IOP-lowering effect was observed among the groups up to 1 year after treatment [21].

De Keyser et al., in their prospective, randomized clinical trial, evaluated 66 patients with either POAG, NTG, or OH following bilateral 360° SLT, who in one eye used indomethacin 0.1% (35 eyes) or dexamethasone 0.1% (31 eyes) three times daily for 1 week; the other eye did not receive any anti-inflammatory treatment [23]. No significant difference in anterior chamber reaction, conjunctival redness, reported pain, or IOP-lowering effect between groups after all time points with a follow-up of 6 months was found [23].

Groth et al., in their randomized, double-masked, placebo-controlled clinical trial, evaluated 96 eyes with either POAG (72 eyes), PXFG (4 eyes), or OHT (20 eyes) following 180° SLT (34 eyes), 270° SLT (11 eyes), or 360° SLT (50 eyes) [24]. Of these, 28 eyes (20 POAG, 8 OHT) were treated with ketorolac 0.5%, 37 eyes (28 POAG, 3 PXFG, 6 OHT) with prednisolone 1%, or 31 eyes (24 POAG, 1 PXFG, 6 OHT) with placebo four times per day for 5 days after SLT [24]. No significant difference in IOP decrease among groups was observed at week 6 of follow-up; both the nonsteroidal anti-inflammatory drug and steroid groups showed a significantly greater decrease in IOP at week 12 of follow-up compared with the placebo group [24].

Thrane et al., in their randomized, placebo-controlled clinical trial, evaluated 39 eyes with either POAG (10 eyes), PXFG (8 eyes), OHT (8 eyes), or NTG (13 eyes) following 360° SLT [25]. Of these, 19 eyes (6 POAG, 4 PXFG, 3 OHT, 6 NTG) were treated with diclofenac 0.1%, and 20 eyes with placebo (4 POAG, 4 PXFG, 5 OHT, 7 NTG) 4 times per day for 5 days after SLT [25]. No significant difference in IOP-lowering effect was observed among the groups after a follow-up of 6 months [25].

In the first SLT surgical technique protocol described by Latina et al. the use of short-term topical steroid therapy fourtimes a day for 7 days as postoperative management after SLT was postulated [1]. Most of the published studies until 2006 followed the prescribed operative SLT protocol, including our reports [1,6–14,19]. The mechanism by which SLT lowers IOP was investigated by many studies [26–37]. According to these findings, the short-term topical anti-inflammatory therapy after SLT became questionable. In many later studies the use of the short-term topical anti-inflammatory therapy after SLT was given on, including ours [15–17]. Therefore, we decided to evaluate whether short-term use of topical steroid therapy after SLT affected the efficacy of SLT in a retrospective chart review, in which we included POAG patients treated 2004, who were using short-term topical steroid therapy after SLT and compared the results with POAG patients treated 2014, who received no topical steroids or nonsteroidal anti-inflammatory agents after SLT.

In our retrospective chart review we evaluated 49 eyes with POAG following 180° SLT. Of these, 25 eyes were treated with dexamethasone 0.1% four times per day for 7 days after SLT and 24 eyes did not receive any topical steroids or nonsteroidal anti-inflammatory agents after SLT. No significant difference was found between the two groups in IOP reductions during whole follow-up period, with a follow-up of 24 months. Moreover, no significant difference was found between the two groups in success rate after a follow-up of 24 months. Short-term use of topical steroid therapy in our study had no impact on the efficacy of SLT for POAG.

Because of differences in age, gender, ocular history, type of antiglaucoma medications, amount of glaucomatous optic neuropathy, SLT treatment parameters, amount of included eyes, follow-up time, assessment of IOP reduction, study design, assessment, and statistical analysis of the results, a comparison of the mentioned studies is difficult and its possibility limited. The results of our study, where we evaluated whether short-term use of topical steroid therapy affected the efficacy of SLT for POAG, are similar to those previously reported [20–24]. The follow-up in our study was 24 months, therefore longer than in reported studies, where the follow-up was 3 to 12 months [20–24]. As in other published studies, our study with longer follow-up found the use of short-term topical anti-inflammatory medication after SLT for POAG makes no difference [20–24]. We also conclude that the IOP reduction is not influenced by the use of short-term topical anti-inflammatory medication after SLT.

No consensus statement exists regarding the postoperative management of patients after SLT. Larger additional long-term outcome studies that include a variety of glaucoma subtypes and different surgical techniques may be necessary to further investigate this issue.

Funding: This research received no external funding.

Institutional Review Board Statement: Ethical review and approval were waived for this study, due to its retrospective design.

Informed Consent Statement: Informed consent was obtained from all subjects involved in the study.

Data Availability Statement: The data presented in this study are available on request from the corresponding author on reasonable request.

Conflicts of Interest: The authors declare no conflict of interest.

References

1. Latina, M.A.; Sibayan, S.A.; Shin, D.H.; Noecker, R.J.; Marcellino, G. Q-switched 532-nm Nd:YAG laser trabeculoplasty (selective laser trabeculoplasty). *Ophthalmology* **1998**, *105*, 2082–2090. [CrossRef]
2. Li, X.; Wang, W.; Zhang, X. Meta-analysis of selective laser trabeculoplasty versus topical medication in the treatment of open-angle glaucoma. *BMC Ophthalmol.* **2015**, *15*, 107. [CrossRef]
3. Wong, M.O.; Lee, J.W.; Choy, B.N.; Chan, J.C.; Lali, J.S. Systematic review and meta-analysis on the efficacy of selective laser trabeculoplasty in open-angle glaucoma. *Surv. Ophthalmol.* **2015**, *6*, 1935–1940. [CrossRef] [PubMed]
4. Schlote, T. Stellenwert der selektiven Lasertrabekuloplastik (SLT). *Klin. Monatsbl. Augenheilkd.* **2017**, *234*, 1362–1371. [CrossRef] [PubMed]
5. Garg, A.; Gazzard, G. Seleciv laser trabeculoplasty: Past, present, and future. *Eye* **2018**, *32*, 863–876. [CrossRef] [PubMed]
6. Kim, Y.J.; Moon, C.S. One-year follow-up of laser trabeculoplasty using Q-switched frequency-doubled Nd:YAG laser of 532 nm wavelenght. *Ophthalmic Surg. Lasers* **2000**, *31*, 394–399. [CrossRef] [PubMed]
7. Gračner, T. Intraocular pressure response to selective laser trabeculoplasty in the treatment of primary open-angle glaucoma. *Ophthalmologica* **2001**, *215*, 267–270. [CrossRef]
8. Gračner, T. Intraocular pressure response of capsular glaucoma and primary open-angle glaucoma to selective Nd:YAG laser trabeculoplasty: A prospective, comparative clinical trial. *Eur. J. Ophthalmol.* **2002**, *12*, 287–292. [CrossRef] [PubMed]
9. Gračner, T.; Pahor, D.; Gračner, B. Wirksamkeit der selektiven Lasertrabekuloplastik bei der Behandlung von primärem Offenwinkelglaukom. *Klin. Monatsbl. Augenheilkd.* **2003**, *220*, 848–852.
10. Cvenkel, B. One-year follow-up of selective laser trabeculoplasty in open-angle glaucoma. *Ophthalmologica* **2004**, *218*, 20–25. [CrossRef]
11. Juzych, M.S.; Chopra, V.; Banitt, M.R.; Hughes, B.A.; Kim, C.; Goulas, M.T.; Shin, D.H. Comparison of long-term outcomes of selective laser trabeculoplasty versus argon laser trabeculoplasty in open-angle glaucoma. *Ophthalmology* **2004**, *111*, 1853–1859. [CrossRef]
12. Lai, J.S.; Chua, J.K.; Tham, C.C.; Lam, D.S. Five-year follow-up of selective laser trabeculoplasty in Chinese eyes. *Clin. Experiment. Ophthalmol.* **2004**, *32*, 368–372. [CrossRef] [PubMed]
13. Gračner, T.; Falež, M.; Gračner, B.; Pahor, D. Langfristige Nachbeobachtung der selektiven Lasertrabekuloplastik primärem Offenwinkelglaukom. *Klin. Monatsbl. Augenheilkd.* **2006**, *223*, 743–747. [CrossRef] [PubMed]
14. Weinand, F.S.; Althen, F. Long-term clinical results of selective laser trabeculoplasty in the treatment of primary open angle glaucoma. *Eur. J. Ophthalmol.* **2006**, *16*, 100–104. [CrossRef] [PubMed]
15. Woo, D.M.; Healey, P.R.; Graham, S.L.; Goldberg, I. Intraocular pressure-lowering medications and long-term outcomes of selective laser trabeculoplasty. *Clin. Exp. Ophthalmol.* **2015**, *43*, 320–327. [CrossRef] [PubMed]
16. Gračner, T. Comparative study of the efficacy of selective laser trabeculoplasty as initial or adjunctive treatment for primary open-angle glaucoma. *Eur. J. Ophthalmol.* **2019**, *29*, 524–531. [CrossRef]
17. Gazzard, G.; Konstantakopoulou, E.; Garway-Heath, D.; Garg, A.; Vickerstaf, V.; Hunter, R.; Ambler, G.; Bunce, C.; Wormald, R.; Nathwani, N.; et al. Selective laser trabeculoplasty versus eye drops for first-line treatment of ocular hypertension and glaucoma (LiGHT): A multicentre randomised controlled trial. *Lancet* **2019**, *393*, 1505–1516. [CrossRef]
18. *European Glaucoma Society: Terminology and Guidelines for Glaucoma*, 5th ed.; Editrice Dogma: Savona, Italy, 2020.
19. Nagar, M.; Ogunyomade, A.; O'Bart, D.P.; Howes, F.; Marshall, J. A randomised, prospective study comparing selective laser trabeculoplasty with latanoprost for the control of intraocular pressure in ocular hypertension and open angle glaucoma. *Br. J. Ophthalmol.* **2005**, *89*, 1413–1417. [CrossRef]
20. Realini, T.; Charlton, J.; Hettlinger, M. The impact o fanti-inflammatory therapy on untraocular pressure reduction following selective laser trabeculoplasty. *Ophthalmic Surg. Lasers Imaging* **2010**, *41*, 100–103. [CrossRef]
21. Jinapriya, D.; DSouza, M.; Hollands, H.; El-Defrawry, S.R.; Irrcher, I.; Smallman, D.; Farmer, J.P.; Cheung, J.; Urton, T.; Day, A.; et al. Anti-inflammatory therapy after selective laser trabeculoplasty. *Ophthalmology* **2014**, *121*, 2356–2361. [CrossRef] [PubMed]
22. Realini, T.; Shillingford-Ricketts, H.; Burt, D.; Balasubramani, G.K. Weast Indies Glaucoma Laser Study (WIGLS) 3. Anterior chamber inflammation following selective laser trabeculoplasty in Afro-Caribbeans with open-angle glaucoma. *J. Glaucoma* **2019**, *28*, 622–625. [CrossRef]
23. De Keyser, M.; De Belder, M.; De Groot, V. Randomized prospective study of the use of afanti-inflammatory drops after selective laser trabeculoplasty. *J. Glaucoma* **2017**, *26*, 22–29. [CrossRef]
24. Groth, S.L.; Albeiruti, E.; Nunez, M.; Fajardo, R.; Sharpsten, L.; Loewen, N.; Schuman, J.S.; Goldberg, J.L. SALT trial: Steroids after laser trabeculoplasty. *Ophthalmology* **2019**, *126*, 1511–1516. [CrossRef]
25. Thrane, V.R.; Thrane, A.S.; Bergo, C.; Halvorsen, H.; Krohn, J. Effect of apraclonidine and diclofenac on early changes in intraocular pressure after selective laser trabeculoplasty. *J. Glaucoma* **2020**, *29*, 280–286. [CrossRef]
26. Latina, M.A.; Park, C. Selective targeting of trabecular meshwork cells: In vitro studies of pulsed and cw laser interactions. *Exp. Eye Res.* **1995**, *60*, 359–372. [CrossRef]
27. Noecker, R.J.; Kramer, T.R.; Latina, M.; Marcellino, G. Comparison of acute morphologic changes after selective laser trabeculoplasty and argon laser trabeculoplasty by electron microscopic evaluation. *Investig. Ophthalmol. Vis. Sci.* **1998**, *39*, S472.

28. Kramer, T.R.; Noecker, R.J. Comparison of the morphologic changes after selective laser trabeculoplasty and argon laser trabeculoplasty in human eye bank eyes. *Ophthalmology* **2001**, *108*, 773–779. [CrossRef]
29. Cvenkel, B.; Hvala, A.; Drnovšek-Olup, B.; Gale, N. Acute ultrastructural changes of the trabecular meshwork after selective laser trabeculoplasty and low power argon laser trabeculoplasty. *Lasers Surg. Med.* **2003**, *33*, 204–208. [CrossRef] [PubMed]
30. SooHoo, J.R.; Seibold, L.K.; Ammar, D.A.; Kahook, M.Y. Ultrastructural changes in human trabeculer meshwork tissue after laser trabeculoplasty. *J. Ophthalmol.* **2015**, *2015*, 476138. [CrossRef] [PubMed]
31. Latina, M.A.; Tumbocon, J.A.J. Selective laser trabeculoplasty: A new treatment option for open angle glaucoma. *Curr. Opin. Ophthalmol.* **2002**, *13*, 94–96. [CrossRef]
32. Alvorado, J.A.; Murphy, C.G. Outflow obstruction in pigmentary and primary open glaucoma. *Arch. Ophthalmol.* **1992**, *110*, 1769–1778. [CrossRef]
33. Izzotti, A.; Longobardi, M.; Cartiglia, C.; Rathschuler, F.; Saccà, S.C. Trabecular meshwork gene expression after selective laser trabeculoplasty. *PLoS ONE* **2011**, *6*, e20110. [CrossRef]
34. Bradley, J.M.B.; Anderssohn, A.M.; Colvis, C.M.; Parshley, D.E.; Zhu, X.; Ruddat, M.S.; Samples, J.R.; Acott, T.S. Mediation of laser trabeculoplasty-induced matrix metalloproteinase expression by IL-1beta and TNFalpha. *Investig. Ophthalmol. Vis. Sci.* **2000**, *41*, 422–430.
35. Guzey, M.; Vural, H.; Satici, A. Endothelin-1 increase in aqueous humour caused by frequency-doubled Nd:YAG laser trabeculoplasty in rabbits. *Eye* **2001**, *15*, 781–785. [CrossRef] [PubMed]
36. Guzey, M.; Vural, H.; Satici, A.; Karadede, S.; Dogan, Z. Increase of free oxygen radicals in aqueous humour induced by frequency-doubled Nd:YAG laser trabeculoplasty in rabbit. *Eur. J. Ophthalmol.* **2001**, *11*, 47–52. [CrossRef] [PubMed]
37. Alvorado, J.A.; Katz, L.J.; Trivedi, S.; Shifera, A.S. Monocyte modulation of aqueous outflow and recruitment to the trabecular meshwork following selective laser trabeculoplasty. *Arch. Ophthalmol.* **2010**, *128*, 731–737. [CrossRef] [PubMed]
38. Lee, J.Y.; Kagan, D.B.; Roumeliotis, G.; Liu, H.; Hutnik, C.M. Secretion of matrix metalloproteinase-3 by co-cultured pigment and non-pigmented human trabecular meshwork cells following selective laser trabeculoplasty. *Clin. Exp. Ophthalmol.* **2016**, *44*, 33–42. [CrossRef]
39. Gulati, V.; Fan, S.; Gardner, B.J.; Havens, S.J.; Schaaf, M.T.; Neely, D.G.; Toris, C.B. Mechanism of action of selective laser trabeculoplasty and predictors of response. *Investig. Ophthalmol. Vis. Sci.* **2017**, *58*, 1462–1468. [CrossRef]

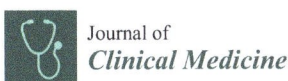

Article

Influence of Overhanging Bleb on Corneal Higher-Order Aberrations after Trabeculectomy

Yu Mizuno *, Kazuyuki Hirooka and Yoshiaki Kiuchi

Department of Ophthalmology and Visual Science, Hiroshima University, 1-2-3 Kasumi Minamiku, Hiroshima 734-8551, Japan; kazuyk@hiroshima-u.ac.jp (K.H.); ykiuchi@hiroshima-u.ac.jp (Y.K.)
* Correspondence: ymizuno@hiroshima-u.ac.jp; Tel.: +81-82-257-5247

Abstract: Recent advances in ocular aberrometry have revealed that ocular surgery increases ocular and corneal higher-order aberrations. This retrospective single-center study aimed to examine the effects of the overhanging bleb on corneal higher-order aberrations using a wavefront analyzer. We included 61 eyes from 50 patients with overhanging bleb after trabeculectomy with a fornix-based conjunctival flap using mitomycin C (overhanging bleb group) and 65 eyes from 54 glaucoma patients with no history of glaucoma surgery (control group). Corneal higher-order aberrations (total higher-order aberrations, coma aberrations, coma-like aberrations, spherical aberrations, and spherical-like aberrations) on a 4 mm pupil diameter were measured using the TOPCON KR-1W wavefront analyzer. Corneal coma aberrations were higher in the overhanging bleb group than in the control group (0.16 ± 0.13 µm and 0.10 ± 0.05 µm, respectively; p = 0.042). Corneal coma-like aberrations were also higher in the overhanging bleb group than in the control group (0.31 ± 0.32 µm and 0.16 ± 0.09 µm, respectively; p = 0.022). With an increasing ratio of cornea covered by the bleb to the entire cornea, all corneal higher-order aberrations increased except for corneal coma-like aberrations. Overhanging bleb after trabeculectomy with a fornix-based conjunctival flap using mitomycin C and its size influenced corneal higher-order aberrations.

Keywords: glaucoma; overhanging bleb; higher-order aberrations; trabeculectomy; mitomycin C

1. Introduction

Glaucoma is an optic neuropathy characterized by gradual progressive morphological changes in the optic disc and visual field loss [1]. Trabeculectomy (TLE) is an effective surgical technique for lowering the intraocular pressure to slow the progression of visual field loss in glaucoma patients [2]. Antimetabolites in TLE, such as mitomycin C (MMC), have significantly improved the success rate of TLE. MMC inhibits the proliferation of fibroblasts, thereby preventing excessive postoperative scarring and enhancing the growth of the large bleb [3]. However, following TLE, patients occasionally complain of foreign body sensation, excessive tearing, sensitivity to light, and vision changes. Some of these patients may have overhanging blebs (OHBs), which are defined as oversized filtering blebs that cover part of the cornea and are caused by tear film instability [4]. Their incidence appears to be increasing with the introduction of antimetabolites [5,6]. In addition, several studies have shown that TLE results in changes in corneal keratometry and topography, and also astigmatism, which leads to a decline in visual acuity [7,8].

Recently, advances in ocular aberrometry have revealed that ocular surface disease or surgeries increase ocular and corneal higher-order aberrations (HOAs) [9,10]. Several studies have revealed that ocular surface diseases such as pterygium, the growth of conjunctival tissue covered in the cornea, affected the HOAs of the cornea [11–13]. Since OHB shares features with pterygium, we hypothesized that OHB might also be associated with corneal HOAs. However, changes in corneal HOAs in OHB after trabeculectomy with a fornix-based conjunctival flap using MMC have not yet been investigated. Here, we examined the effect of OHB on corneal HOAs.

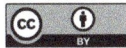

2. Materials and Methods

In this retrospective, cross-sectional study, patients who attended the Department of Ophthalmology, Hiroshima University Hospital, Japan, were evaluated between April 2017 and November 2018. The study received approval from the institution's ethics committee (E—797), and the research adhered to the tenets of the Declaration of Helsinki.

Sixty-one eyes from 50 patients with OHB who had undergone TLE with a fornix-based conjunctival flap using MMC at least 3 months prior to entry were analyzed in this study (OHB group). The eyes with multiple glaucoma surgery were also included in the OHB group. Sixty-five control eyes from 54 glaucoma patients who had no history of prior surgical intervention, except uncomplicated cataract surgery at least 3 months prior to their entry, were concurrently recruited during a similar period (control group). Best-corrected visual acuity (BCVA) and intraocular pressure (IOP; Goldman Applanation Tonometer, Haag-Streit, Köniz, Switzerland) were measured. The anterior segment was observed using slit lamp microscopy. In addition, all eyes with IOLs were using monofocal lenses.

The TOPCON KR-1W wavefront analyzer (Tokyo, Japan) can calculate "corneal" HOAs from the shape of the cornea as well as HOAs of the entire eye. We used the TOPCON KR-1W wavefront analyzer to measure corneal HOAs for a 4 mm pupil diameter without dilating the pupil, and the data were expanded to Zernike polynomials. The magnitude was demonstrated as the mean root square (RMS). Based on our reports, we evaluated corneal wavefront aberrations for coma (C^{-1}_3 and C^1_3), spherical aberrations (C^0_4), the RMS of the third-order, fourth-order, and total HOAs. The RMS of the third-order Zernike coefficients (the square root of the sum of the squared coefficients of C^{-3}_3, C^{-1}_3, C^1_3, and C^3_3) was considered a coma-like aberration. The RMS of the fourth-order Zernike coefficients (the square root of the sum of the squared coefficients of C^{-4}_4, C^{-2}_4, C^0_4, C^2_4, and C^4_4) was considered a spherical-like aberration. Finally, the total of HOAs was defined as the RMS of the magnitudes for the third- to fourth-order aberrations. All patients had BCVA of $\geq$20/40, which was enough to allow fixation on the target of the wavefront analyzer. Aberrometry measurements were automatically measured three times.

For clinical photographic images, we used the TOPCON SL-D8Z slit lamp mounted camera (Tokyo, Japan) to evaluate the anterior ocular segment ($\times$10) from 40 degrees on the temporal side using a diffuser by 50–75 Ws (Watt seconds). OHB was diagnosed if the cornea was covered with bleb under the slit lamp. The dimensional parameters in clinical photographic images were calculated using the NIH image J software (Image J, National Institute of Health, Bethesda, Maryland, USA). The entire corneal area and the area of the bleb over the cornea were measured each as pixels. The ratio of cornea covered by bleb, the ratio of cornea covered by bleb to the entire cornea was calculated as the ratio of the OHB area in the cornea relative to the entire corneal area (Figure 1). We calculated the ratio of the cornea covered by the bleb as follows.

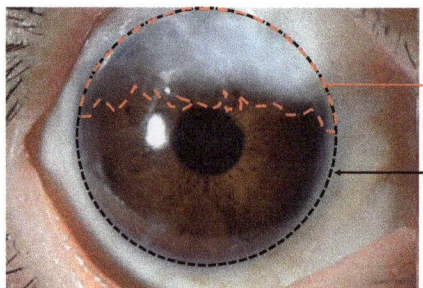

Figure 1. Clinical photographic image using slit lamp mounted camera and dimensions measured using NIH image J software. The ratio of cornea covered by bleb is the ratio of area of the cornea covered by bleb to entire cornea area. The red and black lines are the cornea covered by bleb area and entire cornea area, respectively.

The cornea covered by bleb area (pixels)/the entire cornea (pixels) × 100 (%)

The exclusion criteria were BCVA <20/40 and patients with any history of ocular surgery (other than uncomplicated cataract surgery) for the control group. Patients of the OHB group were not excluded for having had glaucoma surgery several times. Additionally, patients of corneal, conjunctival ocular disease observed on a slit-lamp microscopy were also excluded (e.g., pterygium, superficial punctate keratopathy, corneal opacity, and corneal erosion).

Statistical Analysis

Data were entered in an Excel spreadsheet (Microsoft Corp. Redmond, WA, USA) and analyzed using JMP software (ver. 14, SAS, Inc., Cary, NC, USA). Measurement data were expressed as the mean ± standard deviation with a 95% confidence interval. Continuous data from the two groups were analyzed by an independent t-test, whereas discrete data were analyzed using Pearson's chi-square test. The influence of age, IOP, and the ratio of bleb area on aberrations was analyzed using multiple linear regression. BCVA was converted into logMAR units for analysis. Differences were statistically significant when the p-value was <0.05.

3. Results

The study included 126 eyes from 104 patients who were eligible. The control group comprised 65 eyes with a mean age of 66.23 ± 19.32 years (range, 20–89 years). The OHB group, which included patients with at least one TLE with a fornix-based conjunctival flap using MMC, comprised 61 eyes with a mean age of 67.47 ± 11.11 years (range, 25–90 years). There was no age or gender difference between the two groups. The mean BCVA in logMAR was −0.0086 ± 0.14 and 0.16 ± 0.30 in the control and OHB groups, respectively ($p < 0.0001$). The mean IOP was 14.00 ± 3.66 and 11.60 ± 4.43 in the control and OHB groups, respectively ($p = 0.0012$), which was significantly lower in the OHB group. However, spherical equivalents were −2.25 ± 3.65 and −2.98 ± 2.87 in the control and OHB groups, respectively ($p = 0.22$), and there was no difference between the groups (Table 1).

Table 1. Demographic data of participants included in the study.

	Control (n = 65)	OHB (n = 61)	p
Age (years)	66.23 ± 19.32	67.47 ± 11.11	0.66
Gender (Male/Female)	42/23	34/27	0.31
BCVA (logMAR)	−0.0086 ± 0.14	0.16 ± 0.30	<0.0001
IOP (mmHg)	14.00 ± 3.66	11.60 ± 4.43	0.0012
Lens status (phakic/IOL)	43/22	27/34	0.013
Spherical equivalents	−2.25 ± 3.65	−2.98 ± 2.87	0.22

OHB: overhanging bleb, BCVA: best-corrected visual acuity, IOP: intra ocular pressure.

There were 46 eyes with primary open-angle glaucoma (POAG), five eyes with exfoliation glaucoma, four eyes with primary angle-closure glaucoma (PACG), four eyes with secondary glaucoma (three eyes with uvetic glaucoma, one eye with rubeotic glaucoma), and two eyes with childhood glaucoma in the OHB group. TLE was the most common surgical procedure (86.89%), followed by TLE + PEA + IOL (TLE, phacoemulsification and aspiration, and intraocular lens implantation). The average number of TLE surgeries was 1.33 ± 0.85 times (range, 1–5 times); 51 eyes had experienced only one surgery (83.61%), but a few eyes needed several TLE surgeries. The average period from the last surgery to the examination was 3.18 ± 3.81 years (range 0.25–20.76 years) (Table 2).

Table 2. Clinical characteristics of control and overhanging bleb eyes.

	Control (n = 65)	OHB (n = 61)
Type of glaucoma		
PACG (%)	3 (4.6)	4 (6.6)
POAG (%)	37 (56.9)	46 (75.4)
Exfoliation G (%)	4 (6.2)	5 (8.2)
Uveitic G (%)	0 (0)	3 (4.9)
Rubeotic G (%)	1 (0)	1 (1.6)
Childhood G (%)	2 (3.1)	2 (3.3)
Steroid-induced G (%)	3 (3.1)	0 (0)
PPG (%)	16 (24.6)	0 (0)
PAC (%)	1 (1.5)	0 (0)
Operation (First time)		
TLE (%)	-	53 (86.89)
TLE + PEA + IOL (%)	-	6 (9.84)
Ex-PRESS (%)	-	2 (3.28)
Average number of TLE surgeries	-	1.33 ± 0.85
1st time (%)	-	51 (83.61)
2nd time (%)	-	4 (6.56)
3rd time or more (%)	-	6 (9.84)
Period after the last surgery (year)	-	3.18 ± 3.81

OHB: overhanging bleb, PACG: primary angle-closure glaucoma, POAG: primary open-angle glaucoma, PPG: preperimetric glaucoma, PAC: primary angle closure, G: glaucoma, TLE: trabeculectomy, PEA + IOL: phacoemulsification and aspiration + intraocular lens implantation.

Table 3 shows the association of corneal aberrations in control and OHB groups. Corneal coma aberrations were statistically higher in the OHB group than in the control group (0.16 ± 0.13 µm and 0.10 ± 0.05 µm; p = 0.042). Corneal coma-like aberrations were also higher in the OHB group (0.31 ± 0.32 µm and 0.16 ± 0.09 µm; p = 0.022). However, corneal total HOAs, spherical aberrations, and spherical-like aberrations were not different between the control and OHB groups (0.26 ± 0.14 µm and 0.36 ± 0.40 µm; p = 0.47, 0.04 ± 0.62 µm and 0.04 ± 0.07 µm; p = 0.72, 0.09 ± 0.71 µm and 0.16 ± 0.21 µm; p = 0.11, respectively). Analyzed for eyes with multiple glaucoma surgeries in the OHB group, corneal coma aberrations, corneal coma-like aberrations, and spherical-like aberrations were higher in the OHB group (0.23 ± 0.20 µm and 0.10 ± 0.05 µm; p = 0.0016, 0.37 ± 0.23 µm and 0.16 ± 0.09 µm; p = 0.0006, 0.22 ± 0.24 µm and 0.09 ± 0.71 µm; p = 0.0013, respectively). However, corneal total HOAs and spherical aberrations were not different between the control and the eyes with multiple glaucoma surgeries in the OHB group (0.26 ± 0.14 µm and 0.55 ± 0.57; p = 0.054, 0.04 ± 0.62 µm and 0.06 ± 0.11 µm; p = 0.57, respectively).

Table 3. Corneal aberrations in control and overhanging bleb eyes.

	Control (n = 65)	OHB (n = 61)	p
Corneal total higher-order aberrations (µm, RMS)	0.26 ± 0.14	0.36 ± 0.40	0.47
Corneal coma aberrations (µm, RMS)	0.10 ± 0.05	0.16 ± 0.13	0.042
Corneal spherical aberrations (µm, RMS)	0.04 ± 0.62	0.04 ± 0.07	0.72
Corneal coma-like aberrations (µm, RMS)	0.16 ± 0.09	0.31 ± 0.32	0.022
Corneal spherical-like aberrations (µm, RMS)	0.09 ± 0.71	0.16 ± 0.21	0.11

OHB: overhanging bleb, Total higher-order: magnitude of the third to sixth order, coma-like: third-order Zernike coefficients, sphericcal-like: fourth-order Zernicke coefficients. The influence of BCVA, IOP and lens status on aberrations were analyzed using multiple linear regression.

We measured the range of infiltration area of the bleb to the cornea and entire cornea using image J. The average ratio of cornea covered by bleb was 6.20 ± 5.46% (range 0.59–31.96%). Figure 2 shows the relationship between the ratio of cornea covered by bleb and corneal HOAs. There was a positive correlation between the ratio of bleb area and corneal total HOAs, corneal coma aberrations, corneal spherical aberrations, and corneal spherical-like aberrations (r = 0.38; p = 0.0026, r = 0.39; p = 0.0018, r = 0.34; p = 0.0071, r = 0.30; p = 0.021, respectively). Analyzed for eyes with multiple glaucoma surgeries in the OHB group, there was a positive correlation between the ratio of cornea covered by bleb and corneal total HOAs, corneal coma aberrations, corneal spherical aberrations, corneal coma-like aberrations, and corneal spherical-like aberrations (r = 0.83; p = 0.0027, r = 0.78; p = 0.0083, r = 0.85; p = 0.0020, r = 0.75; p = 0.013, r = 0.83; p = 0.0030, respectively).

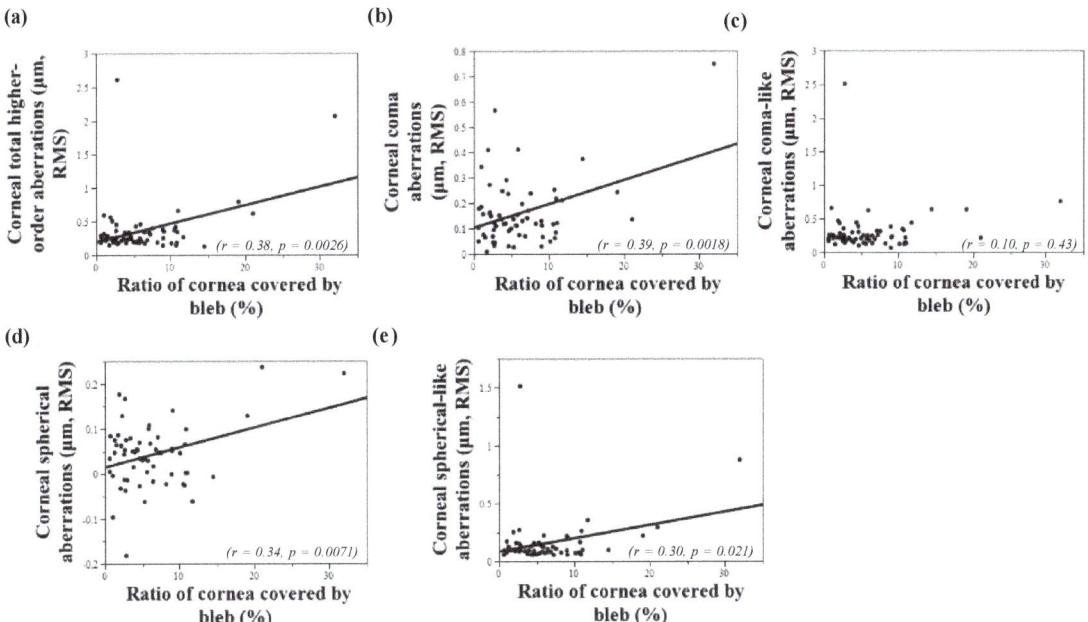

Figure 2. A linear regression comparison of the ratio of cornea covered by bleb with values of corneal higher-order aberrations (HOAs). (**a**) There is a positive correlation between the ratio of cornea covered by bleb and corneal total HOAs (r = 0.38; p = 0.0026). (**b**) There is a positive correlation between the ratio of cornea covered by bleb and corneal coma aberrations (r = 0.39; p = 0.0018). (**c**) Corneal coma-like aberrations showed no correlation between the ratio of cornea covered by bleb (r = 0.10; p = 0.43). (**d**) There is a positive correlation between the ratio of cornea covered by bleb and corneal spherical aberrations (r = 0.34; p = 0.0071). (**e**) There is a positive correlation between the ratio of cornea covered by bleb and corneal spherical-like aberrations (r = 0.30; p = 0.021).

Univariate regression revealed a significant positive relationship between the ratio of cornea covered by bleb for corneal total HOAs, corneal coma aberrations, corneal spherical aberrations, and corneal spherical-like aberrations (β = 0.38; p = 0.0026, β = 0.39; p = 0.0018, β = 0.34; p = 0.0071, β = 0.30; p = 0.02, respectively) (Table 4). Number of TLE surgeries also showed a positive relationship between corneal total HOAs and corneal coma aberrations (β = 0.28; p = 0.027, β = 0.28; p = 0.026, respectively). Univariate regression analysis demonstrated that there was no relationship between IOP <8 mmHg and corneal total HOAs, corneal spherical aberrations, corneal coma aberrations, corneal spherical aberrations corneal coma-like aberrations, and corneal spherical-like aberrations (β = −0.54; p = 0.17, β = −0.31; p = 0.45, β = −0.16; p = 0.71, β = −0.48; p = 0.23, β = −0.03; p = 0.94, respectively). Analyzed for eyes with multiple glaucoma surgeries in the OHB group, univariate regression revealed a significant positive relationship between the ratio of cornea covered by bleb for corneal total HOAs, corneal spherical aberrations, corneal coma-like aberrations, and corneal spherical-like aberrations (β = 0.83; p = 0.0027, β = 0.85; p = 0.0020, β = 0.75; p = 0.0030, β = 0.83; p = 0.0027, respectively). Multivariate regression analysis demonstrated a significant relationship with the ratio of cornea covered by bleb for corneal total HOAs, corneal coma aberrations, corneal spherical aberrations, and corneal spherical-like aberrations (β = 0.37; p = 0.0034, β = 0.40; p = 0.0013, β = 0.34; p = 0.0084, β = 0.28; p = 0.03, respectively) (Table 5). Multivariate regression analysis demonstrated that there was no relationship between <8 mmHg and corneal total HOAs, corneal spherical aberrations, corneal coma aberrations, corneal spherical aberrations corneal coma-like aberrations, and corneal spherical-like aberrations (β = −0.51; p = 0.12, β = −0.45; p = 0.43, β = −0.18; p = 0.69, β = −0.33; p = 0.52, β = −0.0031; p = 0.99, respectively). Analyzed for eyes with multiple glaucoma surgeries in the OHB group, multivariate regression revealed a significant positive relationship between ratio of cornea covered by bleb for corneal total HOAs, corneal spherical aberrations, corneal coma aberrations, corneal spherical aberrations corneal coma-like aberrations, and corneal spherical-like aberrations (β = 1.01; p = 0.0099, β = 1.13; p = 0.0039, β = 0.57; p = 0.016, β = 1.08; p = 0.0095, β = 1.00; p = 0.0098, respectively). Univariate regression analysis and multivariate regression analysis demonstrated there was no relationship between corneal HOAs and IOP <8 mmHg.

Table 4. Univariate regression analysis of corneal higher-order aberrations with associated factors in overhanging bleb eyes.

	Corneal Total Higher-Order Aberrations (μm, RMS)		Corneal Coma Aberrations (μm, RMS)		Corneal Spherical Aberrations (μm, RMS)		Corneal Coma-Like Aberrations (μm, RMS)		Corneal Spherical-Like Aberrations (μm, RMS)	
	β	p	β	p	β	p	β	p	β	p
Ratio of cornea covered by bleb	0.38	0.0026	0.39	0.0018	0.34	0.0071	0.10	0.43	0.30	0.021
Number of TLE ≥ 2	0.21	0.11	0.24	0.061	0.099	0.45	0.077	0.56	0.13	0.31
IOP < 8	−0.54	0.17	−0.31	0.45	−0.16	0.71	−0.48	0.23	−0.03	0.94
Age	v0.03	0.84	0.14	0.28	0.0067	0.96	−0.046	0.73	−0.12	0.36

IOP: intra ocular pressure, TLE: trabeculectomy.

Table 5. Multivariate regression analysis of corneal higher-order aberrations with associated factors in overhanging bleb eyes.

	Corneal Total Higher-Order Aberrations (μm, RMS)			Corneal Coma Aberrations (μm, RMS)			Corneal Spherical Aberrations (μm, RMS)			Corneal Coma-Like Aberrations (μm, RMS)			Corneal Spherical-Like Aberrations (μm, RMS)		
	β	p	VIF	β	p	VIF	β	p	VIF	β	p	VIF	β	p	VIF
Ratio of cornea covered by bleb	0.37	0.0034	1.01	0.40	0.0013	1.01	0.34	0.0084	1.01	0.093	0.48	1.01	0.28	0.03	1.01
Number of TLE ≥ 2	0.038	0.78	1.29	0.048	0.72	1.29	−0.085	0.55	1.29	0.038	0.80	1.29	0.0035	0.98	1.29
IOP < 8	−0.51	0.12	1.25	−0.45	0.43	1.25	−0.18	0.69	1.25	−0.33	0.52	1.25	−0.0031	0.99	1.25
Age	−0.025	0.84	1.02	0.20	0.11	1.02	0.0056	0.65	1.02	−0.024	0.86	1.02	−0.072	0.57	1.02

IOP: intra ocular pressure, TLE: trabeculectomy, VIF: varianceinflation factor.

Figure 3 shows the relationship between the duration of time period after the last TLE and corneal HOAs. There was a positive correlation between the duration of time period after last TLE and corneal total HOAs, corneal coma aberrations, corneal spherical aberrations, and corneal spherical-like aberrations (r = 0.42; p = 0.0007, r = 0.57; p < 0.0001, r = 0.42; p = 0.0007, r = 0.33; p = 0.0089, respectively). Also, the duration of the time period after the last TLE demonstrated positive correlation with the ratio of cornea covered by bleb (r = 0.33; p = 0.0089). Analyzed for eyes with multiple glaucoma surgeries in the OHB group, there was a positive correlation between the duration of the time period after the last TLE and the ratio of the cornea covered by the bleb (r = 1.00; $p < 0.0001$).

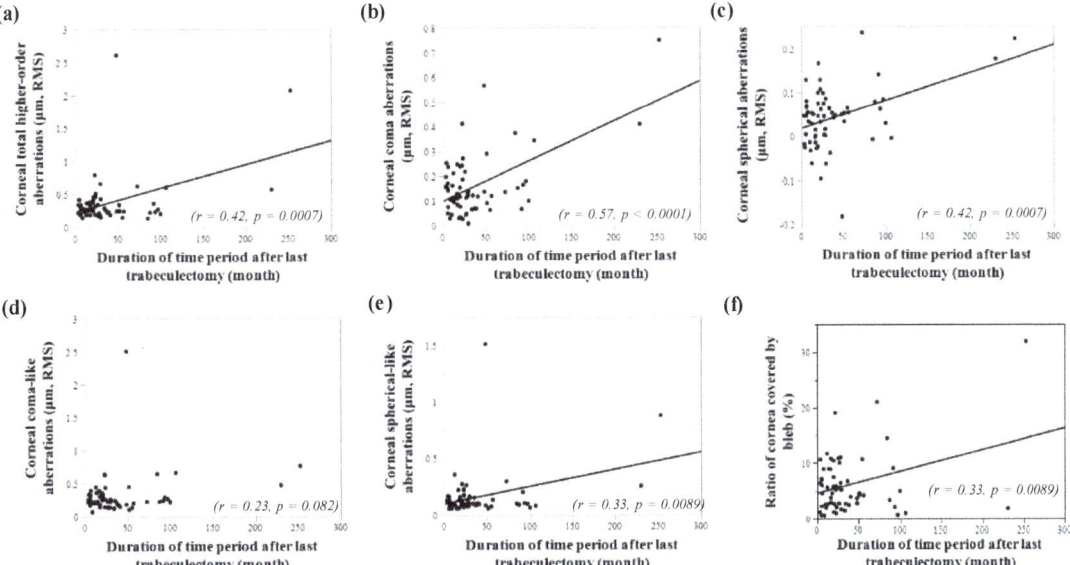

Figure 3. A linear regression comparison of the duration of time period after last TLE and corneal higher-order aberrations (HOAs). (**a**) There is a positive correlation between duration of time period after last TLE and corneal total HOAs (r = 0.42; $p = 0.0007$). (**b**) There is a positive correlation between duration of time period after last TLE and corneal coma aberrations (r = 0.57; $p < 0.0001$). (**c**) There is a positive correlation between duration of time period after the last TLE and corneal spherical aberrations (r = 0.42; $p = 0.0007$). (**d**) Corneal coma-like aberrations showed no correlation between duration of time period after the last TLE (r = 0.23; $p = 0.0082$). (**e**) There is a positive correlation between duration of time period after the last TLE and corneal spherical-like aberrations (r = 0.33; $p = 0.0089$). (**f**) There is a positive correlation between duration of time period after last TLE and the ratio of cornea covered by bleb (r = 0.33; $p = 0.0089$).

4. Discussion

TLE is a standard surgery for uncontrolled glaucoma; patients may expect to control glaucoma progression by lowering the IOP. Additionally, OHBs are a rare complication after TLE, and the mechanism underlying their formation is complex. Several factors, such as gravity on the OHB, the action of the eyelid, scar hyperplasia, and excessive aqueous over-filtration, may contribute to the formation of OHBs [14,15]. Different therapeutic methods (dissection, neodymium YAG laser, and autologous blood injection and compression suture) have been used to deal with these problems [14,16–18]. Following TLE, patients with OHB sometimes complain about vision change and dysesthesia, dry eye, and excessive tearing [19]. However, the mechanism that changes vision has not yet been fully understood. Several studies have revealed that ocular surgeries, such as intraocular lens implantation and cataract extraction [20–22] and scleral buckling [23], lead to a strong effect on corneal or ocular HOAs. Several studies have demonstrated changes in the refractive state or HOAs before and early post-TLE surgery [7,8,24,25]. In addition, some of these studies revealed that corneal or ocular HOAs were changed for 1 week–1 month after TLE, but they had returned to normal levels by 3 months [7,8].

In the present study, consistent with previous reports, we revealed a relationship between OHB on corneal HOAs. Pterygium is a degenerative condition of the conjunctiva with the subconjunctival tissue invading the cornea by destroying superficial layers of stroma and Bowman's membrane [26]. The histopathology of OHB revealed tight connections with corneal tissues or the corneoscleral limbus and multiloculated cystic, rather than simply leaning on the cornea, suggesting that OHB induces changes in the ocular surface [4,27]. Therefore, we consider that OHB, in which the conjunctiva invades the cornea, similar to the pterygium, may also influence corneal HOAs. We previously reported case series to demonstrate changes in the refractive state before and after resection of OHB [28]. In those cases, removal of OHB reduced the symptoms of dysesthesia or corneal HOAs. Several studies showed that pterygium is associated with wavefront aberrations, and excision of pterygium reduces wavefront aberrations, indicating amelioration in visual function [10,13]. Therefore, we assume that the excision of OHBs may reduce wavefront aberrations.

OHB is usually located in the superior quadrant (at least in all our cases it was) and covered part of the cornea. In our study, the analysis demonstrated that corneal coma aberrations and corneal coma-like aberrations were significantly higher in the OHB group than in the control group. Therefore, we believe that the result may support the assertion that OHB caused asymmetric optical distortion in the eyes.

The mechanism of OHB is not completely understood. Several factors, such as gravity on the OHB, the action of the eyelid, scar hyperplasia, and excessive aqueous over-filtration may contribute to the formation of OHBs [14,15]. These factors may cause the OHB to become larger over time. In this study, there was a positive correlation between the duration of time period after TLE and the ratio of corneal area encroached by OHB. Additionally, the duration of time period after TLE demonstrated a positive correlation with corneal total HOAs, corneal coma aberrations, corneal spherical aberrations, and corneal spherical-like aberrations. Based on our findings, the longer period after TLE may worsen OHB, and it seems to be correlated with exacerbation of corneal HOAs, except corneal coma-like aberrations.

During the first 3 months there are typically important changes in IOP, post-operative manipulations (e.g., injections, suture lysis) and important changes in bleb anatomy and configuration due to the scarring process. These changes as potential causes of the corneal aberrations have been reported in ocular or corneal aberrations, except spherical aberrations that were increased at 1–4 weeks after TLE, but they returned to control levels at 1–3 months [8,25]. The authors concluded that temporary ciliary body edema following TLE could change the thickness and position of the lens, and ACD induced the disturbance in ocular HOAs. However, changes of ocular HOAs returned by 3 months, suggesting that those changes in ciliary body edema may return to the control levels by 3 months after TLE surgeries. Because OHB is one of the late complications, in our study, all cases were analyzed 3 months or more after TLE. Like cataract surgery, as for small-incision cataract surgery, changes in corneal aberrations may occur early after surgery; however, these changes gradually returned to preoperative values by 2 or 3 months after surgery [29–31]. In our study, all cataract surgeries were performed with small incisions using a phacoemulsification platform, and all cataract surgery cases were measured 3 months or more after cataract surgery. Therefore, we considered that the effects of TLE surgery and cataract surgery themselves are negligible in our study. In the current study, the duration of the time period after the last TLE showed an association with corneal HOAs (except corneal coma-like aberrations) and the ratio of bleb to the cornea. It was speculated that increases in the duration may affect permanent stable changes in corneal HOAs after glaucoma surgery, especially in the OHB eyes.

Therefore, although, the mechanism underlying OHBs formation is complex, for example, for preventing excessive aqueous over-filtration, it may be useful to ensure an adequate amount of aqueous humor to the conjunctiva, or if OHBs would once occur, it might be useful for resecting them earlier to prevent corneal HOAs, causing visual disturbance.

Our study has several limitations. First, it includes few participants and a lack of anterior chamber depth measurement (ACD). He [32] reported that corneal asphericity and ACD play important roles in determining peripheral wavefront aberrations. However, Jo et al. [33] suggested that the total HOAs change showed no correlation with ACD change before and after TLE using MMC. Further research on ACD and corneal aberrations is required. Second, the tear film fluctuation and OHB heights were not measured in our study. Numerous studies [34–36] have shown that the tear film instability led to wavefront HOA changes, and Ji et al. [19] reported that TLE, especially bleb height, was related to ocular surface instability. OHB may cause ocular surface instability to corneal aberrations. In our study, we excluded from the OHB group patients with corneal damage observed with slit-lamp microscopy, but did not fully investigate whether there was a dry eye or excessive tears such as tear film instability and the effect of eye drops. Further research to study the correlation between ocular stability and corneal aberrations in OHB eyes must address this problem. Third, in this study, we did not assess change of corneal HOAs or symptoms of dysesthesia before and after resection of OHB. Previously, we reported a case series in which surgical removal of OHB reduced the corneal HOAs and symptoms of dysesthesia [28]. However, in order to provide useful information about the benefit of resecting OHB, further research to evaluate the relation between corneal HOAs and symptoms before and after resection of OHB is needed.

In conclusion, OHBs after TLE with a fornix-based conjunctival flap using MMC increased corneal coma aberrations and coma-like aberrations. The ratio of the cornea covered by the bleb positively correlated with the duration of the time period after TLE and corneal HOAs, except for coma-like aberrations. We conclude that increases in the proportion of OHB in the cornea may worsen corneal HOAs, causing visual disturbances in the late period after TLE with a fornix-based conjunctival flap using MMC.

Author Contributions: Conceptualization, Y.M. and Y.K.; methodology, Y.M.; software, Y.M.; validation, Y.M., K.H. and Y.K.; formal analysis, Y.M.; investigation, Y.M.; resources, Y.M.; data curation, Y.M.; writing—original draft preparation, Y.M.; writing—review and editing, K.H. and Y.K.; visualization, Y.M.; supervision, K.H. and Y.K.; project administration, Y.M. All authors have read and agreed to the published version of the manuscript.

Funding: This research received no external funding.

Institutional Review Board Statement: The study was conducted according to the guidelines of the Declaration of Helsinki, and approved by the Institutional Review Board of Hiroshima University (protocol code E-797, 12 June 2017).

Informed Consent Statement: Informed consent was obtained from all subjects involved in the study.

Data Availability Statement: The data analyzed in this study are available from the corresponding author on reasonable request.

Conflicts of Interest: The authors declare no conflict of interest.

References

1. Quigley, H.A.; Addicks, E.M.; Green, W.R.; Maumenee, A.E. Optic nerve damage in human glaucoma. *Arch. Ophthalmol.* **1981**, *99*, 635–649. [CrossRef] [PubMed]
2. Cairns, J.E. Trabeculectomy. Preliminary report of a new method. *Am. J. Ophthalmol.* **1968**, *66*, 673–679. [CrossRef]
3. Lama, P.J.; Fechtner, R.D. Antifibrotics and wound healing in glaucoma surgery. *Surv. Ophthalmol.* **2003**, *48*, 314–346. [CrossRef]
4. Ou-Yang, P.B.; Qi, X.; Duan, X.C. Histopathology and treatment of a huge overhanging filtering bleb. *BMC Ophthalmol.* **2016**, *16*, 175. [CrossRef]
5. Desai, K.; Krishna, R. Surgical management of a dysfunctional filtering bleb. *Ophthal. Surg. Lasers* **2002**, *33*, 501–503. [CrossRef]
6. Lanzl, I.M.; Katz, L.J.; Shindler, R.L.; Spaeth, G.L. Surgical management of overhanging blebs after filtering procedures. *J. Glaucoma* **1999**, *8*, 247–249. [CrossRef]
7. Claridge, K.G.; Galbraith, J.K.; Karmel, V.; Bates, A.K. The effect of trabeculectomy on refraction, keratometry and corneal topography. *Eye* **1995**, *9*, 292–298. [CrossRef]
8. Fukuoka, S.; Amano, S.; Honda, N.; Mimura, T.; Usui, T.; Araie, M. Effect of trabeculectomy on ocular and corneal higher-order aberrations. *JPN J. Ophthalmol.* **2011**, *55*, 460–466. [CrossRef]
9. Pesudovs, K.; Coster, D.J. Penetrating keratoplasty for keratoconus: The nexus between corneal wavefront aberrations and visual performance. *J. Refract. Surg.* **2006**, *22*, 926–931. [CrossRef]

10. Pesudovs, K.; Figueiredo, F.C. Corneal first surface wavefront aberrations before and after pterygium surgery. *J. Refract. Surg.* **2006**, *22*, 921–925. [CrossRef]
11. Gumus, K.; Erkilic, K.; Topaktas, D.; Colin, J. Effect of pterygia on refractive indices, corneal topography, and ocular aberrations. *Cornea* **2011**, *30*, 24–29. [CrossRef]
12. Minami, K.; Tokunaga, T.; Okamoto, K.; Miyata, K.; Oshika, T. Influence of pterygium size on corneal higher-order aberration evaluated using anterior-segment optical coherence tomography. *BMC Ophthalmol.* **2018**, *18*, 166. [CrossRef]
13. Miyata, K.; Minami, K.; Otani, A.; Tokunaga, T.; Tokuda, S.; Amano, S. Proposal for a novel severity grading system for Pterygia based on corneal topographic data. *Cornea* **2017**, *36*, 834–840. [CrossRef]
14. Scheie, H.G.; Guehl, J.J. Surgical management of overhanging blebs after filtering procedures. *Arch. Ophthalmol.* **1979**, *97*, 325–326. [CrossRef]
15. Ulrich, G.G.; Proia, A.D.; Shields, M.B. Clinicopathologic features and surgical management of dissecting glaucoma filtering blebs. *Ophthalmic. Surg. Lasers* **1997**, *28*, 151–155. [CrossRef]
16. Wilson, M.R.; Kotas-Neumann, R. Free conjunctival patch for repair of persistent late bleb leak. *Am. J. Ophthalmol.* **1994**, *117*, 569–574. [CrossRef]
17. Geyer, O. Management of large, leaking, and inadvertent filtering blebs with the neodymium: YAG laser. *Ophthalmology* **1998**, *105*, 983–987. [CrossRef]
18. Ng, D.S.C.; Ching, R.H.Y.; Yam, J.C.S.; Chan, C.W.N. Safe excision of a large overhanging cystic bleb following autologous blood injection and compression suture. *Korean J. Ophthalmol.* **2013**, *27*, 145–148. [CrossRef]
19. Ji, H.; Zhu, Y.; Zhang, Y.; Li, Z.; Ge, J.; Zhuo, Y. Dry eye disease in patients with functioning filtering blebs after trabeculectomy. *PLoS ONE* **2016**, *11*, e0152696. [CrossRef]
20. Mojzis, P.; Majerova, K.; Plaza-Puche, A.B.; Hrckova, L.; Alio, J.L. Visual outcomes of a new toric trifocal diffractive intraocular lens. *J. Cataract. Refract. Surg.* **2015**, *41*, 2695–2706. [CrossRef]
21. Song, I.S.; Park, J.H.; Park, J.H.; Yoon, S.Y.; Kim, J.Y.; Kim, M.J.; Tchah, H. Corneal coma and trefoil changes associated with incision location in cataract surgery. *J. Cataract. Refract. Surg.* **2015**, *41*, 2145–2151. [CrossRef]
22. Oshika, T.; Sugita, G.; Miyata, K.; Tokunaga, T.; Samejima, T.; Okamoto, C.; Ishii, Y. Influence of tilt and decentration of scleral-sutured intraocular lens on ocular higher-order wavefront aberration. *Br. J. Ophthalmol.* **2007**, *91*, 185–188. [CrossRef]
23. Okamoto, F.; Yamane, N.; Okamoto, C.; Hiraoka, T.; Oshika, T. Changes in higher-order aberrations after scleral buckling surgery for rhegmatogenous retinal detachment. *Ophthalmology* **2008**, *115*, 1216–1221. [CrossRef]
24. Dietze, P.J.; Oram, O.; Kohnen, T.; Feldman, R.M.; Koch, D.D.; Gross, R.L. Visual function following trabeculectomy, effect on corneal topography and contrast sensitivity. *J. Glaucoma* **1997**, *6*, 99–103. [CrossRef]
25. Fard, A.M.; Sorkhabi, R.D.; Nasiri, K.; Tajlil, A. Effect of trabeculectomy on ocular higher-order aberrations in patients with open angle glaucoma. *North. Clin. Istanb.* **2018**, *5*, 54–57. [CrossRef]
26. Weale, R.A. Pterygium. In *Epidemiology of Eye Disease*, 2nd ed.; Johnson, G.J., Minassian, D.C., Weale, R.A., West, S.K., Eds.; Arnold Publishers: London, UK, 2003.
27. Grostern, R.J.; Torczynski, E.; Brown, S.V. Surgical repair and histopathologic features of a dissecting glaucoma filtration bleb. *Arch. Ophthalmol.* **1999**, *117*, 1566–1567. [CrossRef]
28. Mizuno, Y.; Hirota, K.; Hirooka, K.; Kiuchi, Y. Improvements in optical characteristics after excision of an overhanging bleb developed following trabeculectomy. *Case Rep. Ophthalmol. Med.* **2021**, *4*, 7433987. [CrossRef]
29. Ye, H.; Zhang, K.; Yang, J.; Lu, Y. Changes of corneal higher-order aberrations after cataract surgery. *Optom. Vis. Sci.* **2014**, *91*, 1244–1250. [CrossRef]
30. Villegas, E.A.; Alcón, E.; Rubio, E.; Marín, J.M.; Artal, P. One-year follow-up of changes in refraction and aberrations induced by corneal incision. *PLoS ONE* **2019**, *14*, e0224823. [CrossRef]
31. Montés-Micó, R.; Cáliz, A.; Alió, J.L. Wavefront analysis of higher-order aberrations in dry eye patients. *J. Refract. Surg.* **2004**, *20*, 243–247. [CrossRef]
32. He, J.C. Theoretical model of the contributions of corneal asphericity and anterior chamber depth to peripheral wavefront aberrations. *Ophthalmic. Physiol. Opt.* **2014**, *34*, 321–330. [CrossRef] [PubMed]
33. Jo, S.H.; Seo, J.H. Short-term change in higher-order aberrations after mitomycin-C-augmented trabeculectomy. *Int. Ophthalmol.* **2019**, *39*, 175–188. [CrossRef] [PubMed]
34. Wang, Y.; Xu, J.; Sun, X.; Chu, R.; Zhuang, H.; He, J.C. Dynamic wavefront aberrations and visual acuity in control and dry eyes. *Clin. Exp. Optom.* **2009**, *92*, 267–273. [CrossRef] [PubMed]
35. Koh, S.; Maeda, N.; Hori, Y.; Inoue, T.; Watanabe, H.; Hirohara, Y.; Mihashi, T.; Fujikado, T.; Tano, Y. Effects of suppression of blinking on quality of vision in borderline cases of evaporative dry eye. *Cornea* **2008**, *27*, 275–278. [CrossRef]
36. Denoyer, A.; Rabut, G.; Baudouin, C. Tear film aberration dynamics and vision-related quality of life in patients with dry eye disease. *Ophthalmology* **2012**, *119*, 1811–1818. [CrossRef]

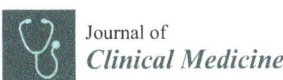

Article

Comparison of Glaucoma-Relevant Transcriptomic Datasets Identifies Novel Drug Targets for Retinal Ganglion Cell Neuroprotection

Tim J. Enz [†], James R. Tribble [†] and Pete A. Williams *

Department of Clinical Neuroscience, Division of Eye and Vision, St. Erik Eye Hospital, Karolinska Institutet, 171 64 Stockholm, Sweden; tim.enz@aol.com (T.J.E.); james.tribble@ki.se (J.R.T.)
* Correspondence: pete.williams@ki.se
† Contributed equally to this work.

Abstract: Glaucoma is a leading cause of blindness and is characterized by the progressive dysfunction and irreversible death of retinal ganglion cells. We aimed to identify shared differentially expressed genes (DE genes) between different glaucoma relevant models of retinal ganglion cell injury using existing RNA-sequencing data, thereby discovering targets for neuroprotective therapies. A comparison of DE genes from publicly available transcriptomic datasets identified 12 shared DE genes. The Comparative Toxicogenomics Database (CTD) was screened for compounds targeting a significant proportion of the identified DE genes. Forty compounds were identified in the CTD that interact with >50% of these shared DE genes. We next validated this approach by testing select compounds for an effect on retinal ganglion cell survival using a mouse retinal explant model. Folic acid, genistein, SB-431542, valproic acid, and WY-14643 (pirinixic acid) were tested. Folic acid, valproic acid, and WY-14643 demonstrated significant protection against retinal ganglion cell death in this model. The increasing prevalence of open access-omics data presents a resource to discover targets for future therapeutic investigation.

Keywords: glaucoma; retinal ganglion cells; RNA-sequencing; neuroprotection; drug discovery

1. Introduction

Glaucoma is a common neurodegenerative disease characterized by the progressive dysfunction and loss of retinal ganglion cells (RGCs), the major output neurons of the retina. The disease clinically manifests with deterioration of visual sensitivity and progressive visual field deficits. The major risk factors for glaucoma are age, genetics, and elevated intraocular pressure (IOP). Despite extensive research, IOP management remains the only clinically available therapy and, to date, there are no clinically available neuroprotective strategies for glaucoma. Despite continuing attempts to lower IOP pharmacologically and surgically, a significant percentage of patients ultimately progress to blindness in one or both eyes [1]. Affecting ~80 million patients worldwide, glaucoma is the most common irreversible blinding disease, constituting a substantial health and economic burden [2]. Thus, efficient neuroprotective therapies would be of great value.

The underlying mechanisms of RGC degeneration that lead to glaucomatous optic neuropathy have been studied broadly using a number of animal-based models, of which controlled optic nerve crush [3] or transection [4], bead models of ocular hypertension [5,6], and the DBA/2J mouse model of glaucoma [7] have been commonly used. Although these models vary in their pathology and mechanism of neural insult, some intrinsic cellular degenerative mechanisms and genetic pathways might be inherent to glaucomatous RGC death. Such mechanisms and genetic pathways would be of particular value as targets for therapeutic interventions.

Recently, RNA-sequencing has been utilized to investigate the molecular mechanisms that drive RGC death in these models, allowing for the identification of differentially expressed genes (DE genes) and pathways. Comparing these across models could provide important data for the discovery of common cellular mechanisms and new insights into the pathophysiology of glaucoma. The identified molecules might be targeted by novel or pre-existing pharmaceutical compounds, which would represent a new data-driven approach to discovering potential glaucoma therapeutics, especially when combined with models that allow for rapid testing of drug candidates.

In this study, we identify compounds that could act on altered genes/proteins common to RGC insult using publicly available transcriptomic datasets and validate these using the mouse retinal explant model of RGC degeneration.

2. Materials and Methods

2.1. RNA-Sequencing Comparison and Identification of Compounds via the Comparative Toxicogenomics Database

Previous results of RNA-sequencing from three different animal models (mouse controlled optic nerve crush [3], DBA/2J mouse model of glaucoma [8], and rat optic nerve transection [4]) were examined. Matrices of DE genes were analyzed at a false discovery rate (FDR, q) of 0.05 (0.10 for the mouse controlled optic nerve crush, as reported in the original study). Gene lists were compared in a three-way analysis in R showing a number of shared DE genes between each model. Pathway analysis was performed (Ingenuity pathway analysis, Qiagen, Hilden, Germany) on shared DE genes between comparisons. The shared DE gene list common to all three models was queried in the Comparative Toxicogenomics Database (CTD), which compiles known gene/protein interactions with chemicals based on published data, and compounds targeting a significant proportion of the identified DE genes (>50% occurrence) were identified. Compounds for neuroprotective testing were selected based on previous neuroprotective literature support and novelty to glaucoma.

2.2. Animal Strain and Husbandry

All breeding and experimental procedures were performed in accordance with the Association for Research for Vision and Ophthalmology Statement for the Use of Animals in Ophthalmic and Research. Individual study protocols were approved by Stockholm's Committee for Ethical Animal Research (10389-2018). All mice were housed and fed in a 12 h light/12 h dark cycle with food and drinking water available *ad libitum*. C57BL/6J and B6.Cg-Tg(Thy1-CFP)23Jrs/J (JAX stock number #003710; CFP + RGCs) mouse strains were purchased from The Jackson Laboratory (Bar Harbor, ME, USA) and bred and maintained in-house. All mice were used at 12–20 weeks of age.

2.3. Retina Axotomy Explant Model

Compounds were tested using a retinal axotomy model that has been previously described [9]. Mice were euthanized by cervical dislocation, and eyes were enucleated immediately. Subsequently, retinas were dissected free in cold HBSS and either fixed immediately with PFA for 1 h (0 days ex vivo; control) or flat mounted on cell culture inserts (Millicell 0.4 μm pore; Merck, Kenilworth, NJ, USA) and maintained in culture (37 °C, 5% CO_2) with Neurobasal-A media supplemented by 2 mM L-glutamate (GlutaMAX, Gibco, Thermo Fisher Scientific, Waltham, MA, USA), 1% N-2 supplement, 2% B-27 supplement, and 1% penicillin/streptomycin (all Gibco) in six-well culture plates (3 days ex vivo). For treated retinas, valproic acid (1 mM), folic acid (50 μg/mL), SB-431542 (10 μM), WY-14,463 (100 μM), and genistein (10 μM) were dissolved in the culture media (all drugs from Merck). Half of the media volume was replaced at 48 h. After 72 h (3 days ex vivo), the retinas were removed from culture, fixed in 3.7% PFA for 30 min, and immunolabelled as detailed below.

2.4. Immunofluorescent Labelling

Retinas were transferred to slides and isolated using a hydrophobic barrier pen (VWR, Radnor, PA, USA). Subsequently, the tissue was permeabilized with 0.5% Triton

X-100 (VWR) in 1 M PBS for 60 min and blocked in 2% bovine serum albumin (Thermo Fisher Scientific) in 1 M PBS for 60 min. Primary antibodies were applied and maintained overnight at 4 °C (detailed in Table 1). Retinas were washed five times for 5 min in 1 M PBS before the secondary antibodies were applied and maintained for 4 h at room temperature. All tissue was washed again five times for 5 min with PBS, and TOPRO-3 nuclear stain (1 µM in 1 M PBS) was applied and maintained at room temperature for 10 min. Tissue was then washed once in PBS and mounted using Fluoromount-G and glass coverslips (Thermo Fisher Scientific). Slides were sealed with nail varnish.

Table 1. Antibodies used.

Antibody	Target	Host	Stock Conc.	Working Conc.	Dilution	Details
anti-RBPMS	RNA-binding protein, RGC specific in the retina	Rabbit	660 µg/mL	1.32 µg/mL	1:500	Novusbio NBP2-20112
anti-GFP	XFPs (e.g., CFP)	Chicken	10 mg/mL	20 µg/mL	1:500	Abcam ab13970
Goat-anti Rabbit Alexa Fluor 568	Rabbit primary antibody	Goat	2 mg/mL	4 µg/mL	1:500	Invitrogen A11011
Goat-anti Chick Alexa Fluor 488	Chick primary antibody	Goat	2 mg/mL	4 µg/mL	1:500	Invitrogen A11039

2.5. Analysis of Retinal Ganglion Cell Degeneration

RGC loss and shrinkage of nuclei were evaluated by CFP, RBPMS, and TOPRO-3 labelling of flat mounted tissue. All images were acquired on a Leica DMi8 microscope with a CoolLED pE-300white LED-based light source and a Leica DFC7000 T fluorescence color camera (all Leica, Wetzlar, Germany). In each retina, six images (40× magnification, 0.55 NA) were taken at 0, 2, 4, 6, 8, and 10 o'clock equidistantly, about a superior to inferior line through the optic disc (~1000 µm eccentricity). All images were cropped to 0.01 mm^2. CFP+ cells, RBPMS+ cells, and TO-PRO-3+ nuclei were counted using the cell counter plugin for Fiji [10]. Cell counts and nuclei counts were averaged across the six images in each retina and expressed as a density per 0.01 mm^2. To assess nuclear shrinkage, the nuclear diameter was measured in >30 nuclei belonging to RBPMS+ cells (per cropped image) using the in-built line tool, giving an average nuclear diameter per image. These values were averaged across the six images of each retina to produce a final average nuclear diameter per retina.

2.6. Statistical Analysis

All statistical analysis was performed in R. Data were tested for normality with a *Shapiro Wilk* test. Normally distributed data were analyzed by *Student's t*-test or *ANOVA* (with *Tukey's HSD*). Non-normally distributed data were transformed using squared transforms; data that remained non-normally distributed were analyzed by a *Kruskal–Wallis* test followed by *Dunn's* tests with *Benjamini and Hochberg* correction. Unless otherwise stated, * = $p < 0.05$, ** = $p < 0.01$, *** $p < 0.001$, NS = non-significant ($p > 0.05$). For box plots, the center hinge represents the median, with the upper and lower hinges representing the first and third quartiles; whiskers represent 1.5 times the interquartile range.

3. Results

3.1. Comparison of Glaucoma-Relevant Transcriptomic Datasets Identifies Common Genes for Therapeutic Targeting

Publicly available transcriptomic datasets from three different animal models relevant to glaucoma (mouse controlled optic nerve crush [3], DBA/2J mouse model of glaucoma [8], and rat optic nerve transection [4]) were analyzed to identify common pathways and shared gene expression profiles. Comparison of the DE genes revealed commonality between models with ~30–40 DE genes shared between individual comparisons (comparisons are displayed in Figure 1 and DE gene lists are detailed in Supplementary Table S1). Three-way comparison of differentially expressed genes identified 12 shared DE genes between all three models (Figure 1 and Supplementary Table S1). The identity and role of these genes are detailed in Supplementary Table S2. Pathway analysis revealed a role of these shared DE genes predominantly in the immune system, neuroinflammatory signaling, and amino acid biosynthesis pathways (Table 2). However, the majority of pathways had a low number of gene hits (pathway hit %), demonstrating that these identified DE genes do not collectively belong to a single or conserved pathway of RGC degeneration.

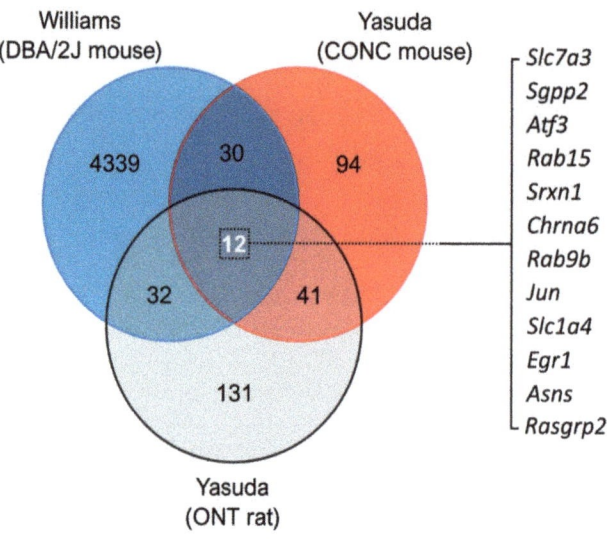

Figure 1. Comparison of RNA-sequencing data identifies gene changes common to models of retinal ganglion cell injury. DE gene lists were compiled from publicly available RNA-sequencing datasets from the DBA/2J mouse model of glaucoma (Williams et al., 2017 [8]), mouse controlled optic nerve crush model (CONC; Yasuda et al., 2014 [3]), and rat optic nerve transection model (ONT; Yasuda et al., 2016 [4]). The results are displayed as a Venn diagram showing the total number of DE genes by dataset, and overlap demonstrating shared DE genes. A three-way comparison identified 12 common genes (listed to right) that may represent gene changes conserved to RGC injury, and thus useful therapeutic targets.

We then used the CTD to screen for compounds that interact with these shared DE genes in order to identify potential novel therapeutics. Screening revealed 40 compounds that interact with >50% of these shared genes (Supplementary Table S3). A number of these are chemical by-products or inorganic compounds tested in toxicity assays (e.g., for carcinogenic effects) and as such are not suitable therapeutics. Other compounds had known neurodegenerative or anti-neuroprotective properties/responses (e.g., LPS and genistein). We identified eight compounds that may be suitable therapeutics based on a literature search (Supplementary Table S3), as they are either hormonal compounds, simple dietary compounds, or compounds that have already been tested in neurodegenerative contexts. These eight compounds were valproic acid, SB-431542 (an inhibitor of TGF-Beta Type I Receptor/ALK5, ALK4 & ALK7), progesterone, estradiol, choline, folic acid, WY-14643 (pirinixic acid, a peroxisome proliferator-activated receptor alpha (PPARα) agonist), and rosiglitazone.

Table 2. Pathway analysis of shared differentially expressed genes between RNA-sequencing experiments.

Comparison	Ingenuity Canonical Pathways	−log(p) *	Molecules	Pathway Hits (%)
D2+ vs. Mouse CONC	Complement System	6.22	ITGAM,C1QA,C1QC,C1QB	10.8
	Neuroinflammation Signaling Pathway	5.87	JUN,AGER,TYROBP,HLA-A,KCNJ5,ATF4,CX3CR1	2.25
	Dendritic Cell Maturation	4.59	TYROBP,HLA-A,FCER1G,ATF4,PLCB1	2.59
	PI3K Signaling in B Lymphocytes	4.04	ATF3,JUN,ATF4,PLCB1	3.08
	GNRH Signaling	3.87	JUN,EGR1,ATF4,PLCB1	2.78
	Role of NFAT in Regulation of the Immune Response	3.44	JUN,HLA-A,FCER1G,PLCB1	2.15
	OX40 Signaling Pathway	3.21	JUN,HLA-A,FCER1G	3.3
	Type I Diabetes Mellitus Signaling	2.96	HLA-A,FCER1G,PTPRN	2.7
	Cytotoxic T Lymphocyte-Mediated Apoptosis of Target Cells	2.81	HLA-A,FCER1G	6.25
	Phagosome Formation	2.77	ITGAM,FCER1G,PLCB1	2.31
D2+ vs. Rat ONT	Glutamate Receptor Signaling	3.72	GRIN2A,SLC1A4,GRIK3	5.26
	Amyotrophic Lateral Sclerosis Signaling	2.87	PRPH,GRIN2A,GRIK3	2.7
	Asparagine Biosynthesis I	2.71	ASNS	100
	MIF Regulation of Innate Immunity	2.49	JUN,PLA2G5	4.65
	Serotonin Receptor Signaling	2.49	HTR5A,HTR1D	4.65
	ATM Signaling	1.8	JUN,GADD45G	2.04
	Sphingosine and Sphingosine-1-Phosphate Metabolism	1.76	SGPP2	11.1
	IGF-1 Signaling	1.73	JUN,YWHAH	1.89
	p53 Signaling	1.7	JUN,GADD45G	1.8
	Neuroinflammation Signaling Pathway	1.64	GRIN2A,JUN,PLA2G5	0.965

Comparison	Ingenuity Canonical Pathways	−log(p) *	Molecules	Pathway Hits (%)
Mouse CONC vs. Rat ONT	AMPK Signaling	2.76	RAB9B,CHRNA6,CDKN1A,CHRNB3	1.85
	Asparagine Biosynthesis I	2.62	ASNS	100
	PI3K Signaling in B Lymphocytes	2.43	ATF3,JUN,ATF5	2.31
	CXCR4 Signaling	2.14	RHOQ,JUN,EGR1	1.82
	eNOS Signaling	2.09	CHRNA6,SLC7A1,CHRNB3	1.74
	Heme Degradation	2.02	HMOX1	25
	IL-8 Signaling	1.93	HMOX1,RHOQ,JUN	1.52
	IL-10 Signaling	1.93	HMOX1,JUN	2.9
	Tetrahydrofolate Salvage from 5,10-Methenyltetrahydrofolate	1.93	MTHFD2	20
	Serine Biosynthesis	1.93	PHGDH	1.85

Table 2. Cont.

Three-way comparison	Asparagine Biosynthesis I	3.25	ASNS	100
	PI3K Signaling in B Lymphocytes	2.63	ATF3,JUN	1.54
	GNRH Signaling	2.55	JUN,EGR1	1.39
	CXCR4 Signaling	2.43	JUN,EGR1	1.21
	B Cell Receptor Signaling	2.31	JUN,EGR1	1.05
	Sphingosine and Sphingosine-1-Phosphate Metabolism	2.3	SGPP2	11.1
	AMPK Signaling	2.2	RAB9B,CHRNA6	0.926
	IL-17A Signaling in Gastric Cells	1.86	JUN	4
	TNFR2 Signaling	1.78	JUN	3.33
	4-1BB Signaling in T Lymphocytes	1.75	JUN	3.12

* $-\log(p) > 1.301029996 = p < 0.05$; † D2 = DBA/2J.

3.2. Retinal Explant Model Provides a Platform to Rapidly Test Candidate Neuroprotective Therapeutics

Axotomy of the RGC axon results in RGC degeneration. In the retina explant model [9,11], severing of the optic nerve leads to RGC axotomy, and results in 30–50% RGC loss over 3–5 days in the mouse. We utilized this model to identify compounds for an RGC neuroprotective effect (Figure 2). Valproic acid, SB-431542, folic acid, and WY-14643 were selected for testing because an established literature already exists for progesterone, choline, and estradiol (see discussion). Following axotomy and maintenance in culture ex vivo for 3 days, retinas exhibited a marked loss of RGCs as identified by significant reduction in the number of CFP+ cells (40% loss, $p < 0.05$) and RBPMS+ cells (39% loss, $p < 0.001$). Nuclear density was variable and was not significantly reduced at this time point, likely reflecting a combination of neuronal loss and glial proliferation. Surviving RGCs had significantly reduced nuclear diameter (14% smaller, $p < 0.001$), indicating significant cellular stress.

Three of the tested compounds conferred significant neuroprotection when dissolved in the culture media. Survival of CFP+ RGCs was best promoted by folic acid (1.75-fold survival from untreated, $p < 0.05$), followed by valproic acid (1.59-fold survival from untreated, $p < 0.05$), and was significant, but highly variable with SB-341542 (1.65-fold survival from untreated, $p < 0.05$). RBPMS+ cell counts were highest in retinas treated with valproic acid (1.47-fold survival from untreated, $p < 0.01$; 11% loss compared with control, $p > 0.05$), followed by WY-14643 (1.4-fold survival from untreated, $p < 0.01$; 11% loss compared with control, $p > 0.05$). RGC loss assessed by RBPMS+ counts was reduced for folic acid treated retinas relative to control (21% loss compared with control, $p > 0.05$), but was not significantly different from untreated retinas, demonstrating variable protection (1.3 fold survival from untreated, $p > 0.05$). Only WY-14643 demonstrated significant protection against nuclear shrinkage (1.11-fold larger diameter compared with untreated, $p < 0.05$; 4.5% loss compared with control, $p < 0.05$). Folic acid and valproic acid demonstrated a less severe nuclear shrinkage relative to control (10% loss, $p < 0.01$; and 9.7% loss, $p < 0.01$, respectively). SB-341542, despite showing some protection to CFP+ RGCs, did not demonstrate significant neuroprotection to RBPMS+ RGCs (1.08-fold survival from untreated, $p > 0.05$; 35% loss compared with control, $p < 0.001$), or against nuclear shrinkage (0.98-fold survival from untreated, $p > 0.05$; 15% loss compared with control, $p < 0.001$), suggestive of a possible RGC subtype bias or preferential protection of healthier cells (i.e., those able to maintain CFP expression) [12].

As further validation of this approach, we selected an identified compound that should not enhance RGC survival (as the CTD returns interactions based only on literature link, irrespective of context). We tested the effects of supplementing the culture media with genistein as it has been demonstrated to influence a number of neuroprotective effects. Genistein had no effect on RGC survival compared with untreated retinas, as assessed by CFP+ counts ($p > 0.05$), RBPMS+ counts ($p > 0.05$), TOPRO-3+ counts ($p > 0.05$), or nuclear diameter ($p > 0.05$). Density of TOPRO-3+ nuclei was actually significantly reduced from control in only genistein-treated retinas (15% loss from control, $p < 0.05$).

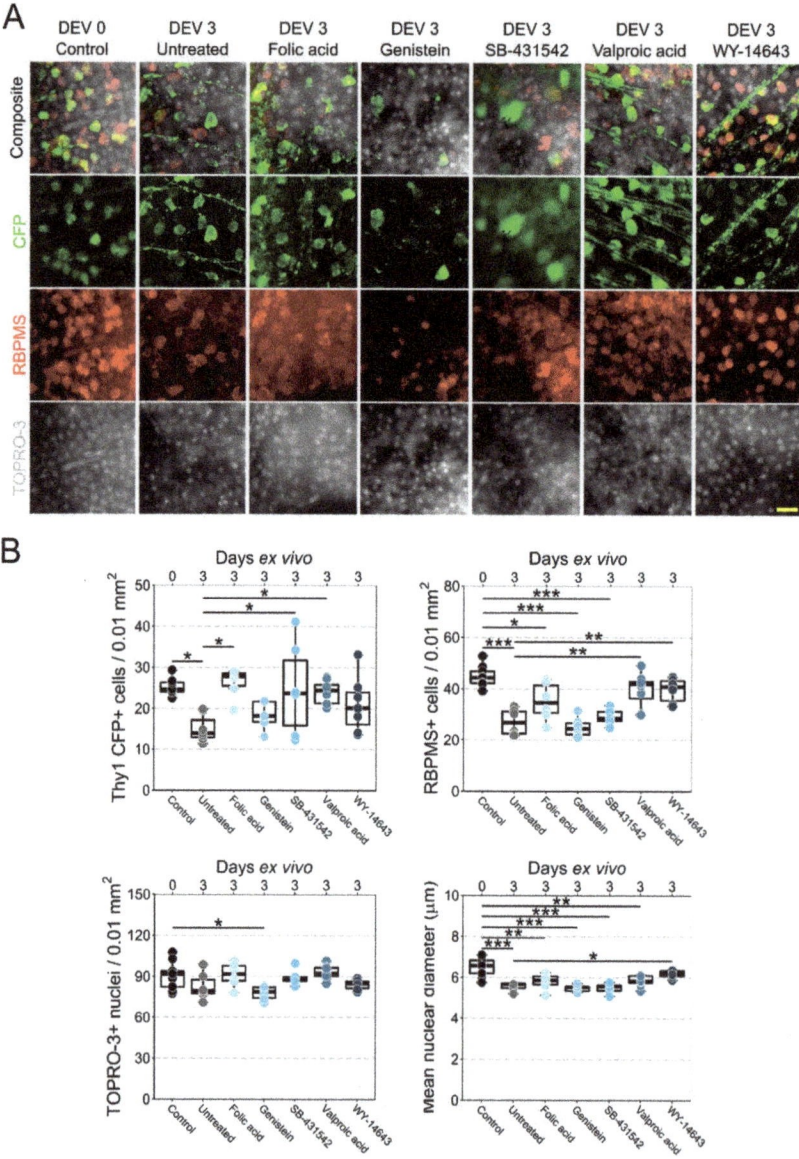

Figure 2. Sequencing data and drug database screening successfully identifies therapeutic candidates that provide retinal ganglion cell neuroprotection. Retina from B6.Cg-Tg(Thy1-CFP)23Jrs/J mice were explanted into tissue culture and maintained for 3 days ex vivo (DEV) with candidate drugs supplemented in the media (in addition to controls: 0 DEV and 3 DEV untreated). (**A**) Retinas were labelled for CFP (anti-GFP), RBPMS, and TOPRO-3 before imaging. (**B**) CFP+ cell density was significantly reduced at 3 DEV in untreated retinas and this was significantly improved in folic acid, SB-431542, and valproic acid treated retinas. RBPMS+ RGC density was significantly reduced at 3 DEV in untreated retinas and this was significantly improved in valproic acid and WY-14643 treated retinas, with moderate protection from folic acid. TOPRO-3+ round nuclei were not significantly altered with the exception of genistein, supporting its lack of protection and possible neurotoxic effects. Mean nuclear diameter was significantly smaller at 3 DEV, and this was significantly improved by WY-14643. Overall, these data support valproic acid, folic acid, and WY-14643 as neuroprotective against acute RGC injury. This validates the approach of identifying potential neuroprotective therapeutics from existing -omics data. Scale bar in A = 20 μm. * $p < 0.05$, ** $p < 0.01$, *** $p < 0.001$.

4. Discussion

The key defining characteristic of glaucomatous optic neuropathy is the progressive loss and dysfunction of RGCs and is one of the only shared features across the pathophysiological spectrum in human glaucomatous disease and animal models of glaucoma. The pathophysiology of RGC degeneration in different animal models is likely to vary. There may be shared intrinsic RGC degenerative mechanisms across all glaucoma models as well as human glaucoma, which can be identified and explored. The purpose of this study was to identify commonalities between RGC injury models (rather than to individually analyze distinct models of glaucoma) with which to identify neuroprotective treatments that may be applicable across the heterogeneity of glaucoma (in animal models and human glaucoma patients).

In this study, we used three publicly available RNA-sequencing datasets of animal models of glaucoma. The DBA/2J mouse is one of the most frequently used glaucoma models in research. In DBA/2J mice, mutations in two genes ($Gpnmb^{R150X}$ and $Tyrp1^b$) drive an iris disease with features of human iris atrophy and pigment dispersion. Pigment disperses from the iris and induces damage in the drainage structures of the eye. This inhibits aqueous humor outflow and leads to an increase in IOP. By 9 months of age, IOP is high in the majority of eyes and transcriptomic and metabolic datasets demonstrate mitochondrial and metabolic dysfunction in RGCs [12]. In the mouse controlled optic nerve crush model, axonal injury is induced mechanically by a temporary compression of the distal optic nerve, resulting in RGC death [3]. Similarly, in the optic nerve transection model, axonal injury triggers axon degeneration, leading to a rapid RGC degeneration [4].

With the increased prevalence of -omics technologies, there is a wealth of open data within the field of glaucoma for researchers to explore and utilize. The aim of the present study was to unbiasedly test a conserved gene set between three publicly available RNA-sequencing datasets. Typically, pathway analysis and ranking of changed genes/proteins/metabolites reveal multiple potential mechanistic avenues for exploration, but practical (funding and publication limits) and narrative/hypothesis limitations leave many of these unexplored. Comparison of datasets to identify common changes can be a powerful method to identify conserved pathological processes in optic nerve injury, as has been demonstrated by previous comprehensive comparisons including the DBA/2J mouse model, optic nerve crush/axotomy models across multiple species, and other CNS neurodegenerations [13,14]. These studies identified commonality and enrichment predominantly within neuroinflammatory and innate immune responses. With the growth of this approach, the field can form data-driven hypotheses to identify and test new mechanisms of neurodegeneration/neuroprotection.

In this study, we compared common gene changes in transcriptomic datasets from RGC injury models and screened these against the Comparative Toxicogenomics Database to identify novel therapeutics. Using a retinal explant model to rapidly test a number of these compounds, we demonstrate the therapeutic potential of drugs identified in this way. Multiple drugs identified had established literature support for RGC and neuronal protection, further supporting this method of identifying potential therapeutics. The ex vivo retinal explant model is ideal as a first-pass model for assessing neurodegenerative events and testing neurodegenerative or neuroprotective drug candidates. In this model, RGCs are axotomized, leading to RGC degeneration [9,11]. As 100% of RGCs are axotomized, the insult is controlled, and maintenance in tissue culture removes the influence of systemic events (e.g., infiltration of myeloid-derived cells) and tightly controls tissue conditions. Only small amounts of a drug is required for testing as it can be directly dissolved in the media. This overcomes any need to test or assess systemic metabolism and bioavailability in the first round of studies, thus keeping the cost of drug and animals low. Further to this, in many research-centric countries (e.g., EU, USA, Australia), additional animal ethical permits are not required to perform this model, increasing its availability to labs that might not have significant animal housing and testing resources.

Screening the shared DE genes between the three glaucoma models against the Comparative Toxicogenomics Database identified valproic acid as the drug that interacted with the most gene products (11/12; the exception was *Chrna6*), followed by SB-431542, progesterone, estradiol, choline, folic acid, WY-14643, and rosiglitazone (see Supplementary Table S3). Valproic acid is an FDA-approved anti-epileptic and migraine drug. Valproic acid's mechanism of action is proposed to be through modulating histone deacetylases activity, which has a well-established literature of limiting RGC degeneration in models of normal-tension and ocular-hypertensive glaucoma [15,16].

Progesterone and estradiol are both endogenous steroids and sex hormones. An extensive literature exists on their possible potential as neuroprotectors and multiple different mechanisms of action are proposed (e.g., regulation of mitochondrial calcium and *Bcl-2* expression, affecting the phosphatidylinositol 3-kinase/Akt signal pathway or preventing caspase-3 activation). A number of studies have been performed to explore the potential of progesterone and estradiol as neuroprotectors in animal models of photoreceptor and retinal ganglion cell loss [17–25]. Given the evidence that RGCs express estrogen receptors, lower estradiol levels are linked with primary open-angle glaucoma (POAG) [26], and that β-estradiol can protect from RGC death [23,27,28], an estrogen analogue-based therapy may be of benefit in many glaucoma patients.

Choline is a quaternary amine, the precursor of many cell components and signaling molecules (e.g., acetylcholine), and an essential nutrient for humans. It is further processed to citicholine and phosphatidylcholine in vivo. Both choline and citicoline are thought to have a neuroprotective effect, possibly by preserving sphingomyelin and cardiolipin and by promoting glutathione synthesis. The literature contains a number of studies suggesting a favorable effect on retinal cell survival, as assessed in various neurodegenerative animal models [15–19].

Folic acid is an essential nutrient and B vitamin which plays a crucial role in the biosynthesis of DNA and RNA. The vitamin is also indispensable for erythrocyte maturation. Clinically, folic acid is mainly used to prevent neural tube defects in the developing fetus. Yet, it has been shown to be protective against certain dysplasia and to reduce gingival inflammation [29]. A number of studies examined the effect of folic acid on microglia and astrocytes in animal models of cellular stress responses, and reported positive results [30,31]. However, to the best of our knowledge, a possible neuroprotective effect in glaucoma has not been previously investigated.

As an established antidiabetic drug of the thiazolidinedione class, Rosiglitazone functions as an insulin sensitizer. The drug binds to the peroxisome proliferator-activated receptors in adipocytes and renders the cells more responsive to insulin. The neuroprotective effect of Rosiglitazone and other thiazolidinediones has been studied extensively and a beneficial effect has been suggested through inhibition of inflammatory responses, pro-apoptotic cascades, and mitochondrial metamorphosis [32–34].

The TGF-β type 1 receptor inhibitor SB-431542 is a drug candidate proposed for the treatment of osteosarcomas in humans. The agent acts through binding the activin receptor-like kinase (ALK) receptors ALK5, ALK4, and ALK7. It has also been shown to promote the transformation of astrocytes into neurons [35]. Two studies found evidence for a possible protective effect from NMDA-induced retinal degeneration in rats and from N-methyl-N-nitrosourea (MNU)-induced rod photoreceptor degeneration in zebrafish [36,37].

Pirinixic acid, also known as WY-14643, is a synthetic drug candidate for prevention of severe cardiac dysfunction, cardiomyopathy, and heart failure as a result of lipid accumulation within cardiac myocytes. Its mechanism of action is through binding the peroxisome proliferator-activated receptor alpha (PPARα), thereby affecting cell proliferation and differentiation, lipid metabolism, and inflammatory signaling cascades. WY-14463 has the potential to protect neurons by modulating mitochondrial fusion and fission [38]. However, the drug's potential neuroprotective effect has not previously been explored in glaucoma models. In summary, our screen identified a number of neuroprotective compounds novel to RGC survival. Valproic acid, folic acid, and WY-14643 performed best in terms of neuroprotection, while treatment with SB-431542 led to variable results.

As a further test of this drug discovery method, we sought to also test identified drugs that, based on literature, would not produce a neuroprotective effect. Genistein is a naturally occurring phytoestrogen and isoflavone. The compound is found in soybeans, flava beans, coffee beans, and others. Genistein is known to inhibit protein-tyrosine kinase and topoisomerase-II, affecting the process of cell differentiation and proliferation, and promoting DNA fragmentation and apoptosis [39,40]. It has been hypothesized that genistein could be used to treat different types of cancer through its antioxidant and antiangiogenetic effects. However, in various animal neurodegenerative models, genistein has been shown to block the neuroprotective effect of agents such as carbamylcholine, forskolin, and veratridine [41–43]. In the explant model, genistein had no effect on RGC survival, thus supporting the applicability of this method for identifying disease modifying compounds.

5. Conclusions

Glaucoma is a complex neurodegenerative disease in which the only shared and clinically defined feature is the progressive dysfunction and degeneration of RGCs (although age, genetic risk, and high IOP are all common risk factors, glaucoma can still occur in the absence of one or more of these risk factors). Many models of glaucoma-related stress have been developed in a wide array of animal species, which recapitulate some of the features of human glaucoma. Comparison of these models to identify common changes can be a powerful method to identify conserved pathological processes in RGC injury. Publicly available -omics datasets such as those from RNA-sequencing represent a data-rich resource for identifying these potential critical pathogenic changes. We identified gene changes common to three modes of RGC injury and screened these against the Comparative Toxicogenomics Database to identify novel therapeutic agents for testing. We demonstrated the validity of this approach by testing the identified compounds using another independent model of RGC injury.

Our drug discovery and analysis platform used only publicly available tools and datasets and an ex vivo model widely amenable to the majority of research-intensive countries that does not require additional animal ethical permits, while keeping drug treatment costs low. This platform is a practical means to utilize the increasing wealth of open access -omics data generated by the glaucoma field in order to move forward towards identifying new therapeutics.

Supplementary Materials: The following are available online at https://www.mdpi.com/article/10.3390/jcm10173938/s1, Table S1: Shared differentially expressed genes between glaucoma RNA-sequencing datasets, Table S2: Roles of shared differentially expressed genes, Table S3: Compounds with known interactions with differentially expressed genes common to all three RNA-sequencing datasets.

Author Contributions: T.J.E. performed experiments, analyzed data, and wrote the manuscript; J.R.T. designed and performed experiments, analyzed data, and wrote the manuscript; P.A.W. conceived and designed experiments, analyzed data, and wrote the manuscript. All authors have read and agreed to the published version of the manuscript.

Funding: This research was funded by Vetenskapsrådet 2018-02124, Ögonfonden (P.A.W.), and Ögonfonden (J.R.T.). The APC was funded by Vetenskapsrådet 2018-02124. Pete Williams is supported by Karolinska Institutet in the form of a Board of Research Faculty Funded Career Position and by St. Erik Eye Hospital philanthropic donations.

Institutional Review Board Statement: All breeding and experimental procedures were performed according to the tenets of the Association for Research for Vision and Ophthalmology Statement for the Use of Animals in Ophthalmic and Research. Individual study protocols were approved by Stockholm's Committee for Ethical Animal Research (10389-2018).

Informed Consent Statement: Not applicable.

Data Availability Statement: All data generated or analyzed during this study are included in this published article.

Acknowledgments: The authors would like to thank Diana Rydholm for assistance with animal husbandry and maintenance; Melissa Jöe, Elizabeth Kastanaki, and Amin Otmani for assistance with immunofluorescent labelling and imaging; St. Erik Eye Hospital for financial support for research space and animal facilities.

Conflicts of Interest: The authors declare no conflict of interest. The funders had no role in the design of the study; in the collection, analyses, or interpretation of data; in the writing of the manuscript; or in the decision to publish the results.

References

1. Stein, J.D.; Khawaja, A.P.; Weizer, J.S. Glaucoma in adults-screening, diagnosis, and management: A review. *JAMA J. Am. Med. Assoc.* **2021**, *325*, 164–174. [CrossRef]
2. Tham, Y.-C.; Li, X.; Wong, T.Y.; Quigley, H.A.; Aung, T.; Cheng, C.-Y. Global prevalence of glaucoma and projections of glaucoma burden through 2040: A systematic review and meta-analysis. *Ophthalmology* **2014**, *121*, 2081–2090. Available online: https://www.ncbi.nlm.nih.gov/pubmed/24974815 (accessed on 26 August 2021). [CrossRef] [PubMed]
3. Yasuda, M.; Tanaka, Y.; Ryu, M.; Tsuda, S.; Nakazawa, T. Rna sequence reveals mouse retinal transcriptome changes early after axonal injury. *PLoS ONE* **2014**, *9*, e93258. Available online: https://www.ncbi.nlm.nih.gov/pubmed/24676137 (accessed on 26 August 2021). [CrossRef] [PubMed]
4. Yasuda, M.; Tanaka, Y.; Omodaka, K.; Nishiguchi, K.M.; Nakamura, O.; Tsuda, S.; Nakazawa, T. Transcriptome profiling of the rat retina after optic nerve transection. *Sci. Rep.* **2016**, *6*, 28736. Available online: https://www.ncbi.nlm.nih.gov/pubmed/27353354 (accessed on 26 August 2021). [CrossRef]
5. Morgan, E.J.; Tribble, J.R. Microbead models in glaucoma. *Exp. Eye Res.* **2015**, *141*, 9–14. Available online: https://www.ncbi.nlm.nih.gov/pubmed/26116904 (accessed on 26 August 2021). [CrossRef]
6. Tribble, R.J.; Otmani, A.; Kokkali, E.; Lardner, E.; Morgan, J.E.; Williams, P.A. Retinal ganglion cell degeneration in a rat magnetic bead model of ocular hypertensive glaucoma. *Transl. Vis. Sci. Technol.* **2021**, *10*, 21. Available online: https://www.ncbi.nlm.nih.gov/pubmed/33510960 (accessed on 26 August 2021). [CrossRef]
7. Williams, P.A.; Marsh-Armstrong, N.; Howell, G.R.; Bosco, A.; Danias, J.; Simon, J.; Di Polo, A.; Kuehn, M.; Przedborski, S.; Raff, M.; et al. Neuroinflammation in glaucoma: A new opportunity. *Exp. Eye Res.* **2017**, *157*, 20–27. Available online: https://www.ncbi.nlm.nih.gov/pubmed/28242160 (accessed on 26 August 2021). [CrossRef] [PubMed]
8. Williams, A.P.; Harder, J.M.; Foxworth, N.E.; Cochran, K.E.; Philip, V.M.; Porciatti, V.; Smithies, O.; John, S.W. Vitamin b. *Science* **2017**, *355*, 756–760. Available online: https://www.ncbi.nlm.nih.gov/pubmed/28209901 (accessed on 26 August 2021). [CrossRef]
9. Tribble, R.J.; Otmani, A.; Sun, S.; Ellis, S.A.; Cimaglia, G.; Vohra, R.; Jöe, M.; Lardner, E.; Venkataraman, A.P.; Domínguez-Vicent, A.; et al. Nicotinamide provides neuroprotection in glaucoma by protecting against mitochondrial and metabolic dysfunction. *Redox Biol.* **2021**, *43*, 101988. Available online: https://www.ncbi.nlm.nih.gov/pubmed/33932867 (accessed on 26 August 2021). [CrossRef]
10. Schindelin, J.; Arganda-Carreras, I.; Frise, E.; Kaynig, V.; Longair, M.; Pietzsch, T.; Preibisch, S.; Rueden, C.; Saalfeld, S.; Schmid, B.; et al. Fiji: An open-source platform for biological-image analysis. *Nat. Methods* **2012**, *9*, 676–682. Available online: https://www.ncbi.nlm.nih.gov/pubmed/22743772 (accessed on 26 August 2021). [CrossRef]
11. Bull, D.N.; Johnson, T.V.; Welsapar, G.; DeKorver, N.W.; Tomarev, S.I.; Martin, K.R. Use of an adult rat retinal explant model for screening of potential retinal ganglion cell neuroprotective therapies. *Investig. Ophthalmol. Vis. Sci.* **2011**, *52*, 3309–3320. Available online: https://www.ncbi.nlm.nih.gov/pubmed/21345987 (accessed on 26 August 2021). [CrossRef] [PubMed]
12. Williams, A.P.; Howell, G.R.; Barbay, J.M.; Braine, C.E.; Sousa, G.L.; John, S.W.; Morgan, J.E. Retinal ganglion cell dendritic atrophy in dba/2j glaucoma. *PLoS ONE* **2013**, *8*, e72282. Available online: https://www.ncbi.nlm.nih.gov/pubmed/23977271 (accessed on 26 August 2021). [CrossRef]
13. Donahue, J.R.; Moller-Trane, R.; Nickells, R.W. Meta-analysis of transcriptomic changes in optic nerve injury and neurodegenerative models reveals a fundamental response to injury throughout the central nervous system. *Mol. Vis.* **2017**, *23*, 987–1005. Available online: https://www.ncbi.nlm.nih.gov/pubmed/29386873 (accessed on 26 August 2021).
14. Wang, J.; Struebing, F.L.; Geisert, E.E. Commonalities of optic nerve injury and glaucoma-induced neurodegeneration: Insights from transcriptome-wide studies. *Exp. Eye Res.* **2021**, *207*, 108571. Available online: https://www.ncbi.nlm.nih.gov/pubmed/33844961 (accessed on 26 August 2021). [CrossRef]
15. Biermann, J.; Grieshaber, P.; Goebel, U.; Martin, G.; Thanos, S.; di Giovanni, S.; Lagrèze, W.A. Valproic acid-mediated neuroprotection and regeneration in injured retinal ganglion cells. *Investig. Ophthalmol. Vis. Sci.* **2010**, *51*, 526–534. Available online: https://www.ncbi.nlm.nih.gov/pubmed/19628741 (accessed on 26 August 2021). [CrossRef]
16. Kimura, A.; Guo, X.; Noro, T.; Harada, C.; Tanaka, K.; Namekata, K.; Harada, T. Valproic acid prevents retinal degeneration in a murine model of normal tension glaucoma. *Neurosci. Lett.* **2015**, *588*, 108–113. Available online: https://www.ncbi.nlm.nih.gov/pubmed/25555796 (accessed on 26 August 2021). [CrossRef] [PubMed]

17. Lindsey, D.J.; Weinreb, R.N. Survival and differentiation of purified retinal ganglion cells in a chemically defined microenvironment. *Investig. Ophthalmol. Vis. Sci.* **1994**, *35*, 3640–3648. Available online: https://www.ncbi.nlm.nih.gov/pubmed/7916337 (accessed on 26 August 2021).
18. Allen, S.R.; Olsen, T.W.; Sayeed, I.; Cale, H.A.; Morrison, K.C.; Oumarbaeva, Y.; Lucaciu, I.; Boatright, J.H.; Pardue, M.T.; Stein, D.G. Progesterone treatment in two rat models of ocular ischemia. *Investig. Ophthalmol. Vis. Sci.* **2015**, *56*, 2880–2891. Available online: https://www.ncbi.nlm.nih.gov/pubmed/26024074 (accessed on 26 August 2021). [CrossRef] [PubMed]
19. Jackson, C.A.; Roche, S.L.; Byrne, A.M.; Ruiz-Lopez, A.M.; Cotter, T.G. Progesterone receptor signalling in retinal photoreceptor neuroprotection. *J. Neurochem.* **2016**, *136*, 63–77. Available online: https://www.ncbi.nlm.nih.gov/pubmed/26447367 (accessed on 26 August 2021). [CrossRef]
20. Jiang, M.; Ma, X.; Zhao, Q.; Li, Y.; Xing, Y.; Deng, Q.; Shen, Y. The neuroprotective effects of novel estrogen receptor gper1 in mouse retinal ganglion cell degeneration. *Exp. Eye Res.* **2019**, *189*, 107826. Available online: https://www.ncbi.nlm.nih.gov/pubmed/31586450 (accessed on 26 August 2021). [CrossRef]
21. Means, C.J.; Lopez, A.A.; Koulen, P. Estrogen protects optic nerve head astrocytes against oxidative stress by preventing caspase-3 activation, tau dephosphorylation at ser. *Cell Mol. Neurobiol.* **2021**, *41*, 449–458. Available online: https://www.ncbi.nlm.nih.gov/pubmed/32385548 (accessed on 26 August 2021). [CrossRef]
22. Hao, M.; Li, Y.; Lin, W.; Xu, Q.; Shao, N.; Zhang, Y.; Kuang, H. Estrogen prevents high-glucose-induced damage of retinal ganglion cells via mitochondrial pathway. *Graefes Arch. Clin. Exp. Ophthalmol.* **2015**, *253*, 83–90. Available online: https://www.ncbi.nlm.nih.gov/pubmed/25216739 (accessed on 26 August 2021). [CrossRef] [PubMed]
23. Prokai-Tatrai, K.; Xin, H.; Nguyen, V.; Szarka, S.; Blazics, B.; Prokai, L.; Koulen, P. 17β-estradiol eye drops protect the retinal ganglion cell layer and preserve visual function in an in vivo model of glaucoma. *Mol. Pharm.* **2013**, *10*, 3253–3261. Available online: https://www.ncbi.nlm.nih.gov/pubmed/23841874 (accessed on 26 August 2021). [CrossRef]
24. Li, H.; Wang, B.; Zhu, C.; Feng, Y.; Wang, S.; Shahzad, M.; Hu, C.; Mo, M.; Du, F.; Yu, X. 17β-estradiol impedes bax-involved mitochondrial apoptosis of retinal nerve cells induced by oxidative damage via the phosphatidylinositol 3-kinase/akt signal pathway. *J. Mol. Neurosci.* **2013**, *50*, 482–493. Available online: https://www.ncbi.nlm.nih.gov/pubmed/23361188 (accessed on 26 August 2021). [CrossRef]
25. Yu, X.; Rajala, R.V.; McGinnis, J.F.; Li, F.; Anderson, R.E.; Yan, X.; Li, S.; Elias, R.V.; Knapp, R.R.; Zhou, X.; et al. Involvement of insulin/phosphoinositide 3-kinase/akt signal pathway in 17 beta-estradiol-mediated neuroprotection. *J. Biol. Chem.* **2004**, *279*, 13086–13094. Available online: https://www.ncbi.nlm.nih.gov/pubmed/14711819 (accessed on 26 August 2021). [CrossRef] [PubMed]
26. Newman-Casey, A.P.; Talwar, N.; Nan, B.; Musch, D.C.; Pasquale, L.R.; Stein, J.D. The potential association between postmenopausal hormone use and primary open-angle glaucoma. *JAMA Ophthalmol.* **2014**, *132*, 298–303. Available online: https://www.ncbi.nlm.nih.gov/pubmed/24481323 (accessed on 26 August 2021). [CrossRef] [PubMed]
27. Kumar, M.D.; Perez, E.; Cai, Z.Y.; Aoun, P.; Brun-Zinkernagel, A.M.; Covey, D.F.; Simpkins, J.W.; Agarwal, N. Role of nonfeminizing estrogen analogues in neuroprotection of rat retinal ganglion cells against glutamate-induced cytotoxicity. *Free Radic. Biol. Med.* **2005**, *38*, 1152–1163. Available online: https://www.ncbi.nlm.nih.gov/pubmed/15808412 (accessed on 26 August 2021). [CrossRef]
28. Zhou, X.; Li, F.; Ge, J.; Sarkisian, S.R.; Tomita, H.; Zaharia, A.; Chodosh, J.; Cao, W. Retinal ganglion cell protection by 17-beta-estradiol in a mouse model of inherited glaucoma. *Dev. Neurobiol.* **2007**, *67*, 603–616. Available online: https://www.ncbi.nlm.nih.gov/pubmed/17443811 (accessed on 26 August 2021). [CrossRef]
29. Merrell, B.J.; McMurry, J.P. Folic Acid. In *StatPearls*; StatPearls Publishing: Treasure Island, FL, USA, January 2021. Available online: https://www.ncbi.nlm.nih.gov/books/NBK554487/ (accessed on 26 August 2021).
30. Cianciulli, A.; Salvatore, R.; Porro, C.; Trotta, T.; Panaro, M.A. Folic acid is able to polarize the inflammatory response in lps activated microglia by regulating multiple signaling pathways. *Mediat. Inflamm.* **2016**, *2016*, 5240127. Available online: https://www.ncbi.nlm.nih.gov/pubmed/27738387 (accessed on 26 August 2021). [CrossRef]
31. Li, W.; Ma, Y.; Li, Z.; Lv, X.; Wang, X.; Zhou, D.; Luo, S.; Wilson, J.X.; Huang, G. Folic acid decreases astrocyte apoptosis by preventing oxidative stress-induced telomere attrition. *Int. J. Mol. Sci.* **2019**, *21*, 62. Available online: https://www.ncbi.nlm.nih.gov/pubmed/31861819 (accessed on 26 August 2021). [CrossRef]
32. Meng, Q.Q.; Lei, W.; Chen, H.; Feng, Z.C.; Hu, L.Q.; Zhang, X.L.; Li, S. Combined rosiglitazone and forskolin have neuroprotective effects in sd rats after spinal cord injury. *PPAR Res.* **2018**, *2018*, 3897478. Available online: https://www.ncbi.nlm.nih.gov/pubmed/30034460 (accessed on 26 August 2021). [CrossRef] [PubMed]
33. He, X.; Feng, L.; Meng, H.; Wang, X.; Liu, S. Rosiglitazone protects dopaminergic neurons against lipopolysaccharide-induced neurotoxicity through inhibition of microglia activation. *Int. J. Neurosci.* **2012**, *122*, 532–540. Available online: https://www.ncbi.nlm.nih.gov/pubmed/22524690 (accessed on 26 August 2021). [CrossRef]
34. Li, P.; Xu, X.; Zheng, Z.; Zhu, B.; Shi, Y.; Liu, K. Protective effects of rosiglitazone on retinal neuronal damage in diabetic rats. *Curr. Eye Res.* **2011**, *36*, 673–679. Available online: https://www.ncbi.nlm.nih.gov/pubmed/21599458 (accessed on 26 August 2021). [CrossRef] [PubMed]
35. Yin, C.J.; Zhang, L.; Ma, N.X.; Wang, Y.; Lee, G.; Hou, X.Y.; Lei, Z.F.; Zhang, F.Y.; Dong, F.P.; Wu, G.Y.; et al. Chemical conversion of human fetal astrocytes into neurons through modulation of multiple signaling pathways. *Stem. Cell Rep.* **2019**, *12*, 488–501. Available online: https://www.ncbi.nlm.nih.gov/pubmed/30745031 (accessed on 26 August 2021). [CrossRef] [PubMed]

36. Ueda, K.; Nakahara, T.; Mori, A.; Sakamoto, K.; Ishii, K. Protective effects of tgf-β inhibitors in a rat model of nmda-induced retinal degeneration. *Eur. J. Pharm.* **2013**, *699*, 188–193. Available online: https://www.ncbi.nlm.nih.gov/pubmed/23220705 (accessed on 26 August 2021). [CrossRef]
37. Tappeiner, C.; Maurer, E.; Sallin, P.; Bise, T.; Enzmann, V.; Tschopp, M. Inhibition of the tgfβ pathway enhances retinal regeneration in adult zebrafish. *PLoS ONE* **2016**, *11*, e0167073. Available online: https://www.ncbi.nlm.nih.gov/pubmed/27880821 (accessed on 26 August 2021). [CrossRef]
38. Zolezzi, M.J.; Silva-Alvarez, C.; Ordenes, D.; Godoy, J.A.; Carvajal, F.J.; Santos, M.J.; Inestrosa, N.C. Peroxisome proliferator-activated receptor (ppar) γ and pparα agonists modulate mitochondrial fusion-fission dynamics: Relevance to reactive oxygen species (ros)-related neurodegenerative disorders? *PLoS ONE* **2013**, *8*, e64019. Available online: https://www.ncbi.nlm.nih.gov/pubmed/23675519 (accessed on 26 August 2021). [CrossRef]
39. Yakisich, S.J.; Lindblom, I.O.; Siden, A.; Cruz, M.H. Rapid inhibition of ongoing dna synthesis in human glioma tissue by genistein. *Oncol. Rep.* **2009**, *22*, 569–574. Available online: https://www.ncbi.nlm.nih.gov/pubmed/19639205 (accessed on 26 August 2021). [CrossRef]
40. Markovits, J.; Larsen, A.K.; Ségal-Bendirdjian, E.; Fossé, P.; Saucier, J.M.; Gazit, A.; Levitzki, A.; Umezawa, K.; Jacquemin-Sablon, A. Inhibition of dna topoisomerases i and ii and induction of apoptosis by erbstatin and tyrphostin derivatives. *Biochem. Pharmacol.* **1994**, *48*, 549–560. Available online: https://www.ncbi.nlm.nih.gov/pubmed/8068042 (accessed on 26 August 2021). [CrossRef]
41. Pereira, P.S.; Medina, S.V.; Araujo, E.G. Cholinergic activity modulates the survival of retinal ganglion cells in culture: The role of m1 muscarinic receptors. *Int. J. Dev. Neurosci.* **2001**, *19*, 559–567. Available online: https://www.ncbi.nlm.nih.gov/pubmed/11600318 (accessed on 26 August 2021). [CrossRef]
42. Santos, C.R.; Araujo, E.G. Cyclic amp increases the survival of ganglion cells in mixed retinal cell cultures in the absence of exogenous neurotrophic molecules, an effect that involves cholinergic activity. *Braz. J. Med. Biol. Res.* **2001**, *34*, 1585–1593. Available online: https://www.ncbi.nlm.nih.gov/pubmed/11717712 (accessed on 26 August 2021). [CrossRef] [PubMed]
43. Pereira, S.F.P.; de Araujo, E.G. Chronic depolarization induced by veratridine increases the survival of rat retinal ganglion cells 'in vitro'. *Int. J. Dev. Neurosci.* **2000**, *18*, 773–780. Available online: https://www.ncbi.nlm.nih.gov/pubmed/11154846 (accessed on 26 August 2021). [CrossRef]

MDPI
St. Alban-Anlage 66
4052 Basel
Switzerland
www.mdpi.com

Journal of Clinical Medicine Editorial Office
E-mail: jcm@mdpi.com
www.mdpi.com/journal/jcm

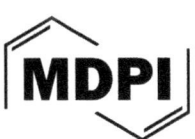

Disclaimer/Publisher's Note: The statements, opinions and data contained in all publications are solely those of the individual author(s) and contributor(s) and not of MDPI and/or the editor(s). MDPI and/or the editor(s) disclaim responsibility for any injury to people or property resulting from any ideas, methods, instructions or products referred to in the content.